♪❋ The Lady Named Thunder

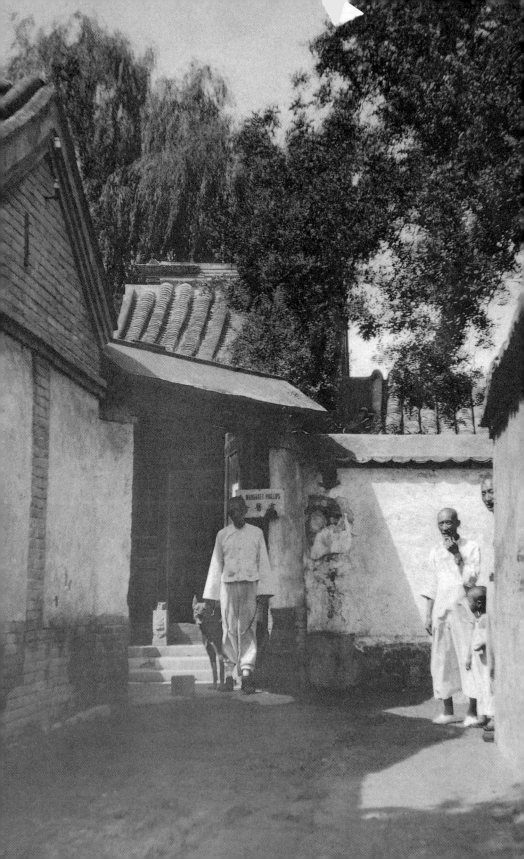

Clifford H. Phillips (Lei Houtian)

ﬔ **The Lady
Named Thunder**

A BIOGRAPHY OF
DR. ETHEL MARGARET PHILLIPS
(1876–1951)

The University of Alberta Press

Published by
The University of Alberta Press
Ring House 2
Edmonton, Alberta   T6G 2E1

Copyright © The University of Alberta Press 2003

NATIONAL LIBRARY OF CANADA CATALOGUING IN PUBLICATION DATA

Phillips, Clifford H., 1920–
    The lady named Thunder : a biography of Dr. Ethel Margaret Phillips (1876–1951) /
    Clifford H. Phillips (Lei Houtian).

Includes index.
ISBN 0–88864–408–6 (bound).—ISBN 0–88864–417–5 (pbk.)

    1. Phillips, Ethel Margaret, 1876–1951. 2. Missions, Medical—China. 3. Missionaries, Medical—
China—Biography. 4. Physicians—China—Biography. 5. Physicians—England—Biography. I. Title.

R722.32.P49P49 2003   610'.92   C2003–905032–7

Printed and bound in Canada by Houghton Boston Printers, Saskatoon, Saskatchewan.
First edition, first printing, 2003.
Editing by Jill Fallis.
Maps by Wendy Johnson.
Book design by Alan Brownoff.

The University of Alberta Press is committed to protecting our natural environment. As part of our
efforts, this book is printed on New Leaf paper: it contains 100% post-consumer recycled fibres and is
acid- and chlorine-free.

The University of Alberta Press gratefully acknowledges the financial support received for its publishing
program from The Canada Council for the Arts. In addition, we also gratefully acknowledge the
financial support of the Government of Canada through the Book Publishing Industry Development
Program (BPDIP) and from the Alberta Foundation for the Arts for our publishing activities.

Canadä

THE CANADA COUNCIL | LE CONSEIL DES ARTS
FOR THE ARTS | DU CANADA
SINCE 1957 | DEPUIS 1957

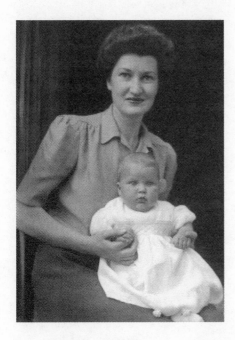

Margaret's daughter-in-law Enid and grandaughter Lesley Margaret c. 1946.

ℐ❋ *To my wife, Enid, who came to love Margaret as much as I did.*

"God moves in a mysterious way His wonders to perform."

—WILLIAM COWPER

THE GREAT WALL

Great Dragon of the hills—for centuries have you lain
Sprawling across the mountain tops,
Guarding the fertile plains of fair Cathay.
Old and weather-worn
Evidence of man's industry and determination.
A symbol of endurance
God's hills, man's mark
Man's work upon God's hills.

—ETHEL MARGARET PHILLIPS

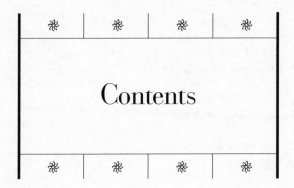

Contents

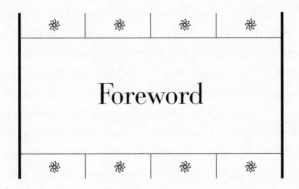

Foreword

♪❋ CLIFFORD PHILLIPS was not quite two when he first met his mother. She was a doctor, a medical missionary and single. The year was 1921 and the place Shanghai, where Cliff had just arrived by ship from England. As he was to learn, his mother was exceptional, and nearly unstoppable. In the following pages he recreates the life of this extraordinary woman, who the Chinese knew as "The Lady Named Thunder."

Ethel Margaret Phillips was forty-five when she gained her son. She had already seen and accomplished enough to fulfill the lives of a dozen persons her age. Her childhood and early womanhood in north-west England is the stuff of Victorian novels. Bright, combative and increasingly aware of the inequalities of the sexes, she enrolled in honours chemistry at the University of Manchester—an exceptional course for a young woman to pursue in 1900. Indeed, the university had only recently begun to admit women. Later she transferred to medicine, a choice made economically possible by a scholarship from the Society for Promoting Christian Knowledge, which was interested in the training of doctors who were willing to go abroad as medical missionaries.

In August 1905, Margaret graduated with a bachelor of medicine and surgery, becoming the third woman to graduate in medicine from the University of Manchester. One month later she sailed for Peking to take up medical mission work in China, leaving England on the day that the treaty ending the Russo-Japanese War was signed. Margaret, it seems, was destined, as the Chinese say, "to live in interesting times."

Margaret Phillips arrived in China as the Qing dynasty (1644–1911) was in its final throes, having already suffered sixty-five years of foreign invasion and internal revolt. The latest humiliation had come with the suppression of the Boxer Uprising in 1901 and the "liberation" of Peking by an eight-nation expeditionary force that had occupied the city and looted the imperial palaces. Foreign troops remained in Peking as legation guards, and the Qing government was saddled with a crippling indemnity.

She had entered a world of foreign privilege that had been gained, and maintained, by the use or threat of military force. Chinese people were generally anti-foreign, opposed to foreign ideas on religion and medicine. Chinese society put little value on the abilities of women. Missionaries were unwelcome; they had to win respect through hard work, good works and by their example. Margaret Phillips was well up to the task.

In the telling of his mother's life, Clifford Phillips has produced more than a simple biography. He gives us insights into Victorian family life, into the mind of a woman pioneer in medical studies, and into the struggles and triumphs of a single woman who fought to bring effective medical treatment to China during tumultuous years of revolution, warlordism, civil strife and foreign invasion. As a bonus, we learn something about Cliff himself, whose own story is worthy of a separate volume. Peking and Edmonton bracket a life that includes an extraordinary childhood in China, "sensitive" wartime service in His Majesty's forces and a post-war career as a brilliant teacher of Chinese language and as an author. In describing his mother, he has sought the wings rather than the spotlight.

This compelling portrait of Ethel Margaret Phillips is of particular interest to those who wish to know more about the Victorian family, the history of medicine, the history of women, the history of medical missions, the history of China and the history of Chinese–Western relations.

The Lady Named Thunder could not have known, when she collected her young son at the Shanghai waterfront, that she had welcomed her future biographer. Readers of this remarkable story will come to appreciate just how fortunate we are that this meeting took place.

BRIAN L. EVANS
Professor Emeritus, University of Alberta

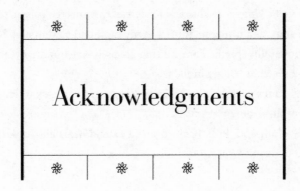

Acknowledgments

♪ I AM MOST GRATEFUL to many of my friends for their encouragement, advice and help with compiling this magnum opus, initially inspired by my family. There are three people in particular who deserve to be named: Corrine Cheng, who read my MS, chapter by chapter, twice over and helped make my efforts more readable from a woman's point of view. This is also an appropriate time to acknowledge the superb job of editing performed by Jill Fallis, a freelance editor engaged by the Press, for the mammoth task of reducing my work by a third. She achieved this virtually seamlessly, having a sensitive feeling for the subject matter. I congratulate her, and again I applaud the woman's touch. Next—last but by no means least—is my wife, Enid, to whom this book is dedicated. Right from the start she read and reread the MS many times over, suggesting suitable changes of wording as can happen in work of this sort.

I am indebted to the Director, Linda Cameron, for her insight regarding the worthiness of the MS and giving the green light to publish this book, and to the team of the University of Alberta Press staff for their input:

Michael Luski and Alethea Adair in editing, Alan Brownoff in design, and Cathie Crooks in marketing.

It is intended that a portion of the proceeds of this biography shall be donated to the University Hospital for research in tuberculosis on the 23rd October 2005, as a fitting memorial to my mother, Dr. Margaret Phillips. I have chosen this specific date, it being precisely one hundred years since she first arrived in Beijing in 1905.

Finally I am grateful to Kay Selin for her generous contribution toward the cost of the Index.

To my old friend, Prof. Brian Evans, I extend heartfelt thanks for his kind and perceptive Foreword.

CLIFFORD PHILLIPS
(LEI HOUTIAN)

Edmonton, Alberta, August, 2003

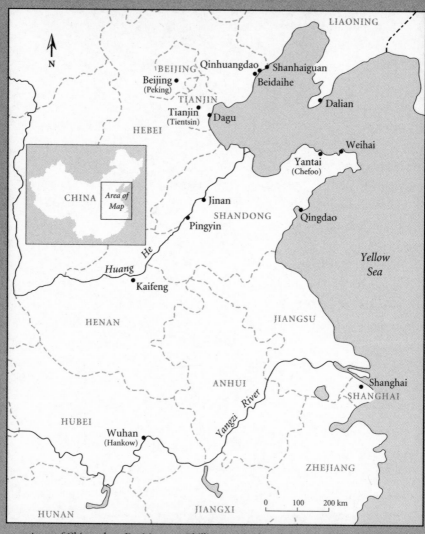

Areas of China where Dr. Margaret Phillips practiced medicine.

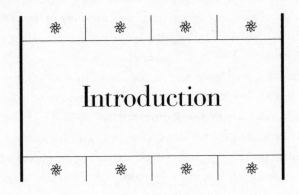

Introduction

♪✻ A FEW YEARS AFTER MY MOTHER DIED, I came into the possession of a suitcase full of papers, which became generally referred to as "Mother's Papers" and accompanied me whenever I moved. Nearly fifty years later, after persistent persuasion from my family, I decided to give the contents my serious attention. I then realized that in my hands lay the account of virtually the whole of my mother's life.

Three large and bulky brown paper wrappers, each with its own clear label—"Medical," "Political" and "Social"—mingled with a smaller clump of newspaper clippings, an assemblage of miscellaneous papers and a selection of poems. I knew that for the last five or six years of her life that my mother had "dabbled," as she put it, and this poetry caused me to settle down to seriously reading her material. There were copies of short articles she had written about Chinese culture, some for publication and others for radio broadcasts, as well as carbon duplicates of her own letters, which surprised me until I realized their purpose. For many years Mother had corresponded with generous friends who funded her work in China, and by duplicating her letters she was able to ensure that she was not needlessly repeating herself. Finally, there were her private diaries and not-so-private journals. Possibly she had intended to write her history, for there were also closely typed pages relating to her girlhood—most of which was news to me. After about a month of reading, I started to develop an overall picture of my mother's life.

The trickiest part lay in sorting the papers so as to relate events in their proper sequence. To convey the times and conditions in which she lived, I felt compelled to describe in detail the day-to-day circumstances in which she worked and the variety of ailments and diseases she handled. I also added passages of political import supporting her documentation. I was persuaded to include my own particulars impinging on her daily life after my adoption, as I became an essential part of her last thirty years. Knowing her observations to be factual and unbiased, I accepted them as objective, thus making it seldom necessary to conduct much further research. Other biographies exist which contain references to Dr. Margaret Phillips, so it is as well that her biography is available for comparison.

Apart from her busy and varied medical practice, Mother exercised a variety of talents: playing violin and piano; singing soprano; painting watercolours; knitting and crochet. Her writings included learned articles for the *British Medical Journal*, lighter pieces for the *Saturday Evening Post*, under the pen-name Philippa King, and a worldwide correspondence with more than two hundred people. Despite all this, she never thought of herself as a workaholic, much less an overachiever.

This feisty maiden lady was known to her friends as Dr. Margaret. Her Christian beliefs nurtured her indomitable spirit, her unyielding standards were high and compromise she invariably considered as weakness. Mediocrity had no place in her work. Her strength of character carried her through many a tough situation. She often endured hardship but seldom complained. She did not suffer fools lightly and, being unfailingly truthful, she could be startlingly blunt in her comments. Her Chinese surname, Lei, meaning "thunder," indicates how well—in their subtle way—the Chinese people accepted her persona and temperament, despite

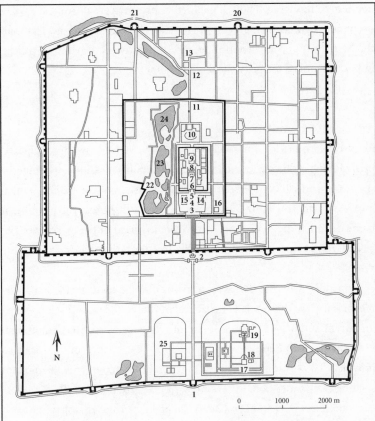

N

| 0 | 1000 | 2000 m |

1 Gate of Everlasting Stability, *Yong Ding Men*
2 Fore Gate, *Qian Men*
3 Gate of Heavenly Peace, *Tian An Men*
4 Gate of Correct Deportment, *Duan Men*
5 Meridian Gate, *Wu Men*
6 Golden Water Stream, *Jin Shui*
7 Gate of Supreme Harmony, *Tai He Men*
8 Halls of Supreme Harmony, *Tai He Dian*,
   Middle Harmony, *Zhong He Dian*,
   Preserving Harmony, *Bao He Dian*
9 Inner Palace Halls
10 Prospect Hill, *Jing Shan*
11 Site of Gate of Earthly Peace, *Di An Men*
   (northern gate of Imperial City)
12 Drum Tower, *Gu Lou*

13 Bell Tower, *Zhong Lou*
14 Imperial Ancestral Temple, *Tai Miao*
15 Altar to the Soil and Grains, *She Ji Tan*
16 Imperial Archives, *Huang Shi Cheng*
17 Altar of Heaven, *Huang Qiu*
18 Imperial Vault of Heaven, *Huang Qiong Yu*
19 Hall for Good Harvests, *Qi Nian Dian*
20 Gate of Peaceful Stability, *An Ding Men*
21 Gate of Victorious Vitrue, *De Sheng Men*
22 South Lake, *Nanhai*
23 Central Lake, *Zhonghai*
24 North Lake, Beihai
25 Temple of Agriculture, *Xian Nong Tan*
   (demolished 1950s)

Map of Peking.

her being a foreigner. Though inclined to present a stern front, she was a deeply caring and loving person. Her standards, requiring no less than the best from anyone around her, did not always endear her to others, but as the soul of integrity she feared no one.

♪※

FOR CENTURIES China's capital city was known by the anglicized name Peking. As a courtesy to the People's Republic of China, the English-speaking world has now recognized the Chinese name Beijing, which means "Northern Capital." However, because Peking was the prominent name during Margaret's time, it is constantly used in this narrative. The city of Hankow, a name also used in this narrative, has since become Wuhan.

Appendix A briefly discusses romanization of the Chinese language; *pinyin* is used in this book. For practical purposes, the narrative is couched in current language, although forms of reference which were traditional until the People's Republic of China became established in 1949 are also provided. These traditional names, in parentheses, accompany the modern spelling at first mention; for example, the Yangzi (Yangtse) River.

Appendices B, C and D relate to Chapters 3, 10 and 12 respectively.

CLIFFORD H. PHILLIPS
January 2002

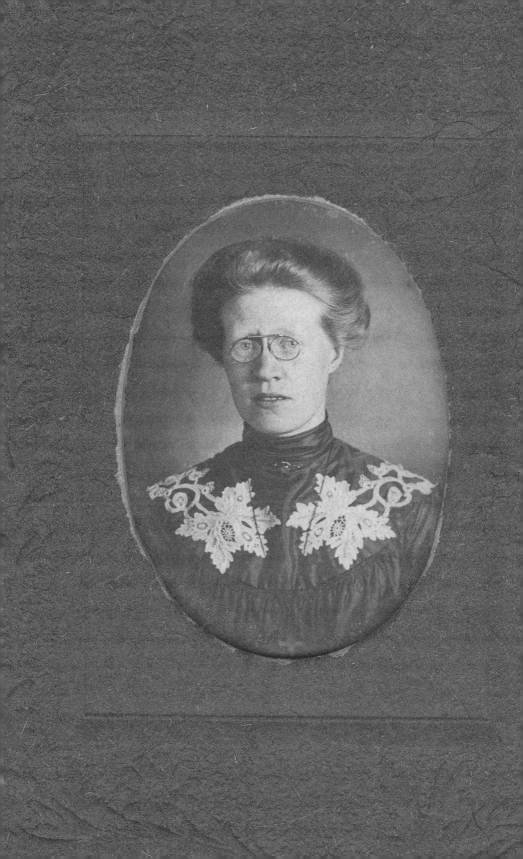

CHAPTER I

Character
in the Making

ℐ✻ ETHEL MARGARET PHILLIPS was only four years old on the day her mother asked, "Would you like to go and see Papa?" Ethel and her sister Annie, fourteen months younger, and her brother Frank, barely two, hailed the suggestion with delight, for they had not seen their father for almost a year. William had developed tuberculosis and, although not hospitalized, had been advised to trade the hard, shut-in life of an engineer for healthier work. Consequently, he moved alone to the adjoining county of Shropshire and started a business manufacturing mineral waters, in the small country town of Bridgnorth. This allowed him to spend more time outdoors, fresh air and rest being the only treatment offered at the time for TB.

That move, however, resulted in Ethel's young mother being left with four young children to care for on her own. To ease the burden, the eldest child, Mamie, had been sent to stay with Grandmother Phillips when Ethel was still a toddler. She hardly remembered the big sister whose role she had assumed. Obedient and dependable, she became her mother's right hand, and the two became very close. Ethel felt proud that she could be entrusted to go to buy a reel of cotton for her mother from the little shop around the corner. Her father was not much in the picture in those days, though she and her mother often talked about him.

The visit to see Papa was to be a surprise. And all the more exciting, the family would travel by train to Bridgnorth—their first train ride. Mrs. Phillips carried baby William Herbert, fondly known as Bertie, in her arms. On arrival, she calmly instructed Ethel to go with Annie and Frank, adding, "Tell Papa that I am going away."

Her siblings were too young to properly understand, but Ethel was rather taken aback. Nonetheless, she obeyed, as always, and led the way to her father's door, while Bertie remained with his mother. Papa was surprised to see them. Upon hearing what Mama had said, he ordered the children to wait inside and rushed up the street after his wife. Later he returned and sadly announced, "Mama would not stay. She has left us and taken baby Bertie with her. I just saw her off on the train."

The family was devastated, especially Ethel, who had been closest to her mother. Any heartache on her mother's part had been well concealed—in those days, the English were prone to present a stiff upper lip in the face of adversity—and to Ethel's mind, any tears shed were hers alone. Years later she wrote about her mother's cold-blooded departure: "That was the end of my happiness. I loved my mother so dearly and missed her very much. It would have been better if she had explained the situation to me, but instead it long remained a mystery."

Attending to her lessons helped to distract her from her pain. At four, Ethel could read easy words, and by the time she was six she could read almost anything. She became quite adept at needlework, and due to her circumstances, she gradually developed an amazing capacity for teaching herself. But soon arrangements were made for the children to leave Papa and stay with Grandmother Phillips, where Mamie lived along with a number of her aunts and uncles, and where Ethel had "always felt rather nervous." Grandmother seemed to be a mischief-maker, and the hostile and unbending atmosphere at her house offered Ethel no comfort. One of the aunts, in particular, treated Ethel rather severely, constantly commenting on her behaviour, insisting that she say "Yes, please" and "Thank you" at the end of almost every sentence, and not allowing her to speak unless spoken to. Ethel and Annie felt utterly rejected, and by way of consoling each other, the girls naturally grew very close. They were inseparable until their adolescence, when they were finally parted by circumstance.

Ethel thought of her mother constantly and prayed for her to come back. As she grew older, she wondered about the desertion—how could her mother possibly have been so gentle and kind, then have repudiated her love for her children? Had Ethel somehow contributed to the circumstances that were so hard for her mother to bear? Years later, when she was grown and met her mother again, Ethel learned that her father had not provided sufficient money to care for their children, while her mother was accused of extravagance. One would have thought that living together was more economical for the family. However, tuberculosis and a new baby added every year would have strained the family resources to the limit, so Ethel concluded that separation probably had been the wiser course. Was this separation an extreme form of birth control? Overall, she believed that to be the main reason. Ethel's parents never did realize what a long-term tragedy this separation was to a little girl. Grandmother Phillips disliked Ethel's mother and forbade any mention of her name in her house.

♪﹡

THE CHILDREN had not long been at their grandmother's house before Ethel and Annie were sent away. Feeling troubled and insecure, they were put on a train to London in the care of the guard. He checked on them every time the train stopped, and the other passengers took a kindly interest in the two wee mites—Ethel not quite five years old, and Annie only three—who were taking such a long journey on their own. In London they lived with two elderly ladies whom they called aunts. Having her younger sister with her provided a steadying effect; Ethel felt responsible for and was very protective of Annie. Initially, arrangements were made for the two girls to attend a nearby day school in London, and later they joined Mamie at the private school kept by the wife of a

Doctor Snodgrass in Southam, a small village in Warwickshire. Not long after their arrival, the doctor died. The girls needed a school where they could remain during the holidays, as they could not go home to Grandmother Phillips, who had a large enough family to contend with, fifteen of whom were still living at home. And so they accompanied the widow Snodgrass on her move to Leamington, where she would establish a larger school. The new house was big with a large garden and many tall trees. Ethel remembered the move, sitting amongst the furniture on the last cart and sleeping on a mattress on the floor for the first night. Little did young Ethel know that she would undertake many such journeys in her life.

Mrs. Snodgrass's spoilt and troublesome son, Anthony, was about Ethel's age. His quick-tempered mother was apt to blame the girls for his pranks, and they were often beaten harshly and unjustly. One day she stormed into the classroom where they were quietly learning their lessons. She told them to hold out their hands while she went round and struck them all painfully with a strong round ruler, unable to discover who had done some wrong thing reported by young Master Anthony. No one knew what all the fuss was about, which only served to further infuriate the woman.

Occasionally Ethel was beaten and shut in a room for something she had not done. In sheer frustration, she would stamp and scream with rage till she fell exhausted to the floor. She was taken by the shoulders and shaken severely, and told she was the worst girl in the school, yet she had no idea what she had done to deserve such abuse. During these two years, Ethel changed from a sweet, happy child to a resentful girl given to extreme tantrums. Invariably truthful, she bitterly resented not being believed. She was particularly offended by young Anthony's lies, and she soon realized that boys often enjoyed preferential treatment. Frank had joined the girls at Leamington, and he too received better treatment from Mrs. Snodgrass. As the first-born son, Frank had inherited a trust fund from his grandmother's parents, with two guardians controlling his education and upbringing.

One of the children's favourite amusements was running along the tops of walls and climbing trees, each vying with the other to climb the highest. Ethel was as much of a daredevil as the rest. One day they were playing a game of Barber's Shop. The game itself was innocent enough, and while scissors played their part in make-believe, Mrs. Snodgrass was enraged, as she strictly forbade the use of these as playthings. To make her point, she cut the girls' beautiful long hair to such devastating effect that, to their great shame, Annie and Ethel looked like boys.

Ethel passed her seventh birthday at Mrs. Snodgrass's school and received the present of a prayer book, which she treasured.

♪※

DISSATISFIED WITH how Mrs. Snodgrass had treated the girls, Grandmother Phillips decided to withdraw them. Frank, now six, remained in Leamington. Once again Ethel was put on a train under the care of the guard, with instructions to ensure that she got off at Small Heath, a suburb of Birmingham. One passenger took a kindly interest in this eight-year-old girl travelling alone. Ethel was small for her age, with an appealing charm which seemed to attract help whenever needed.

Ethel assured the kind lady that her aunts would be there to meet her, but when she got off the train, the platform was empty. The lady watched anxiously from the window, then jumped off the train, saying she would see her home. Ethel could not have been more thankful. The stranger called a cab, and off they went together. Ethel had no idea how to reach her grandmother's house, and it turned out to be quite a distance. When they finally arrived, the lady refused to come in and instructed the cab driver to unload Ethel's trunk. They left before anyone in the house even realized Ethel had arrived.

It transpired that the school had sent Ethel home a day earlier than what was stated in the principal's letter. Her grandmother was upset that Ethel's benefactress had not allowed her the chance to express her thanks. Ethel often wondered about the identity of her kind Samaritan, sometimes fantasizing that this woman was her mother—why else would she not stay to be thanked for her kindness? But years later Ethel's mother assured her that this was not so.

Ethel soon joined Annie and Mamie at a home school in Wolverhampton. An elderly Victorian lady, Miss Lydia Sloper, maintained this small establishment in a terrace house on a quiet street. The neighbourhood, situated on the side of town away from all the ironworks, had easy access to the open countryside. The girls were allowed to go for walks with some small neighbourhood boys and Mamie in charge. They greatly enjoyed these rambles and loved exploring new routes.

The curriculum was typical Victorian fare, as might be expected of an educated lady like Miss Sloper. It consisted of *Little Arthur's History of England* and *The Child's Guide to Knowledge* (questions and answers on a range of subjects), astronomy, geography, grammar and arithmetic. They read books such as *The Peep of Day, Ministering Children* and *Lamplighter* (Ethel's favourite). On Sundays, as a treat, they read John Bunyan's *Pilgrim's Progress.* Every morning, breakfast was followed by family prayers and a reading from the Holy Bible, each taking turns reading verse by verse a whole chapter at a time. Excluding the genealogies, they read the Bible straight through. By the time Ethel left, they were well into reading it for a second time. If anyone had a cold and could not go to church, she had to memorize and recite a whole chapter.

The food at school was plain, mainly porridge, bread and butter, and a dinner of meat and vegetables, plus a pudding. Occasionally the girls were invited to children's parties, but Ethel, being shy, found these to be stiff and formal. Nonetheless, she thoroughly enjoyed such games as Gathering Nuts in May, Oranges and Lemons, and musical chairs. Once the girls went to a party, only to discover that it was for a birthday. They had no gifts, and to Ethel's embarrassment, the young host came up and asked, "Let me see, what present did you give me?"

The girls' greatest excitements were the rare visits by their father. Each would play the piano for Papa to show her progress. For a treat he usually took them for a walk in the park, trying to allow each of his daughters her fair share of walking beside him. Every week they wrote letters to him, each paying for the penny stamp out of her three pennies weekly pocket money. Since a penny was needed for the offertory on Sunday, that left only one penny for sweets. Sometimes they could earn an extra penny for hemming one side of a sheet, and occasionally Miss Sloper would award a penny as a reward for drinking a cup of chamomile tea (said to be much nastier than the latter day's variety) or a mild purgative such as Gregory's powder the day after a party.

One day, to the girls' astonishment, their uncle Arthur visited. He had run away to sea when he was quite young. Uncle Arthur was so jolly he kept the girls in fits of laughter. He took them for a walk and treated them to cakes and sweets and shocked them terribly by dancing the hornpipe in the street. After that he visited whenever he came home from the sea, which was seldom, as he was away for months at a time.

The three sisters remained in Wolverhampton for five years, staying at the school over most holidays but visiting their grandparents at Christmastide. Those Christmas holidays were quite awesome. The girls had fun with their young aunts and uncles—four of school age, and one aunt, May, a year younger than Ethel.

Ethel first saw a Christmas tree when she was eight years old, the first Christmas the three girls spent with Grandmother Phillips. The tree stood in the breakfast room, where most family meals were taken and where the children played. On Christmas morning after breakfast, the children would all march into the dining room. There, laid out on the dining table, were presents from the parents and grandparents. Grandfather handed these to each child rather like a prize-giving. His own present to each grandchild was invariably a bright new silver shilling. Afterwards, the family went off to church. The long walk there and back made everyone appreciative of the sumptuous turkey dinner with plum pudding that followed. Sometimes twenty-one or more people came for Christmas dinner. Ethel and the other small children sat at a separate table for this big event.

Dinner over, the elders retired to sleep off the aftereffects while the younger uncles and aunts and grandchildren went to play football in a nearby field. If the weather was cold enough, they skated on a pond close by. Unfortunately, there were not enough skates to go round, so the smaller children had to make do with one skate each. Later, tea and Christmas crackers were more than welcome, and then followed the ceremony round the Christmas tree, which looked so beautiful when they put out the gas lights and the little candles were lit one by one. Then came more presents: smaller ones hanging on the tree and larger ones beneath it. These gifts the family members gave to each other, many of them handmade. Afterwards, there was usually a brisk game of Snap Dragon, which caused a great deal of mirth as raisins were snatched from a large dish of burning brandy.

The evening ended with a cold supper of ham and pork pie with hot cocoa. The children were allowed to stay up late, and after supper everyone joined in a card game called Speculation. The grandparents never allowed playing for money, but they were allowed to play for hazelnuts—though only for one game.

During the summer the girls spent two weeks at Bridgnorth with their father. They loved this holiday, especially when Frank was there too. They often went for walks in the country, sometimes taking lunch with them and going off for the whole day. Occasionally the girls visited their grandparents in the summer to have their wardrobes renewed. A dressmaker came and sewed all day, making over some of the aunts' clothing for the girls while the aunts taunted them about being the cause of their mother's headaches. Years later, Ethel's father was furious when he heard about the hand-me-downs, insisting that he had always paid enough for the girls to have new clothes.

At age nine, Ethel was walking with a limp. She was made to lie on the dining room carpet at her grandmother's house while the doctor measured her legs. Finding that her left leg was a centimetre (half-inch) shorter than her right, he prescribed a treatment of a large watering can of cold saline solution poured over her leg every morning, followed by a hard rubbing with a rough towel until her leg was warm again. A thicker sole was fitted to her left shoe. Ethel's aunts and uncles never missed an opportunity to adopt an exaggerated limp whenever they saw her, and they were constantly at pains to remind her to walk straight. The treatment proved effective, but by the time Ethel was fifteen, the leg had stopped growing again, so the treatment was repeated. Thankfully the trouble ended then, though her left foot was always noticeably smaller than her right.

Ethel was also having trouble with her eyes, which became red and inflamed. She had to wear a blue veil over her hat when she went out, which she hated, and to stay in a darkened room. The prescribed eye-drops smarted. The long high fence that ran along a footpath by their house created bars of light and shade in the sunlight, which hurt her eyes as she walked by.

Ethel always felt timid and shy with her grandmother, and invariably she was glad to return to school. Miss Sloper had several friends of similar age and style who frequently visited for tea and a chat. Once Ethel heard them discussing the gramophone, Thomas Edison's latest invention, and speculating that someday speaking into a microphone or sending a recorded message by post might be possible.

Around the time of Queen Victoria's jubilee in 1887, when Ethel was eleven, she "gave her heart to Jesus." Miss Sloper, a congregationalist, took the girls to chapel with her on Sunday mornings. In the afternoon, the girls also went to St. Mark's Church, as stipulated by their grandmother. While listening to addresses by E. Digby Everard and a sermon by the London Missionary Society, Ethel conceived of the idea of becoming a missionary when she grew up. This intention remained with her for several years, but as she grew older she realized that shyness and self-consciousness could prevent her from preaching. Subsequently faced with the need to earn a living, she put the idea behind her, though she never quite lost sight of that keen resolve.

At Wolverhampton, Ethel's attitude towards life improved. She still missed her mother badly, and the affection that grew between her and Miss Sloper did much to relieve that lack. Although the teacher was always respectfully referred to as Miss Sloper, she took great pride in the sisters' appearance, especially in their long hair, which she combed and plaited every night. Annie and Ethel were the same height and were dressed alike; they were often taken for twins, although the two were quite different in their features and hair colour. Mamie had left two years earlier to go to school at Kilders in Wales; the girls had a good giggle when she came back with the singsong accent typical of the Welsh.

About two years later Miss Sloper took ill and had to give up her little school. For the remaining weeks of that term Ethel and Annie lived with a kind neighbour whose children had also attended the school. One of the daughters, Muriel, was fourteen, about Ethel's age, and she became her first intimate friend. Ethel told Muriel the story of her mother's desertion, the first time she had ever confided her sadness to anyone. Every Sunday Annie and Ethel visited Miss Sloper in the pleasant rooms where she had gone to live, and they took turns reading aloud from her illustrated copy of *Pilgrim's Progress*. After the girls left Wolverhampton, they corresponded. Ethel once received a valentine in which Miss Sloper spoke of an impending visit by Ethel and sent a motto:

> *I will not easily offend,*
> *Nor be easily offended;*
> *What's amiss I'll strive to mend,*
> *And endure what can't be mended.*

Miss Sloper's last letter was dated June 28, 1890. It eventually dawned on Ethel she had died. Ethel was much saddened to find that her friend had passed away without her knowing, and for some time this worsened her grief.

New arrangements for the girls' education were already in hand. Ethel dreaded the idea of going to school as far away as Mamie, and she begged her father not to send her to Wales. Great was her relief to hear she was to live in Birmingham and share a governess with her young aunt May, although this entailed living in the austere atmosphere of her grandparents' home and her relationship with May was cool. As well, Ethel and Annie would be separated for the first time in their lives, as Annie was to stay with her father.

Ethel's routine started with drawing lessons three mornings a week at the Birmingham School of Art. She was given one shilling a week for her bus fare to the city centre five kilometres (3 miles) away. However, she preferred to save some of that towards sweets, so often she would walk both ways. There were only a few pupils in the morning classes, and Ethel had but one companion, Trixie. They were happy together, but Trixie warned that her grandparents would not allow them to mix if they knew that Ethel's grandfather was in "trade." He was a furrier and owned two shops on New Street, the best part of the city, one for hats and one for furs. The two girls practised freehand and model drawing, and studied geometry and perspective, but the masters left them mostly on their own.

Ethel had to be home for dinner by two o'clock, when May had her music lesson. Then came lessons till five o'clock. On alternate days Ethel had her music lesson at two. As she was studying to be a pupil-teacher, the two free mornings were spent preparing lessons. May's lessons were easier, but Ethel felt the need to push on because she expected to soon be earning her living.

Saturday mornings usually consisted of make-and-mend-type chores. Ethel, in company with her aunts of varying ages, participated in mending their clothes or darning her uncles' socks. Ethel urged her aunts to refuse to mend the old socks and to compel their brothers to buy new ones. However, when the men got home from business, their sisters would usually spoil them instead, waiting on them hand and foot, while her uncles ordered their sisters or wives about, or grumbled and growled about the food. Ethel considered their attitude to be most unjust, and rather lacking any sense of courteous chivalry.

It seemed to Ethel that there was little pleasure in life. The loss of her mother's love and attention still hurt, and she felt vulnerable to "the slings and arrows of outrageous fortune."

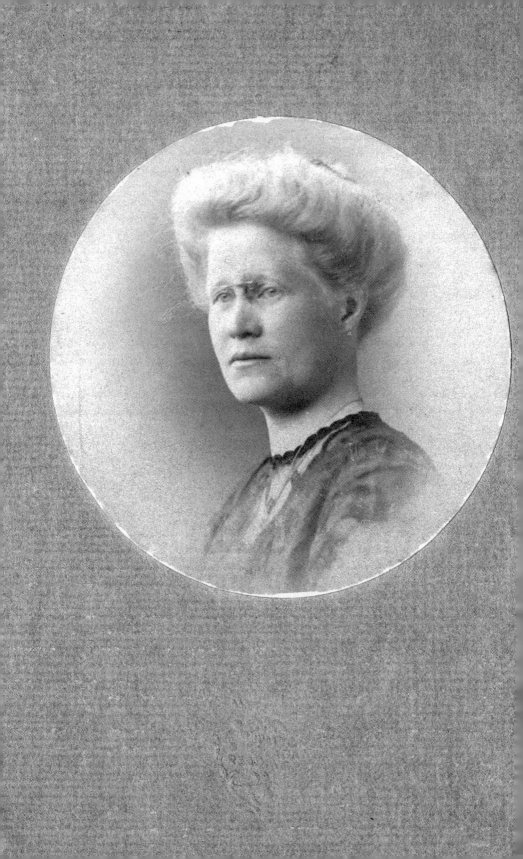

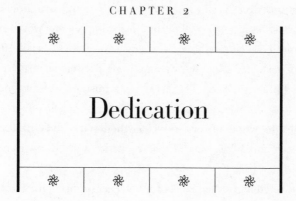

CHAPTER 2

Dedication

♪﹡ ASPIRING TO BECOME INDEPENDENT, Ethel adopted as her motto the words of the contemporary poet W. E. Henley: "I am the master of my fate; / I am the captain of my soul." She also felt called to serve God, and was confident that he would always be there when she needed him.

At age fifteen, she began earning her living. She joined Mamie and Annie at a private school in Kidderminster, Shropshire, which was rather expensive, so arrangements were made for her to make use of her pupil-teacher training. Rushmore College, which was considered very superior, was run by two elderly sisters, Miss Persis and Miss Eliza Friend, who taught the girls the basics of social etiquette. With fifteen to twenty boarders and an equal number of day pupils, they formed a respectably long line, known as a crocodile, when they walked out two by two. Four classes at a time were given in a large schoolroom, another class in a small study and music lessons in the dining room.

Aside from a music mistress and a visiting French teacher, Miss Eliza did the bulk of the teaching, while Ethel taught the youngest children reading, writing and arithmetic, and continued her own classes. Soon she was preparing for the College of Preceptors exams. It was customary to pretend to have exam nerves beforehand and afterwards to say that the questions were hard, a camouflage Ethel found irritating, but her schoolmates thought she was putting on airs when she would not play their game. They chortled hugely when she received a "Failed" in music theory, after she had said it was easy. Exam results were normally accepted, but Miss Eliza, convinced there had been a mistake, wrote to the examiners. It was discovered that Ethel had indeed passed well and placed seventh in the whole of England. Her schoolmates apologized for misjudging her, and Ethel realized that, by sticking to her own principles, she would prevail.

While at Kidderminster, Ethel continued her studies at the Birmingham School of Art—twenty-seven kilometres (17 miles) away—and began passing the exams needed for the art class master's certificate. With the addition of music lessons and practising, there was little time for play. Every Sunday the girls went to church, occupying the first two rows of pews, chiefly because most people disliked being in front. One day Miss Eliza asked if they would help out the boys' choir by mending the torn surplices and hassocks. The girls agreed gladly, but instead of just hassocks, the cassocks—even more in need of repair—also arrived, so they busily stitched them all. The following Sunday, the choir was late, finally entering rather sheepishly, the small boys almost tripping over cassocks far too long for them. The explanation was soon forthcoming: the cassocks had been hung on the wrong pegs with no time to sort them out. For some time this was one of the best school jokes of the year.

Near the school was a poorhouse for paupers or indigent youth, and its residents delighted in annoying the girls by pelting them with pebbles as they marched past. As Miss Eliza thought the best way to stop this was to make friends with the boys, they were invited for tea and some entertainment. The tea was much appreciated but not the entertainment, which the boys did not understand, so they were asked to perform or recite something in return. In the end, the girls were the ones who were entertained as the boys were very funny. The plan worked and the unpleasantness ended.

When Ethel was seventeen and preparing to go home for the summer holidays, Miss Eliza said, "Come back with your hair up and your skirts down." That was an order, for she was being promoted from part-time to full-time teacher. Annie, now sixteen, left the school, as she took no interest in her lessons and her father thought she might as well return home as a companion to Mamie. So it came about that in 1893 Ethel returned to school alone and as a teacher. At first she had difficulty in keeping order with certain pupils who were former classmates, but soon everyone settled into the right relationship. Ethel continued with her studies, studying in her room after supper and going to bed at ten o'clock instead of nine.

A new music mistress, Miss Andrews, joined the staff this term. She was twenty-five, dark, smart in style and quite poised. Ethel was fascinated but thought she was affected. Though they were both teachers, Ethel was allowed to polish up her musical skills with Miss Andrews's help. She was a skilled teacher and Ethel made rapid progress. A warm rapport soon developed, and they became firm friends.

In 1894, while Ethel was staying with her grandparents, her grandfather had a serious operation, performed at home by "the famous Dr. May." Ethel watched the preparations. The kitchen table was used as the operating table. One kidney was removed; the verdict was cancer. The private nurse was a very attractive and charming woman, but Grandmother disapproved of her so she was quickly dismissed. Several aunts helped with the nursing, and Grandfather soon recovered.

Then Ethel began having severe attacks of pain during her menstrual periods. She kept it to herself as long as possible, but her aunts eventually found out and she was taken to see a specialist. He considered her condition urgent, requiring an operation. Ethel was adamant that she could not leave her work before the summer holidays since it would be impossible to find a substitute in the middle of the school year. The doctor, however, so impressed on her aunts the gravity of the situation that they made Ethel promise, in case of another attack, to go straight to his nursing home. Ethel returned to Rushmore and informed Miss Eliza of the situation, but she could not accept that there was anything wrong as Ethel always looked so well. Miss Eliza disapproved of men doctors dealing with women's complaints, and she simply dismissed what she had been told.

About this time Ethel overheard her grandmother talking about her father trying to get a divorce. She considered this strange after so long— more than eighteen years had elapsed since her mother deserted them.

Motorcars and sightseeing coaches began coming into use. Charabancs— as these coaches were called—ran to Leicester. Ethel ventured on one once, but the charabanc came to constant standstills and baulked at the hills, so she decided that train travel was the better choice. In those days people dressed for a car ride in overcoats, bonnets, mufflers and goggles. Motorcycles were in use too, and Uncle Norman's wife disgusted Grandmother Phillips by riding one in Birmingham.

Soon afterwards Ethel received news of her grandmother's death from bronchitis and heart failure. It was the first death in the family and she took it very much to heart, like losing her mother again. She felt that she must get some black clothes, for she now realized that Grandmother had loved her and done a great deal for her. Ethel bought a nice-looking readymade black dress, which needed only slight alterations. It was the best-looking and best-fitting dress she had ever owned.

At the end of the following school term, Ethel, now eighteen, took a position as a private governess to a little girl of eight—which turned out to be an unfortunate experience. Ethel was still young, undeveloped and self-conscious. Gladys was a dear little girl, and she and Ethel became good companions and enjoyed their walks. Mr. and Mrs. de Braith, retired Indian civil servants, were kind and treated Ethel with considera-tion, but she always felt uneasy. Mr. de Braith had his own ideas and theories, and he planned and supervised the lessons minutely.

They lived in the vicarage. The rector lived nearby in his second parish, and he sometimes visited. All the de Braiths had poor appetites, and as Ethel was too shy to eat more than one helping, she was constantly hungry. Some nice biscuits were kept in a glass jar on the sideboard, and occasionally she helped herself to one. Mrs. de Braith evidently noticed that the biscuits got fewer, for she commented one day that the maid must be taking them. That might have been so, but Ethel dared not take any more after that.

Ethel's health was poor then, and perhaps the de Braiths feared she had a tendency to tuberculosis, as they knew her family history. In the end she stayed with them less than three months—a blow to her pride but a relief overall, for she found the situation a strain. One morning she was packed off in a carrier's cart to the station, where she saw herself off to Bridgnorth. A doctor advised her to stay at home for a few months. She continued her studies and her piano practice by herself, once a week going to Kidderminster for music lessons with Miss Andrews. At home she helped with the dusting, but whenever she offered to do any heavier housework she was told to go back to her books. One day Ethel insisted on being allowed to cook the Sunday dinner while everyone else went to church, just to show that she still could. Happily both the roast and the pudding were a success.

It had always been understood that Ethel would earn her own living, so in August she started looking round for another position, and finally she was engaged as a teacher in a small private school in Tenbury (now known as Tenbury Wells), a picturesque village in the county of Worcestershire. Miss Fanshaw's school, The Laurels, was set in a pleasant house with an attractive garden. The other resident mistress, Fanny Higham, was a complete contrast to Ethel. Fanny was very sophisticated and shocked Ethel at once by asking if she flirted, refusing to believe that Ethel, at twenty years old, hardly knew what that meant. Fanny, having marked down the vicar as her prey, began flirting immediately. A scandal soon developed which led to the disappearance, first of Fanny and then the vicar, whereupon Ethel was promoted to senior teacher. The new junior teacher was, Ethel thought, "not nearly so interesting."

Ethel studied in the evenings and continued her violin lessons. During the day, she taught the students music and singing. She passed the Cambridge higher local examinations and began working for the College of Preceptors teacher's certificate, then becoming an Associate of the Royal College of Preceptors (ARCP). She began to teach herself short-hand and took the Pitman's examination, receiving certificates for theory and speed. This use of her leisure time coupled with some practice on a typewriter soon proved to be important.

♪❋

WHILE ETHEL resided at The Laurels, she maintained an extensive journal, recording many of her own philosophical, religious and poetical thoughts, and often quoting from Euripides, Emerson, Spenser, Shakespeare and Milton, or more contemporary writers like Longfellow, Kingsley, Newbolt, Browning and Lord Chesterfield. She was also interested in the works of two women of her time: Elizabeth Barrett Browning and the younger poet Adelaide Ann Proctor, renowned for her poem "The Lost Chord." Excerpts from the various authors and thinkers and biblical verses dutifully included the names and references of each passage. An exception was the omitted source of an item scrawled on the flyleaf of her notebook:

> In reading authors, when you find
>> Bright passages that strike your mind,
> And which perhaps you may have reason
>> To think of at another season,
> Be not contented with the sight,
>> But take it down in black and white;
> Such a respect is wisely shown,
>> It makes another's sense one's own.

Ethel gained considerable solace and inner strength through her spiritual development, and she resolutely strove to follow the words of John Ruskin: "Become a Christ's lady . . . thinking always of herself most as sent to do / His work; and considering at every leisure time what she was to do next." On March 7, the first Sunday in Lent, she recorded the sermons of a visiting missioner of the Hereford diocese, the Reverend H. P. Croushaw. His sermons had a profound effect on her. She continued to attend services regularly at St. Mary's and St. Michael's in

Tenbury. Saturday, March 20, 1897, was a significant day in her life—possibly her confirmation—as this was the date she inscribed with her signature on the flyleaf of the leather-bound Holy Bible that she kept by her for the rest of her life.

♪※

EVENTUALLY THE FAMILY LEARNED that Father's divorce had taken place and that William intended to marry a woman, Laura, he had met at a hotel, who presumably was a barmaid—a terrible blow to the family pride. Ethel was heartbroken, especially as she did not believe in divorce. She heard Laura was a Roman Catholic and that her father would become a Catholic in order to marry her. He moved to Southampton and opened a hotel there, ostensibly for health reasons; this too was considered another blow to the family pride.

Out of the blue Mamie wrote to ask Ethel if she could stay with her at Tenbury. She was engaged to a ship's engineer who had stayed at Father's hotel while in port at Southampton. As they had become engaged after only three days' acquaintance, it was Father's turn to be scandalized. Ethel put the case to Miss Fanshaw, who would do almost anything for Ethel, and she agreed to take Mamie on as an assistant teacher but stipulated that Ethel was still to be the head teacher. Now there were three teachers and the school had as many pupils as it could cater for. Mamie remained on staff for two terms before she got married and eventually took up residence as Mrs. Jones in New York.

Early in 1897, Ethel received a letter from Miss Andrews, imploring her to return to Rushmore as a teacher, since Miss Eliza could not find a suitable person. Ethel wanted more than anything to be with her friend again, yet she worried that she ought not to desert Miss Fanshaw, who set so much store by her. She did not know what to do and turned to Rev. Croushaw, who advised that she inform Miss Fanshaw and leave the decision to her. "The dear old thing set me free, but my mind has never been happy about it," Ethel later wrote, "and I was very sad about leaving her."

By the spring of 1897, Ethel was back at Rushmore, this time sharing the teacher's room with Miss Andrews. She could continue her art classes and violin lessons, despite being busy all day preparing lessons and correcting books. Most of Jubilee Day was spent marking homework, Ethel all the while seething with indignation that she had no time to enjoy herself.

Just before Easter, Ethel had another haemorrhage, this one so severe that it alarmed her. She told Miss Eliza that she was going to her grandparents' home for the Easter holidays, then into the nursing home on Easter Tuesday, but again Miss Eliza appeared to take no notice. Ethel found her grandfather rapidly getting worse. The cancer had returned in the spine and he had attacks of excruciating pain, despite being given morphia repeatedly. On Easter Sunday the pain was unbearable, so in the afternoon Aunt Lilly and Ethel walked to the doctor's house and begged permission to give him an extra dose of morphia. At first he was reluctant, but finally he consented, saying that it did not really matter now. After the injection Grandfather fell into a drowsy condition and did not complain of any further pain. Before leaving, Ethel went to say goodbye, but he seemed half asleep and hardly knew her. She realized she would never see him again.

On Tuesday Ethel checked into the nursing home. The next morning, while she was waiting to have her operation, Sister told her that Miss Eliza had come to see her. The doctor had refused to let her in. Miss Eliza was angry with Ethel for leaving her in the lurch and wanted to compel Ethel to return with her. Ethel assured the doctor that she had told Miss Eliza the state of affairs quite plainly, but she hadn't listened. The doctor gave Ethel the anaesthetic in bed. After the operation, her awakening was very gradual and partial, and she was conscious only at intervals. At first she had two nurses, one for days and one for nights, then later just one who slept in her room. Once Ethel heard them whispering together about whether they should inform her of a letter. They did not, but Ethel knew that her grandfather was dead. A few days later her father visited her. When she asked if Grandfather had died, he confirmed that was why he had come to Manchester.

The fibroid operation was successful, but the patient nearly died. Something was impeding her recovery and she was kept on her back for nearly six weeks. Ethel felt no pain, only great weakness. One day she raised her head from the pillow and saw a white face staring at her—at first she did not recognize herself in the mirror. Another night she sat straight up in bed after a dream; the pain made her cry out, frightening the nurse. Her father visited again before returning to Southampton, and occasionally her aunts came by. She read many books loaned by Dr. Taylor, including Benjamin Kidd's *Social Evolution,* which introduced new ideas to her. When she told Dr. Taylor that she wanted to be a doctor, he replied, "If you go on wanting it hard enough, you will be." But to Ethel that seemed impossible, and she put the thought aside.

At last she was allowed to sit up, and the next day to sit out of bed for half an hour. The nurse placed a glass of water by her side, which Ethel scoffed at, saying, "I never faint," but she was very glad to get back into bed. The following day she walked a little way between two nurses, but her legs did not seem to belong to her. The day after that she was sent home. It was rushing things, but Dr. Taylor knew there were aunts on hand to look after her.

Miss Andrews had promised to take her home, and Ethel was glad to see her arrive with a cab. But just before reaching the house, her friend stopped the cab and walked away. Ethel suspected Miss Eliza had made mischief over the operation and her long absence. She would have liked Miss Andrews to meet the family, but she had no wish to place her friend in an awkward position. Though Ethel was so weak that she could not get out of the cab unaided, it was some time before the aunts came out to help. Even then they did not understand until she had to ask for help to climb the stairs. The next day she was evidently expected to get up for breakfast. She managed to dress and made her bed according to their usual custom, but she was nearly in tears by the time Aunt Lilly came to her rescue. Ethel explained that she had not been given sufficient time to regain her strength. Finally her aunts recognized the need to give her better care.

Aunt May, the youngest, had been sent to a mental home during Grandfather's last illness, but immediately after his death Aunt Kate brought her home again, and she devoted the rest of her life to caring for her weak-minded sister. Oakfield House was up for sale and the aunts were going to take a small house in Yardley. Ethel was forced to look for a job, and her convalescence was cut short.

Once again Ethel was miserable. She longed for love and comfort, and felt that her father had forfeited his children's allegiance. For years Ethel had prayed that her parents would reunite, but now she had to give up that hope. Her thoughts turned to her long-lost mother. Ethel was now twenty-one, and Mamie had always instilled into her siblings that at that age one was free to act as one wished. Ethel wrote her mother a letter in care of a sister, whose address she knew. The response was quick and reassuring; she was overwhelmed with joy. They planned a meeting, but Ethel begged for secrecy and made her mother promise not to contact the rest of the family. Though she felt justified in desiring to meet her mother after so many years apart, she did not want to hurt her father by apparent disloyalty. "For many years I led a double life."

The two met at Worcester. Mrs. Phillips was nice, but Ethel was so weighed down with her sense of her mother's deceit and disloyalty that she was unable to respond as she had hoped. She doubted the reality of her mother's displayed affection. How could she act so resigned to having been without her children for so long? Nevertheless, the day was exciting, and Ethel lost her voice completely.

Ethel was now able to get to know her youngest brother, Bertie, now sixteen, who lived with their mother in a comfortable two-storey cottage. The first time she saw him since he was a baby was at a village near Blandford, where Bertie had been appointed church organist. Mrs. Phillips met Ethel at the station with a smart little donkey cart. The drive back was most amusing as the donkey constantly tried to turn aside and stop by the hedge for tasty mouthfuls. The three had an enjoyable time, and for several years after Ethel visited the pair of them during the school holidays, immensely enjoying being made a fuss of.

Later her mother and Bertie settled in Bridgwater in the county of Somerset, living in a Victorian-style building named Bridge House on the banks of the River Parrett. Mr. P., as Bertie became known, was the parish church organist and taught music and was very involved in other musical activities of the county. Soon Ethel began to feel more relaxed. The three visited places like Weston-Super-Mare, Minehead, and one summer Ethel spent a week in Worcester for the Three Choirs Festival: Gloucester, Worcester and Hereford. She had a blissful time listening to Handel's oratorios, and the organ music meant even more to her as brother Bertie was an organist.

♪✻

ETHEL WAS REALLY SURPRISED to obtain a position at Quorn as mistress in an endowed grammar school, all the other teachers being masters. The Quorn school was endowed in the reign of King Charles II but had lapsed for many years. Now it was being reopened with fine new buildings, made possible by the accumulation of funds, and it was to be coeducational. No boarders were taken, though some pupils took their midday meal at school. This was where Ethel's knowledge of shorthand became an asset and partly obtained her the post, as it would be an extra item on the curriculum. She resided with the headmaster, Mr. Hensham, and his wife, as did the science master, Mr. Brittain. Ethel believed that this arrangement was rather a trial for Mrs. Hensham, especially as she was occupying her guest-room. They had a private dining room, so when they entertained, Ethel and Mr. Brittain had their meal alone. After a year, he found rooms in the village, and Ethel moved into his room, which entailed using the back stairs.

Mr. Hensham was fearfully critical and unpopular with the other masters. At first Ethel appreciated any advice about teaching, but pleasing him seemed impossible, so she found that she had to stand up to him. He relished discovering mistakes that she had overlooked in some boy's exercise. At last Ethel stopped this by collecting all the books she had to correct in a week and taking the pile to him, pointing out the oversights in his own corrections.

At first there were only five girls, and later about fourteen. Ethel taught all subjects, including needlework, and supervised the girls' athletics, for the boys and girls did not play together. As far as time allowed, Ethel continued her studies, which included physics lessons from Mr. Brittain. She wanted to learn more and was advised to go to the technical school in Leicester. This entailed a short train journey and a walk of about one and a half kilometres (1 mile) home at midnight, involving a shortcut across the churchyard. The lecturer, a young master from the Leicester Grammar School, fascinated Ethel. She freely admitted that she had fallen blindly in love with him, and naturally he was somewhat interested in the only woman student in the class. Ethel continued for two terms, then took private lessons from him in organic chemistry; he fondly grinned every time he spoke of ethyl compounds. They corresponded occasionally, and once he invited Ethel to tea at a restaurant in Leicester, but after she left Quorn their letters ended. Ethel feared her adoration was all too evident, and that he was probably too accustomed to it, for he was most attractive.

MOONLIGHT IS FOR LOVE

Come walk with me in the moonlight
And link your arm in mine.
Let us share our inmost feelings
And mystic wonderings.

For moonlight is for fancies
And murmurings of love;
For thoughts of home and friendship
And dreams of youth and joy.

Moonlight is for lovers' trystings,
Sweet embracings, bitter partings;

Daring plans for high adventure,
Vows of steadfastness and trust.

In the magic sheen of moonlight
Ugly things are beautified,
Then emotion casts out wisdom
Making foolishness seem right.

Yet this life is meant for gladness,
And we need not all be wise,
So I will choose the moonshine madness
And leave the sanity for you.

(E. M. P.)

In September 1898, Ethel took the college entrance exam. In the middle of her English paper, she was told that she had entered for nine subjects but only seven were allowed. Which subjects would she prefer to drop? Having to think quickly, she dropped Latin and mechanics, her two self-taught and weakest subjects. Ethel passed the exam but did not win the bursary that would have covered residential expenses, although she did get a smaller bursary of fifteen pounds a term for three years, which was better than nothing. Her father felt encouraged enough to promise to take care of the rest. (The winner of the bursary told Ethel some years later that she had won it because her father was a well-known Manchester doctor; she could not have gone to college without it, but she did not think she had won it fairly.)

What a change came over the Quorn community when they heard Ethel was leaving to go to university. Initially she had accepted their patronizing attitudes philosophically, but now she felt somewhat contemptuous, although she did not refuse any invitations. Even Mrs. Hensham became a little warmer. Mr. Brittain was another matter. A mutual regard had developed between her and the science master who, from the start, was impressed by the academic potential of this young lady staff member.

She was gratified by his encouragement and grateful for his guidance and support in developing her ambitions. Moreover, as her friend and mentor he had endorsed her ability to compete with men in her academic endeavours— in those days, a rare pursuit for a woman.

The university term started in October, so Ethel had a long holiday to enjoy. As finances were tight, she decided to spend it with the family, mostly with Mamie, who now lived in Southampton, preparatory to moving to the United States. Her husband, Owen Jones, was docked in port there. Ethel visited her father just once and his new wife Laura made a good impression on her, certainly much better than expected. If her father had found happiness with Laura, Ethel concluded, it was his own business—except for the divorce, which Ethel considered a sin.

One day Ethel overheard her father telling Mamie that he suspected Ethel was in love. Her sister disagreed; she thought Ethel was so happy to be going to university. Still, Father was right, for there is something about a person in love that cannot be mistaken. In Ethel's case, it was obviously a double happiness.

Mamie had to make a hurried departure for Liverpool as Owen's ship was on a different run, docking farther north in England. Ethel went to stay with Mamie in Liverpool, and Annie, who was there to help with housework and the baby, came to meet her. Annie had no bump of locality. They were to take a certain tram home, but she missed the spot and they got lost. They wandered into some rather slummy streets and came across some drunken women fighting, so they turned back. By enquiring in some shops they finally got the right tram. Mamie's little house appalled Ethel, although it was nicely arranged. She could not help contrasting it with her previous proud notions.

Ethel set out for the University of Manchester with a song in her heart.

COMPLEMENTS

Good is not good without evil,
Wrong is not wrong without right,
Gain is not gain without struggle,
Love is not love without pain.

Love is not always good
As pain is not always bad.
Sorrow can lead to perfect joy
And Hope overcome despair.

(E. M. P.)

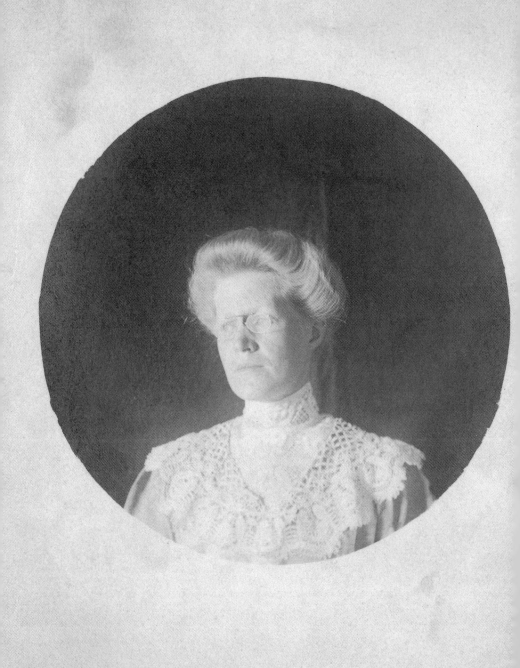

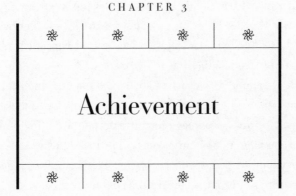

CHAPTER 3

Achievement

♪✳ ETHEL WAS ENROLLED in the chemistry honours course at Victoria University of Manchester, and she was so happy that everyone noticed it. Only recently had women been admitted to the university, in every department except medicine. She lived at Ashburne Hall, a private residence in Victoria Park purchased by the college as a hall of residence for women. She shared a large ground-floor room, divided down the middle by a curtain, with another student, Jane. Miss Stephen, the warden, was aristocratic, shy and proper, and extremely conscientious. She found her task difficult, for the students persisted in flirting with the men. Jane used to slip out at night to talk through the garden railings to the students from the men's hall of residence just across the road.

In January 1901, Queen Victoria died. Ethel had been brought up so much in the Victorian tradition that she felt the loss deeply. Going to see the funeral procession in London was out of the question, but she did go to the town hall square to hear the proclamation of King Edward VII and she attended a memorial service held at Manchester Cathedral, which was the next best thing to going to London.

After a three-storey wing was added onto Ashburne Hall, Ethel got a tiny bed-sitter of her own, a much appreciated luxury. There she could receive her own friends, although sometimes too many. Eventually, to ensure some time for her studies, she put up an ENGAGED notice on her door, only to find one day another sign posted beneath hers, saying CONGRATULATIONS. Ethel was in her element, enjoying simple pleasures such as evening cocoa parties. Poetry was popular, and people liked to cap one another's quotations, an amusement at which Ethel excelled. Sometimes Saturday evenings brought entertainments for students in residence: perhaps an orchestral concert in which Ethel would take part with her violin, or occasionally, a play. Once the students acted out a selection from *Macbeth* with Ethel as one of the witches.

Ethel's first-year subjects for the interned B.Sc. in chemistry honours were inorganic chemistry, practical zoology and botany. At first she continued her studies at the School of Art, and her German classes, but soon these were more than she could manage as there was so much practical work in her three subjects. She enjoyed practical chemistry the most and loved testing the solutions. It was a favourite trick of the demonstrator to give anything but plain water to test. He was disgusted when she quickly found it out, though he could not complain when he saw that she had done the necessary work to exclude substances in solution.

At first Ethel wrote all her chemistry notes in shorthand, but eventually she gave that up as she could not spare the time for transcribing. Her art training was also useful. In zoology and botany, the students drew pictures of their specimens and of the microscopic slides, and coloured them. Seeing the professor absentmindedly handling the frogs as he lectured made Ethel shiver. She had always hated worms and frogs, and needed a strong will to pick them up. The first time she handled these specimens she felt so proud of herself that she left class to tell her new friend, Ethel Lomas, who appeared more contemptuous than amused. At the end of the year she won a prize for the best notebook of diagrams of botany and zoology.

During the second term, the college authorities of the medical school opened their doors to women, the last of the faculties to follow the modern trend of equality for the sexes. It seems it was a grudging consent. Some professors always began their lectures with the greeting "Gentlemen"— ignoring the few women in their classes—whereupon fellow students invariably called out "Ladies" or "Ladies and Gentlemen."

When Ethel discovered that the interned B.Sc. in chemistry honours course coincided with the first-year medical course, it was an opportunity too tempting to ignore for one whose early ambition had been to become a doctor, and she applied to her father again. He agreed to help make up any financial deficit, for this would take at least five years instead of three. She then transferred to the Faculty of Medicine.

Ethel Lomas planned to go to London for hospital training after completing the two years of interned M.B., away from her home in Manchester to enable more strenuous study. One day her bicycle skidded on the tram lines and she fractured her elbow, forcing her to stay at home for several weeks. Ethel cycled over nearly every afternoon after class to take her notes to her, entailing a return journey of about twenty-five kilometres (15 miles). The parents were extremely touched, and the next year they returned this kindness in full measure.

Other good friends included Ethel Elliott and Ethel Robinson. This profusion of Ethels caused our Ethel to resort to her second name, Margaret, which she retained thereafter. Her family still called her Ethel, although her mother and Bert switched to Margaret.

The registrar for women, Miss Edith Wilson, took a kindly interest in Margaret and was always most helpful. When she heard that Margaret wanted to transfer to the medical school, and that it was a question of means, she asked if Margaret had thought of becoming a missionary, as she knew that the Society for Promoting Christian Knowledge (SPCK) gave scholarships to students who were willing to go abroad as missionary medical doctors. This awoke an even earlier wish of Margaret's, her childhood desire to become a missionary. To be both a doctor and a missionary seemed an ideal combination, and she was very happy at the thought.

Miss Wilson promised to give Margaret a recommendation, and she invited her to come to Rochdale for the day to meet her brother, the canon. There they went on the moors for a delightful outing. Margaret was relaxed and gave a good account of herself. Afterwards, the canon wrote a first-hand reference, which certainly helped her to obtain the grant she needed.

She then went to London for a medical inspection and an interview with the SPCK committee. Dr. Scharlieb inspected her from head to toe. When she heard of Margaret's operation, she said it was no barrier and that her chest was sound and condition so good that she would have been proud to have been her surgeon. Afterwards, the doctor took an interest in Margaret, and they corresponded until her death. At the time, however, her stern manner scared Margaret no end.

At her interview with the SPCK committee, Margaret felt nervous, but the sight of a dozen genial-looking elderly men reassured her and she answered their questions calmly. It would be necessary, they said, for Margaret to apply to a missionary society. Margaret replied that she would apply to the Society for the Propagation of the Gospel (SPG) and she would be willing to go to India, which pleased them. They expressed surprise that Dr. Scharlieb had rendered such a good report, as they thought Margaret did not look very strong. However, they understood why when she explained that she was in the middle of exams and would be travelling all night to get back in time for her exam the next day. The result was a grant for seventy-five pounds a year for three years.

The summer vacation lasted three months. For her first "long vacation," as the summer break was known, Margaret visited Aunt Lilly in Guildford, Surrey, to help look after Mary, her niece, aged two, and her nephew, Philip, aged six months. The best part of that holiday was cycling with her uncle. Surrey is a beautiful county and they took some long rides, sometimes stopping for tea and poached eggs at a country inn. Here Margaret's old pain returned, becoming so severe in church that she told Aunt Lilly about it after the service, who sent for the doctor. After a few days in bed, she was all right again. Still, she found pushing two children about in a large perambulator too much for her moderate strength. The net result was that Margaret was none too fit when she returned for her second year at university.

Now she had some new friends, Katherine Clarke, Jessie Clark and Marion Hawcridge, all straight from high school, and they roomed together. Margaret's current subjects were organic chemistry, physics, physiology, histology and anatomy, all with practical courses. The classes were large. It took two years to cover the course, and seniors and juniors studied together. Two women were ahead of Margaret: Catherine Chisholm, who graduated in 1904, and Louisa Corbett, who was just ahead of Margaret in her year. Margaret considered herself fortunate in having such "famous professors" as Professor Dixon for chemistry, Professor Schuster for physics, Professor Gray for anatomy and Professor Stirling for physiology, the course in which she was most interested.

Most students attended classes regularly, but in some subjects the roll-call became a farce, for students would say "Present" to one name, then creep along behind the desks to answer to another. The women never dared to go in if they were late, as they would be greeted with stamping feet, cheers or shocked cries of "Shame."

Margaret found dissecting to be another hurdle; her difficulty was so obvious that the kindly Dr. Gray asked if she could go on. That, of course, pushed her right over the hurdle, for there was nothing like a suggestion of a challenge to put Margaret on her mettle. She had a good memory and worked so hard at anatomy that after the first-year exam Dr. Gray said hers was truly a one-hundred-percent result and he wanted her to become the anatomy demonstrator for the next year's students. He failed to obtain an honorarium for her, but Margaret had the pleasure of helping others. The end of the college year found Margaret with the prize for her histology notebook. From then on there was keen competition in her class. Unfortunately, that year saw a recurrence of her pains, and she travelled to Birmingham to see Dr. Taylor, who could not understand the reason for it.

After Christmas she began the study of obstetrics and embryology under another "famous professor," Sir William Sinclair. These were subjects of which Margaret was entirely ignorant, and she honestly found the huge diagrams on display somewhat disturbing. For certain lectures the women students were asked to stay away. During this term Margaret became ill again and was persuaded to go to Sir William for advice. He was so extremely kind and fatherly and matter-of-fact that she followed his counsel and accepted everything as naturally as possible. He explained that the first operation had been inadequate and should be redone. Margaret's hysterectomy was performed on Good Friday. For six days afterwards she was only semiconscious and vomited persistently.

One day, while the nurse was holding her head over the basin, another nurse put her head round the door and said someone had come to ask how Margaret was. Her nurse replied that she was quite comfortable, but Margaret snorted indignantly, "You can say I am as well as can be expected or going on all right, but *comfortable* is not the right word." She must have begun to turn the corner, and the matron hastened her recovery by telling her she made so much noise that she was disturbing the other patients.

It was now that her kind friend, Mrs. Lomas, Ethel's mother, came to her rescue, taking Margaret to her house for her convalescence. No mother could have been kinder, and ever after that Margaret referred to her as her "Mother-Friend." It was pleasant simply to lounge in their garden on fine days. By Whitsuntide, she was back at the residence hall and allowed to attend classes, on the understanding that she did not work too hard. It came home to her how ill she had been during the annual sports festival in June, in which she did not take part. A visitor to whom she had been offering tea, asked her name, then exclaimed, "I thought you had—"

"No, I did not die," Margaret snapped, "and I'm very well now."

Margaret feared her attendances had been too few to allow her to enter the yearly exams, and that she might have to repeat the year, but the authorities decided to allow her to continue. Then she found that her matric was deficient in two required subjects—the two she had dropped— so she had to cram Latin and mechanics as well. She took private lessons in Latin for six weeks, but her tutor considered her knowledge quite inadequate and held little hope of her passing. When Margaret tried to excuse herself by saying that she was self-taught and that she had never had lessons in Latin before, he snorted, "A little late to begin." That spurred Margaret on, and doubtless to his surprise she passed. Later Dr.

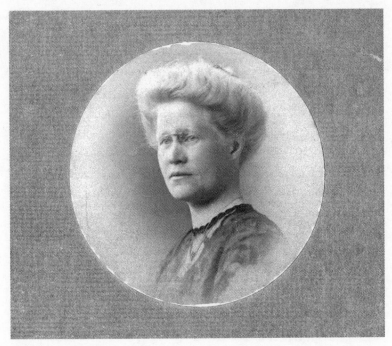

Ethel Margaret Phillips, c. 1903.

Gray told her confidentially that though Latin was not her strong point, the authorities thought she knew enough for the study of medicine.

Margaret's second long vacation was spent at Coniston in the Lake District with her friend Jessie Clark. For the first month the weather was wonderful and the two had many delightful outings, including climbing the Old Man of Coniston and visiting Ruskin's home. The loveliest spot was a pine-fringed tarn called Coniston Water. They also wandered over the Langdale Pikes, a long ridge off to the north-west glorified by Wordsworth more than a hundred years earlier.

∫✳

DURING THE NEXT YEAR, Margaret continued studying anatomy, physiology and obstetrics, as well as attending the outpatients department at the Manchester Royal Infirmary, which in those days was situated right in the heart of the city. Most Manchester streets were paved with cobblestones, and the noise of the traffic—mainly horse-drawn vehicles with ironclad wheels—was tremendous: a cacophony of clopping horses' hooves, steel clashing on stone and occasional shouts. Margaret wondered how the doctors could possibly hear the breath in their patients' lungs. It was always necessary to close the windows first.

In the outpatients department, the students did dressings or listened to the specialists as they examined the patients. One day Margaret was told to extract a man's tooth, because the patient had refused to let men students rather than doctors do it. Imagine his chagrin when he was turned over to a female intern. The doctor showed Margaret how to apply the forceps and to lever, not pull, out the tooth. Luckily, it came out quite satisfactorily.

The timetable allowed no interval for lunches, what with lectures in the morning and practical in the afternoon. Margaret was appointed to approach the dean, Professor Gray, to ask for a lunch break. When she told him that other university departments had a free interval for lunch, he remarked, "Ah, but they don't work on the other side," implying slyly that life in the hospital operated in a different way. How had the men managed, he asked; no complaint had been made before. Margaret suggested that they had practised the fine art of skipping lectures. Anyway, the point was taken and from then on there was a free half-hour between eleven-thirty and noon, when sandwiches were eaten and tea made in the women's common room.

During that year Professor Stirling pointed out the possibility of Margaret getting a science degree en route to the medical one. She could do this in physiology honours if she would take on some extra work in practical physiology. A second subject was necessary and she chose psychology, under Professor Alexander, whose absentmindedness was proverbial. On one occasion he set his students an essay to write, telling them to send the papers to his rooms. When asked for his address he hesitated, and unable to recall it, he advised, "Ask the porter."

This absentmindedness became rather serious for Margaret in her oral exam in practical psychology. As often happened, there was no external examiner. Professor Alexander asked a certain question, which she answered, and he said, "No, think again." Surprised, Margaret tried various answers, all of which were wrong. Finally she reverted to her original answer, and he promptly said, "Right. Why didn't you say that before?"

"But I did!" Margaret replied desperately, and after that they got on all right. When the results were out, he said, "I am sorry it wasn't a first. I'm afraid I am really to blame for that."

In her third long vacation, Margaret joined Ethel Elliott and Ethel Lomas at Lake Windermere. They made many bicycle excursions, and though the hills were too steep to pedal to the top, there were downhill slopes to compensate. They stopped at small inns for tea, at a regulation charge of one shilling.

Margaret's last two years at college were busy, with courses and clinics including pathology, public health, medicine, surgery, diseases of the skin, eye, ear, nose and throat, and midwifery. As an intern student she was more interested in surgery than medicine, because the results were more obvious and encouraging. The many chronic cases in the medical wards discouraged her. But overall she thought the teaching at her school was "distinctly good" and that the women had equal opportunities with the men. The professors did not talk down to them, as she suspected they might have done to a class of women alone.

In the infirmary, the junior and senior intern students (or dressers) in the medical and surgical wards each attended to five or more beds. Patients were examined and their case histories recorded. Unlike most students, who wished to get away in the holidays, Margaret chose to stay at Ashburne Hall, as she was senior intern student in charge of twenty-five beds. One morning she had a new case. After examining the patient, she recorded her diagnosis: cancer of the stomach. The resident surgeon was annoyed as this was to be a "case for diagnosis," and he told her that it was not for her to make a pronouncement. However, he left it there and the patient was duly taken to the operating theatre for an exploratory laparotomy. Professor Thorburn read the notes without comment, and Margaret assisted with the instruments and needles. It proved an inoperable cancer, so the patient was sutured and sent back to the ward. Then Dr. Thorburn remarked dryly, "It seems that the intern was the only one who diagnosed this case."

Margaret was surprised that there had been any doubt, but it appeared that the patient had been on the medical side for some weeks, getting progressively thinner, and no definite diagnosis had been made. She felt rather overwhelmed by the number of questions and comments that came her way. Even the dean of medicine, Dr. Wilkinson, asked her why she had thought it was cancer; her reply was that she could "feel" it.

Another morning Margaret accompanied a patient with a lipoma at the side of the abdomen to the operating theatre, which was filled with students. To her horror, Dr. Thorburn announced, "This operation will be done by the intern student." Perhaps it was a good thing she had no warning. This was to be her first operation and she just had to do the best she could. The operation was an easy one, and Dr. Thorburn was very kind in directing the steps to be taken which helped her to get through. It was a valuable lesson. Often the students suffered from a lack of sufficient practice. They never had the chance even to give a hypodermic injection.

The infirmary also provided training for nurses. The nurses too suffered from a lack of experience, as the medical students helped with the dressings, which normally would have been the nurses' job. The students were glad to leave tidying up to the nurses. The matron was not partial towards women medicals.

The clinics held round the patients' beds were very instructive. Students had to attend a certain number of these. One morning Margaret arrived a little late. A group of students stood round a patient who was holding out a wrist for inspection. As she entered Dr. Collier looked round and said, somewhat sarcastically, "Here is Miss Phillips. She will be able to tell us what it is." Margaret drew nearer but did not touch the patient's hand. Although she had never seen one before, she knew it at once and promptly answered, "It is a ganglion of the wrist."

"A good guess," said Dr. Collier, much to her indignation. When the clinic was over, Margaret told him, "It was really not a guess. I had never seen one before, but I happened to be reading it up just before I came to the clinic."

Nearly all the teachers emphasized that a doctor's first duty was disease prevention, with the cure secondary, especially as this often proved to be palliative. However, Margaret found the course in public health the dullest of all. She was feeling strained with so many subjects and classes, and had almost given up taking notes, which seemed to annoy the lecturer, who commented sarcastically on that fact. This made her work extra hard, and he must have been surprised when she won the bronze medal in the class exam—one of eight she won during her five years at university. Margaret felt that she had an advantage over the other students because she was older and had experience of exams that she actually enjoyed. Her good memory enabled her to cram a subject, and she won several scholarships which helped greatly, for there were many incidentals to be paid for and holidays to be arranged since she no longer had a home.

♪✳

DURING MARGARET'S THIRD LONG VACATION her father had a severe attack of haemoptysis (coughing up blood) as he was walking along the street. He spent several weeks in hospital. Margaret was anxious about him, but she could not afford the fare to visit. Her kind friend, Mrs. Lomas, insisted on giving her the fare, so off she went to Southampton. Her father seemed quite himself and had made a wonderful recovery. He told Margaret he would probably have died had it not happened that he took ill outside the hospital. Margaret pondered whether this was mere chance. Often she too sensed "a scent from afar."

Later her father moved to Bournemouth and took life more quietly, and Margaret visited him during a summer holiday. He had told her he had planned a holiday in Jersey and had bought his ticket already. Margaret insisted that his trip be postponed, as she wished them to have the longest possible time together, and so he delayed going until after her visit. It happened that the ship on which he would have sailed was the ill-fated *Stella* that foundered with a great loss of life.

Once or twice the students persuaded Miss Stephen, the warden, to allow them to hold a dance at the residence hall, though she did not encourage friendships with the men students. One night, soon after dinner, the maid announced that a gentleman had come to visit Margaret. She went downstairs to find Frank waiting in the hallway, and without thinking, she took him straight up to her room on the third floor. He had come to Manchester on business, he said, but had not had time to let her know beforehand. They had a pleasant talk, and she made cocoa for him. At ten o'clock he thought he should leave, so she went downstairs to let him out. Just outside the hall entrance she kissed him goodbye. Then she went inside, only to find Miss Stephen waiting for her.

"Oh, Miss Stephen," said Margaret. "Wasn't that nice? My brother just came to see me. I never expected him."

"Ah, so it was your brother," Miss Stephen replied flatly. On her way upstairs, Margaret called in to see Jess and Marion and Kath, who were lying in wait, simply devoured with curiosity. When she told them that it was her brother who had visited, they rolled about with laughter, saying how Miss Stephen had been running up and down the stairs, waiting for her visitor to go. Had she but known, Margaret said, she would have let Miss Stephen ask more questions before telling her who the male visitor was.

On another occasion Margaret's father and mother both announced that they were coming to see her on the same day. Her problem was how to keep them from seeing each other. Her father had come on business and would drop by in the morning, so she had to tell her mother and Bert, who were making a special trip to visit her, that she would not be free till the afternoon. Margaret wondered why they should all want to come on the same day.

Her father was glad to see how Margaret lived, and they enjoyed a happy time. In the afternoon, her mother and brother arrived and Margaret showed them round the residence hall. This was to be the one opportunity Margaret had to reveal any details of her life to them. They were impressed and, naturally, delighted to see that she had been doing so well. The three then went out to a restaurant for tea and spent as much time together as possible, until Margaret saw them off on the train. She had not talked so much for a long time, yet there always seemed to be more to be said than time allowed.

♪＊

DURING HER FOURTH WINTER, Margaret attended a missionary meeting at the Free Trade Hall and heard Bishop Geoffrey Iliff eloquently speak about his work in the Chinese province of Shandong (Shantung), particularly of the need for doctors in China. He appealed to the medical students of Manchester to volunteer, and Margaret returned to the residence hall with a foreboding that she might have to go to China, though she did not want to.

The following summer she was invited to attend some SPG meetings in London and stayed for three days with Bishop and Mrs. Montgomery. The bishop was the SPG secretary. One afternoon, at a garden party, Margaret was introduced to Bishop Iliff, who immediately appropriated her for Shandong. It was useless her saying that she was booked for India—not that she badly wanted to go to India, since she had always had a secret dread of snakes, so maybe the change would be for the best after all. He sat by her all afternoon until she promised that she would ask the SPG to allow her to go to China.

She was rather surprised to discover that the SPG seemed quite annoyed at her wanting to change, although remaining anxious that Margaret get some missionary training before leaving England. She agreed to spend her last Christmas vacation at St. Andrew's Home in Portsmouth, where the SPG sent their women missionaries for training in parish work. The train journey there took fifteen hours instead of the usual seven, as the whole of England was enveloped in dense fog. The four-wheeler wagon that came to the residence hall to fetch her was late to start with, and a man had to lead the horse all the way. If he got up beside the driver, even for a minute, they were on the sidewalk. Upon finally reaching the station, they had a long wait as the engine was nowhere to be found. At last they were off at a crawl, and a crawl it had to be, as the driver could not see the signals until he was close enough to touch them. After a long wait at one place, someone asked where they were. The answer was, "We think we're outside Oxford, but we do not know for sure."

Margaret shared her packet of sandwiches with a family in the same carriage. No one was able to get out anywhere to get food. When she had to change trains at Reading, she sent a telegram to St. Andrew's Home: "DELAYED. DON'T WAIT FOR ME." There was no certainty of arriving that day.

Slowly the fog lifted, and gradually nearly everyone left the train till Margaret was alone in her compartment. A man from the next carriage came to speak to her during the waits at the wayside stations. He may have meant to be helpful, but she wished he would leave her alone. She assured him that she would be met, though she did not expect it after her telegram. He said he could find a nice hotel where she could stay. She was wondering what to do, for she was supposed to get out at a branch station just before the main Portsmouth station. She had decided to stay on the train till it reached Portsmouth, when suddenly she caught sight of a sister of mercy waiting on the platform. How grateful Margaret felt. She asked if her telegram had been received, and the dear woman said, "Yes, but I would have waited here all night until you came." She took her to the home and gave her a good meal. Margaret finally felt relaxed, at ease and safe.

Mother Emma was very kind, and Margaret enjoyed her stay. There she met Miss Esther Sworder, who would later become a deaconess and sail with her to China, and Marion Service, who was bound for Japan. Margaret went to church several times a day, to lectures and Bible classes, and did a little district visiting with one of the sisters. Mother Emma wanted Margaret to promise to return for a year after she finished her course to give classes to the sisters, but she had already decided that two weeks was all that she could spare.

Actually, Margaret had planned what she wanted to do in the year before her departure for China. Professor Sinclair had promised to give her an internship in midwifery at St. Mary's Hospital, and he had suggested a subject to work on for her M.D. She had applied for a fellowship for one year to help financially and had been told she had a good chance, but it was given to a senior medical student whose father was a college professor. (The next time Margaret was in England, half a dozen years later, she heard this student had applied for a position which he failed to obtain. He committed suicide, as he had threatened to do if unsuccessful.)

In those days students sat for nearly all subjects in their finals. In her practical medicine, Margaret had to examine a patient suffering from pernicious anaemia and she got on quite happily with his case. However, she had a bad time later with her viva voce (oral examination), a case of a man with kidney trouble. Evidently she had not asked the right questions. She knew she had done badly, and later, when the dean asked why she was looking so serious, she told him she had failed her viva. He assured her that could not be and that her examination of the medical case had been very good. Professor Wild in pharmacology also said she had nothing to worry about as her work was all first-class standard.

Happily, Margaret did much better in the surgical oral. When Dr. Carless asked her if she could diagnose a case of appendicitis before there were any symptoms, she promptly answered no, which pleased him. He then went to use up some viva time by telling her how he had once diagnosed such a case without symptoms.

During her last year, money was scarce, and Margaret was glad to get a position teaching physiology and hygiene at a girls' private school in a suburb of Manchester. She went by train, twice a week, for one term, somehow managing to fit it in with her fixed classes. By then she had learned the art of cutting non-essentials and to take fewer notes. She found it hard to study at night and was displaying signs of burnout. Despite this, after hearing that there was much eye trouble and blindness in China, she tried to prepare herself by making extra attendances at the eye hospital.

In anticipation of the religious aspect of her calling, Margaret attended some of Professor Peake's courses in Bible study. He was intrigued that a medical student should attend his lectures and told her that it had been his wish to become a missionary, but his health had prevented it. Knowing she was a poor hand at speaking, Margaret joined the women's debating society, and at every meeting she tried "to say a few words."

During her college course, the proposition arose of dividing the three colleges of Victoria University—Manchester, Liverpool and Leeds—into three universities. The burning question was which college should retain the title of Victoria University, or whether the name should be abandoned. The subject was taken up hotly by the students, and reporters attended the meetings. Margaret wrote her first letter to the editor; for all her diffidence over speaking in public, she had no inhibitions over proclaiming her opinions. Finally, it was decided that Manchester, being the oldest college, should retain the title, and the tumult subsided.

At the end of the college year, a dozen or so male and female students organized a few days' holiday at Grasmere. The county of Cumberland with its Lake District was handy to reach from Manchester, making it a popular choice for students. The women students—Jess, Marion, Kath, Marjorie and Margaret—stayed at the Swan in Grasmere with a young chaperone, while the men slept in a tent in a field across the road. The tranquillity of those idyllic surroundings helped forge lifelong friendships, which in Margaret's case became very significant.

One Sunday during her final exams, Margaret took a day trip to Blackpool to refresh her mind. It seemed amazing to see the sands covered with people, and she wandered about, enjoying herself in a quiet way, realizing that the process of taking leave of her beloved England had begun.

In the middle of the medical final examination, which Margaret sat in July, she received a letter from the SPG saying that plans for her had changed: she was to be ready to sail to China on September 5. She would go to Peking to start language training and to gain some experience at mission hospitals there. They knew this could conflict with her plans but hoped that she would take this in the right way. It never occurred to her to oppose the decision. Had she known what she found out years later, that every medical student in the United States became an M.D. on graduation, and that this custom was to be instituted in China, she would have taken steps to obtain her M.D. first.

The exam result was a great disappointment, though not unexpected after that dreadful viva in medicine, but happily she passed. Sir William Sinclair told her afterwards that the external examiner wanted to fail her altogether, but he was not allowed to have his way. Apparently, there was a struggle over it and Professor Sinclair was angry, for he said that her work in his department was first class, and at least three other professors agreed. Some said the examiner objected to women doctors, for Margaret was the only woman taking the exam that year, as her fellow student had decided to postpone it.

Graduation was thrilling. It had been a strenuous five years, with one year badly messed up by a serious illness and hospitalization. By taking extra classes Margaret obtained a bachelor of science in physiology and in practical psychology (honours). She was awarded the Robert Platt physiology exhibition in 1902 and the Sidney Renshaw exhibition and second-class honours in physiology in 1903. She finished her medical course in 1905, graduating with a bachelor of medicine and surgery.

Afterwards Margaret signed the medical council register and joined the British Medical Association. Since her birth, the number of women doctors in England had grown from a mere twenty-five to more than two hundred by the time she qualified. Not only were women medical practitioners overwhelmingly outnumbered by male doctors, Margaret was concerned over how few women doctors had expertise in female diseases. To her mind, who better than a woman doctor to apply her skills to obstetrics or other problems afflicting women specifically? She maintained that a female patient should be able to exercise her right to consult another woman, if only there was one available. Her experiences with her own operations added particular emphasis to this point.

In July 1905, Dr. Ethel Margaret Phillips became the third woman to graduate in medicine from the University of Manchester. The first was a name hallowed in the annals of the medical school, Dr. Catherine Chisholm, who graduated in July 1904, followed by Dr. Louisa Corbett in March 1905.

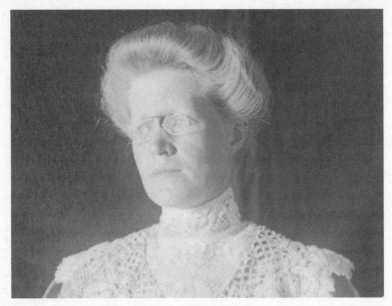

Dr. Ethel Margaret Phillips, upon her graduation in 1905.

The zeal with which Margaret approached much of her duties was based mainly on her conviction that to win souls for God, she needed to follow those precepts manifested in Christ's lifetime. Her motivation lay principally in the relief of suffering in any form.

> *Suffering is a consequence of misapplication or obstruction of Law (the Laws of the Universe, spiritual and natural). The causes are there, though they may not always be evident to us. Wouldn't our lives be very shallow without suffering and difficulty? The response to suffering is the courage of the sufferer, the active kindness and sympathy of the observers, the urge to relieve and put right, and to prevent it from happening to others.*

Margaret had a gift for accurate diagnosis, even in cases of "causes... not always...evident." If any symptoms were atypical of a patient's condition, she would attempt to account for their presence with a logical connection before concluding her diagnosis. The "fly in the ointment," as she called it, sometimes yielded surprising results.

While Margaret resided in Ashburne Hall, which could accommodate up to fifty women students, she proudly became involved with the women's suffrage movement. Not being militant, she preferred to exemplify by precept what women could achieve given the chance, and that did not include antagonizing public opinion.

Over the next few weeks she had to get clothes made to last for the next five years, at least, and she was busy visiting and saying goodbye to friends and relations in England. Near the end she went to London for a farewell service in the SPG chapel. In Birmingham she stayed with Frank and his wife, Frances, for a few days, and said goodbye to her aunts. Aunt Kate remarked, "Well, I never thought it would come to this!" So they had not taken her seriously after all, Margaret thought. She spent a few days at Bournemouth with her father and Laura; saying goodbye there was the hardest, as she felt it was for the last time. Then she went on to Bridgwater to her mother and Bert, and lastly back to Manchester to gather up her things. Jess came to be with her for the last day, and they took a room in a bed-sitter for the night. Jess told Margaret that she was practically engaged to Arthur Skemp, a brilliant young man, already a lecturer and later to become a professor in English literature at Bristol University. Margaret's staunch friend Mary Evans came from Wales and implored her to give up the idea of going to China, for she was afraid that the mission society would let Margaret down.

But Margaret was pledged. It seemed unthinkable that she could draw back, although she sometimes dreaded the thought of going off to China, and often woke up in the night saying to herself, "I can't go!"

Her friends feared for her safety, and her father strongly opposed the idea of her going to China rather than India. As dreadful as the Boxer Uprising had been five years previously, the press was sensationalizing the situation even further, issuing reports that the intervening years still gave grounds for revulsion towards any dealings with China. Yet, remarkably, groups of people persevered in their attempts to alleviate the suffering existing in China.

Dr. Margaret, as she had become known to her friends and close associates, could only have had an inkling of what lay ahead, but she knew that God's hand would guide her through. Particular meaningful to her was the prayer "Just for Today":

Just for today, My Father, give me power
To live to Thee: tomorrow is not mine.
I crave Thy wondrous grace this very hour
 To make the present sweet. The future's Thine
Alone. Prepare me Lord, I pray,
Just for the duties I must meet today.

Margaret saw clearly what she wanted to do. By following the teachings of the Great Healer she aspired to achieve the healing of the bodies and souls of her fellow creatures in his name.

MY PHILOSOPHY

Do you think Adam was happy in his beautiful garden
With loveliness and perfection around him everywhere?
A dear companion to share his days and hold converse,
No work, no duties, no uncertainties or irritations?
I think his days were too monotonous;
There were no contrasts in his life
For all was ease and satiety.
The shady groves, the lovely flowers were always there to see;
Where there was nothing ugly, what was there to admire?
All day they played and ate and slept.
The days were all alike; what could they talk about?

God found out the mistake, so changed His scheme
And made His first decree:—
"Of all the trees mayst thou freely eat, save one,
Of the tree in the midst of the garden, the fruit is not for you."

...
More delicious was the fruit than other trees.
Forbidden fruit always is and Adam found it so.
Think not ill of him; we had not known disobedience
Had he not disobeyed.
I like to think, in after years,
In the joy of effort and achievement Adam was glad he had escaped
From the beautiful Garden of Ease.

(E. M. P.)

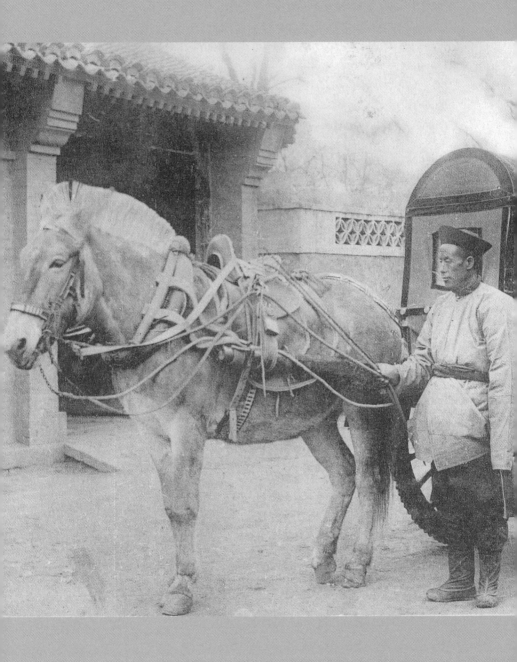

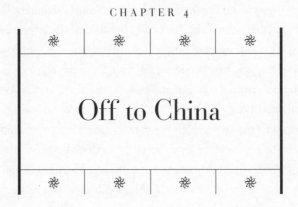

CHAPTER 4

Off to China

ʃ* WITH JUST OVER A MONTH TO PREPARE for what was to be her destiny, Margaret had little time to learn about current conditions in China. Even if faced with a turbulent atmosphere, however, her resolve was to bring solace and better health to the sick and suffering at her posted mission station. Her briefing by the Society for the Propagation of the Gospel (SPG) dealt principally with their missionary interests; little had been said that might deter their new recruit from fulfilling their purposes.

The Chinese have a deep sense of history and a long memory. Their existing hostile feelings for foreigners related to two major occurrences. During the thirteenth century, China was conquered for the first time by an external force, the Mongol hordes, causing a deep-rooted, long-lasting repugnance towards the barbaric outer world surrounding the civilized nation of the Middle Kingdom.[1] The Mongols overran the country, and for almost a century China formed part of the Mongol Empire, giving rise to the Yuan dynasty. The Chinese Ming dynasty that followed restored the flowering of the true spirit of Chinese culture, unprecedented for more than three hundred years previously when the Tang dynasty flourished. For a considerable time East–West trade routes and foreign visitors such as Marco Polo and Jesuit priests (admittedly three hundred years apart) encouraged a more tolerant attitude towards foreigners.

Near the end of the Ming dynasty, at the start of the seventeenth century, the Chinese administration decided, for political reasons, to withdraw from contact with the outside world. The West strongly opposed this decision, primarily for political and commercial purposes, and executed their challenge using traders backed by military force, thus exacerbating Chinese disdain towards foreign pressure. In Chinese culture, shopkeepers and the military formed the lowest levels of society. That these kind sought to impose their will on the nation was considered beneath contempt.

Then came a second blow, the Anglo-Chinese War (often known as the Opium War), culminating in the Treaty of Nanking in 1843. The humiliation of the Chinese was complete. Following China's defeat, a dozen rapacious foreign nations availed themselves, over a long period, of unequal peace treaties to further their own ends. The Chinese could do nothing to protect themselves, compounding the nation's outrage. Matters worsened later when Russia and Japan successively sought to exploit China's weakness. Thus the peace-loving Chinese developed a hatred for the insurgent foreign "barbarians."

Westerners often regarded the Chinese as impassive and inscrutable—largely due to the impenetrable front presented in uncomfortable situations. This attempt at preserving dignity was misinterpreted by the Western powers as deviousness. The result was a mutually scant respect. The Chinese viewed the foreign barbarians as concerned only with their own gain, bereft of decorum and without sufficient intellect to understand the basics of Chinese culture. Although convinced of the need to repel outside pressures, the Chinese, unfortunately, completely lacked the power to do so. Despite China's much vaunted ancient culture, the decadent Qing dynasty ruled over a primitive people who were no match against colonial powers. Even if they had maintained the sea power enjoyed centuries earlier, it is debatable whether the Chinese could have withstood invasion for long.

Basically, the situation was a stand-off, pitting powerful Western arrogance against the Chinese played-out sense of superiority. In practical terms, the contest was hopelessly loaded against the Chinese nation, which, ironically, vastly outnumbered the invaders.

Beneath that Chinese cultural veneer of inscrutability lay a highly emotional and volatile potential for violence, and as matters got out of hand a major exasperation became prevalent. Given this situation, barbarism at Chinese hands well outmatched any the foreign element might have manifested. Accordingly, it became a case of "Come not between the dragon and his wrath."

The thinly disguised Chinese hostility subsequently culminated in the unsuccessful Taiping Rebellion (c. 1850–64), followed nearly fifty years later by the Boxer Uprising, which climaxed with the siege of the Legation Quarter in Peking. It took fifty-five days for a joint force to relieve the beleaguered foreign community. While this alien presence was only one cause of these insurrections, the masses were not loathe to ventilate their hatred of the foreign "occupation" whenever opportunities arose. Often missionaries were victims of this violence, having little more than their faith to protect them. Doing their best to remain true to their beliefs, the missionaries followed military subjugation, only making matters worse. Their stubborn resolve provided further ammunition for propaganda to inflame national resentment. Nor did the Chinese appreciate being regarded as heathens. They had their own spiritual values, which they treasured.

♪*

A CRUEL CHARACTERISTIC typical of most Far Eastern countries was the vast discrepancy between the educated and affluent classes and the remainder, largely the peasantry. In China, most people were distressingly poor, struggling to eke out a bare existence. Eventually, as some benefits of the foreign presence became apparent, the peasants started to come forward, and eagerly missionaries of all denominations reached out to help. Though often misunderstood by the Chinese, the boundless faith supporting people such as Dr. Phillips was impressive, and it provided the inner strength behind the courage needed to take on this immense challenge.

Not only were the efforts of the medical missionaries increasingly affecting the minds of the Chinese people, mission schools were also slowly opening eyes to the benefits of democracy. Both inland and overseas Chinese students realized how necessary it was to discard the yoke of imperial autocracy. The Qing dynasty, well aware of the influence exerted by these foreign elements, was belatedly considering educational reforms as well as a more constitutional form of government. By this time, however, the Manchu domination was in its death throes, and attempts to modernize were overtaken by results.

The mission field was vast, and until commercialism and politics were embroiled in competition for spheres of influence in China, the basic principles of missionary work, apart from evangelism, were exerting a distinct influence. Foreign medical practice was finally being accepted by the masses as effective in relieving their suffering, and it was slowly attracting people to develop an improved quality of life.

As hospitals came into being, so did schools. Recently founded schools had introduced modern subjects such as mathematics, world history and science into their curricula in addition to the Chinese classics—a practical move towards replacing the traditional Hanlin examinations on the Chinese classics, which hitherto had produced a supply of officials for government positions. These classical examinations were held in the provincial capitals and in Peking until abolished by the empress dowager, but again the tide of modern events overtook this belated attempt at reform.

Western methods of education did much to assist China to become a republic, and hundreds of eager students were welcomed abroad to study. However, the rapid decline of the Qing dynasty caught the Chinese nation unprepared as a whole to become a democracy, at least not in the Western meaning of the principle. For that unsettling situation, the Western nations were responsible, however sincere their intentions.

China was, and always had been, an agrarian nation. The farming peasantry considerably outnumbered the urban population. Whether in good times or bad, the Chinese peasant battled famine caused by flood or drought, and the corruption and greed of an autocratic administration. Undeniably, China enjoyed many periods of greatness and posterity, but rarely did the peasantry benefit to any great extent or derive any reprieve from an existence of continuous hardship. Generations of endurance under such harsh conditions resulted in a tough and resilient nation of people.

Widespread poverty meant a constant struggle against pestilence of both natural and man-made causes. While the Chinese culture, based on Confucianism, fashioned the general way of life, the nation was divided in its religious pursuits, principally between Daoism and Buddhism. The country folk, however, adhered primarily to widespread superstition, based on the fear of the devil, attended by ghosts and demons.

Chinese notions of hygiene were woefully lacking compared to Western standards. Sanitation was virtually nonexistent in the villages. Water was drawn by hand and replaced as and when necessary, while flood and drought both adversely affected availability. Unless water was boiled before use, drinking it was never safe; even artesian wells could not be guaranteed to produce potable supplies. Lavatories were of the crudest types: usually an outhouse privy or an earth closet. Sewerage, where it existed at all, consisted of soil pipes leading to fields adjoining the dwellings. For centuries Chinese farmers availed themselves of nature's most prolific biodegradable source of fertilizer: human excrement.

Medical practice not only had dreadful conditions to contend with but also a whole different concept of health as practised under Chinese culture. The Chinese approach was steeped in ancient origins closely linked with traditional methods. Health was defined as a balance of the body's vital *yin* and *yang* energies in harmony with the forces of nature. Herbal medicines, used to fortify the immune system and to ease stress, were purchased from "medicine shops." Margaret found that Chinese doctors would see a patient only when paid up front, and if a cure was not immediate, the patient would proceed to another doctor, then another.

Remarkably, where medicine shops were so plentiful, and their concoctions so freely absorbed, empirical knowledge remained rudimentary and inefficient. The many superstitions attaching to the phenomena and treatment of sickness often contributed adversely to giving relief. All sickness was attributed to the agency of the devil, and many ceremonies were observed by the populace to avoid being claimed as victims.

Understandably, all the major infectious diseases known to man existed in China, with smallpox and tuberculosis among the most prevalent. Although the developed resistance to certain endemic diseases was truly amazing, the toll extracted was tragic. Here was clearly one way the Western approach to medical and surgical methods could ease the agony of illnesses of all sorts, but for one further consideration: a Chinese patient of that era had absolutely no idea of the discipline required with Western treatment. Chinese customs opposed Western practices; whenever any improvement manifested, the patient often simply disappeared.

Western doctors had an unending struggle to persuade their patients to conform with standard medical practice. Being firm was not enough; one also needed a kindly understanding of predominant circumstances, since an insistence on improved living conditions was impractical. Despite the best will in the world, the prevalent domestic conditions offered little chance of success. Equally, hospitalization was not always expedient or pragmatic considering the day-to-day or seasonal demands of country life. Frequently, only sheer misery and desperation overcame the superstitions or distrust of the "foreign barbarians."

To succeed, the missionaries needed to prove that what they were offering was immeasurably better than what was familiar to the peasants. Conditions were difficult enough for missionary workers on secular issues; carrying their challenges into spiritual grounds made great demands of their resolution. The sheer dedication of the evangelists obviously achieved its purpose over time, and revealed the strength of the Christian faith. The love of Christ motivating the missionaries frequently achieved the desired effect in converting the surrounding communities. However, from such a proliferation of denominations, it must have seemed something of a lottery as to which offered the best kind of salvation.

Not for nothing did the term "rice Christian" come into use, and undoubtedly many became converts as a matter of expediency while inwardly retaining their original superstitions; one might suggest they were hedging their bets. Yet others were sincere converts who chose to follow the Light the foreigners sought to show them. The faith of Chinese converts was sorely tested during the Boxer Uprising, when thousands perished at the hands of their own compatriots because of their belief, as well as their foreign associations. The foreigners could give them no support, being themselves grievously oppressed while under siege in the capital during the summer of 1900. Politically speaking, few repercussions were apparent by the time Margaret arrived on the scene, although many missionaries retained harrowing memories of those days only five years earlier. This unsuccessful insurrection resulted in China being forced to make further territorial and economic concessions designed to protect the foreign presence.

Dr. Sun Yat-sen, a leading Chinese nationalist who had continued his education abroad, led an abortive revolt even before the Boxer Uprising and had to flee his country in 1895. In essence the Boxers enjoyed the backing of the empress dowager in an attempt to restore greater Manchu control. This strategy failed, and in 1911 the Father of the Chinese Republic, as Dr. Sun Yat-sen became known, returned to China to become the first provisional president.

This potted history, of the China to which Margaret had dedicated herself, illustrates the atmosphere and conditions she was to face. Whether she was fully aware of the situation is questionable. Her resolve and reactions said much for her faith and her courage.

♪✳

MARGARET KNEW that her introduction to the Chinese people and the Mandarin language would be in Peking. She was to stay at St. Faith's Home, the residence for SPG women missionaries—a sort of Church of England sisterhood, though there were only two nuns, Jessie Ransome and her sister, Edith, who had come to England to take Margaret and

Miss Esther Sworder, a fellow missionary, under her wing. It was suggested that Margaret wear a uniform, but she demurred, saying it could cause her to be mistaken for a nurse. She promised to dress quietly in an inconspicuous grey costume, covering herself from below the ankle to high in the neck, with long sleeves even in summertime. Her dresses were so voluminous that later she made three petticoats out of one.

Margaret travelled from Manchester to London by night train to meet the ship, arriving tired as she could not afford a sleeper and was too excited to sleep. In London she found Frank waiting on the platform. They had breakfast in the railway restaurant, then went on to Waterloo Station and took the special boat train for Southampton docks, where an animated gathering of friends awaited. Margaret linked up with Sister Edith, Miss Sworder and the Reverend Mackwood Stevens, secretary of the North China and Shantung Mission to which Margaret was appointed. It amused Margaret that Miss Sworder's parents put their daughter in her care, for Esther was a year older. Once finally aboard the ship, the three women easily spotted Frank and Rev. Stevens in the crowd waving farewell, as the reverend had tied a handkerchief to his umbrella. Margaret watched till they disappeared from view.

On September 4, the Norddeutscher Lloyd steamer *Princess Alice* left for China, a seven-week voyage. This was Margaret's first time at sea. Ports of call included Genoa, San Nicolo and Naples, where the three travellers enjoyed onshore sightseeing trips. Margaret marvelled at sights such as the Rock of Gibraltar bathed in "the delicate filmy haze of early morning," magnificent paintings at the Jalazzo Durazzo, and Mount Vesuvius with black smoke fuming from its top. During the voyage Sister Edith gave Esther and Margaret basic instruction on the Mandarin dialect.

On October 10, they arrived in Shanghai. As the ship was too large to go upriver—in those days the Yangzi (Yangtse) River had not been dredged, although later most oceangoing ships could proceed upriver as far as Nanjing (Nanking) and Hankow—they were met by the company launch, which brought letters from Bishop Charles Perry Scott: one for Margaret and two for Sister Edith. The letters were welcome until it was realized that they bore sad news. Sister Jessie Ransome had died of dysentery after a short illness. Sister Edith was terribly stricken. She bore up bravely, though the lack of privacy on the launch was hard. The group was thankful when they landed safely in Shanghai.

The women were to stay at the deanery, and Sister Edith was surprised that Dean Walker had not sent anyone to meet them. They left their heavy luggage to be called for, then got into separate rickshaws and were rushed away helter-skelter, presumably towards the address provided by Sister Edith. To Margaret's horror, she saw the nun's rickshaw disappear around a corner. Unable to speak a word of Chinese, she could not persuade their rickshaw men to stop, and the more she tried the faster they ran, never pausing to see whether the third rickshaw was following. They raced through streets, seeing only Chinese buildings and Chinese people till the rickshaw men pulled up with a flourish outside the doors of the Roman Catholic mission. Because of Sister Edith's garb, the rickshaw men had presumed the women were Catholics. A French priest kindly redirected the rickshaw men and off they raced again, finally arriving at the deanery.

Although Dean and Mrs. Walker were kind, Sister Edith longed for privacy to give way to her grief. The wonderful house provided every comfort, but the mosquitoes were fierce and it rained almost every day. The three women spent five days in Shanghai, waiting for one of the better northbound coastal steamers. Once at sea, they ran into rough weather. The small ship rolled and pitched, plunging into deep troughs, then rearing skywards. Margaret and Esther Sworder were hopelessly sick, remaining in their cabins for three days, watching the luggage slide up and down the cabin floor, while their dresses swung almost horizontally from the closet rails.

Margaret felt guilty of neglecting Edith Ransome, though she managed to struggle to her cabin twice. Finally Sister Edith staggered into their cabin, saying, "I think I'm going to die, I feel so weak." That cured Margaret at once, and she got up and fetched some champagne for her, staying with her till she felt better. Near Yantai (then known as Chefoo), they thankfully encountered calmer waters. There the captain decided to anchor for another night, fearing the violence of the storm might have caused floating mines—hangovers from the Russo-Japanese War earlier that year—to drift across their course. Near the end of the voyage, he earnestly advised Deaconess Sworder and Margaret to return home, as China was no place for two young women. They knew his advice was meant kindly, but replied that they were committed and could not go back.

CONTENTMENT

If all were bright and beautiful how dull our lives would be!
How flat a picture looks without its light and shade.
If we know no pain or trouble how shallow we should be.
How feeble our mentality if life were always gay!
If we never knew the joy of helping others
Or the stimulus of friendship and the pain of love;
If we never had to struggle and endure,
If life were always easy, should we really like it so?

(E. M. P.)

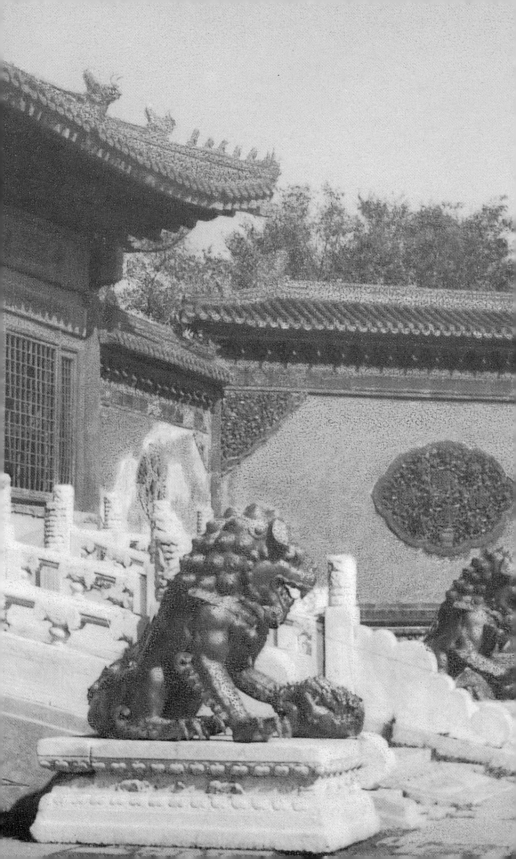

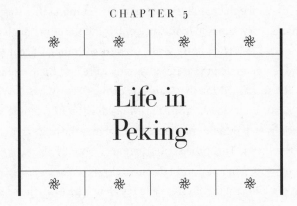

CHAPTER 5

Life in
Peking

♪* THE SHIP DROPPED ANCHOR OFF DAGU (Taku)
Bar on October 23 at nine o'clock in the morning, and Margaret spent
her first ten hours in North China travelling by train to Peking via Tianjin
(Tientsin), the port city to the capital. Bishop Scott, who was waiting at
the dock, accompanied the women for the rest of the journey. The party
travelled the equivalent of first class, which did not compare favourably
even with third class back in England. Chinese trains offered "soft class"
and "hard class," labels that virtually spoke for themselves, but Margaret
looked askance at even the superior level of travel: an open coach train.

Most of journey was through flat, brown, treeless countryside, the
most striking feature being the numerous mounds dotted about all over
the fields, which turned out to be graves. Finally, they reached Peking, and
Margaret felt a surge of excitement when they passed through the city
wall, though it was only the low outer wall of the Chinese City.

Peking basically consisted of three walled cities, one inside the other,
with a fourth walled area to the south. The innermost city was the legendary Forbidden City, then known to the Chinese as *Da Nei* (The Great
Within), its high stone castellated walls surrounding a rectangular area,

where the emperor resided in his palace with its yellow glazed-tiled roofs. The only other occupants were the emperor's concubines and vast staff of eunuchs, hence the name "Forbidden." Surrounding that was a larger quadrangular city, the Imperial City, containing the court, high officials and their families. Thick lofty walls, pierced with magnificent gates on all four sides, encircled the outermost enclosure and main expanse, the Tartar City, so named for the Manchus of the Qing dynasty. When the Qing dynasty took power from the Ming dynasty, the ethnic Chinese population was driven out of the Tartar City into the large area immediately to the south. This broad suburban area, about half the size of the Tartar City, was, generally and tautologically, referred to as the Chinese City, but the Chinese themselves called it *Qian Men Wai,* meaning "outside the Fore Gate."

After winding round inside the Chinese City, through what seemed only wasteland, the train ran along the outer foot of the Tartar City's big wall. The Empress-Dowager had refused to allow the evil spirits of the foreign *huo che* (fire wagons) to disturb the serenity of her celestial city, so the train station had to be built outside the wall. Nevertheless, it was a great convenience to have a railway, as it reduced the travel time between Tianjin and Peking to four hours from two or three days by canal or cart.

It was now dark so the travellers were unable to see much of their surroundings, except countless handheld lanterns. This was Margaret's first glimpse of a genuine Chinese lantern, made of glass and iron, and far more artistic than the paper ones back home. Finally, they arrived and the group was hustled from the crowded station, which seemed to consist of a few railway lines and trains among platforms of mounded earth. Though the new arrivals did not realize it then, this was the famous Watergate Station, where relief forces had broken through and ended the Boxer Uprising on August 15, 1900, freeing the foreign residents after eight weeks' siege.

Led by a servant from the mission who took charge of the luggage, the group jostled their way through the central archway of the Fore Gate (*Qian Men*) to an awaiting mule cart. A blue cloth covered its hooped framework, with a minute window on each side and a blind in front.

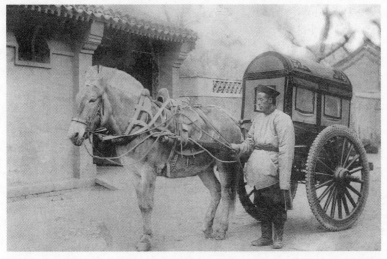

The type of vehicle in which Dr. Margaret may have ridden early on in Peking. It had solid rubber tires and was drawn by a Mongolian pony.

Inside were no seats, simply straw matting covering the rough floorboards. The driver pulled out a small stool from between the shafts to assist Margaret and Sister Edith in climbing into the small two-wheeled cart. Deaconess Sworder, being the tallest, sat on a shaft. Then began a journey of bumps over Peking's rough roads. Margaret was thankful the cart was slightly padded; otherwise, she expected they might have arrived with broken bones. She clutched two cameras in her right hand and held on with her left, sometimes wondering whether her arm might snap and which variety of fracture it would be. Other times she feared, with the next jerk, that her arm might be pushed right through the back of the cart. All that could be seen was the high city wall. Shouts arose above the din as the driver led the mule through the city gate. There appeared to be some difficulty in manœuvring the cart through, the gate being a veritable needle's eye, allowing only one-way traffic.

There seemed to be no roads, merely a number of "ways," and even that term Margaret considered complimentary. Every so often the interminable walls and gates gave way to a wasteland of mounds and rubbish heaps. The mule steadily jolted onward through the darkness, regardless of any slight diversion in the course and quite indifferent to the vehicle behind, rocking and swaying like a yacht in rough seas. Over everything he went, mounds, ditches and all.

The high walls surrounding the Tartar City had nine gate towers for access. Being nighttime, the gates were beginning to close, and long processions of mule carts waited single file in either direction. Once Margaret's cart was through each half-opened gate, their mule seemed to head straight for some high wall, coming so close that she feared it would flatten itself or actually crash through; then suddenly, to her relief, the cart would swing round through an unseen opening. (The newcomers were unaware that the main gates were actually two at right angles, necessitating such sharp manœuvres.)

Margaret could not tell what direction they were taking. Sharp turns in what appeared to be the opposite direction seemed to interrupt any progress. From the station they had made a huge circuitous route, then almost back again. While Sister Edith and Margaret sat inside the cart with their legs straight out in front, Deaconess Sworder perched at the opening with her legs dangling over the shaft. It was considered unseemly for foreign women to be seen on the streets, but as it was dark, she was not too noticeable. From her vantage point, she could dimly see the landmarks and inform her companions when they neared the journey's end. Finally, they reached St. Faith's Mission in the south-west part of the city. After almost an hour of patient suffering, they stood on firm ground again. (In years to come, a rickshaw could do the same trip in twenty minutes.)

Late though it was, quite a band of people awaited their arrival, and the tired and hungry newcomers were cheered by their greeting. Among others, Margaret met Miss Mary Scott, the bishop's niece and housekeeper, Miss Shebbeare, head of the girls' school, Rev. and Mrs. Benham-Brown, and Miss Dorothy Bearder, a nurse who would later accompany Margaret to Shandong.

Margaret and Deaconess Sworder were shown to their quarters to freshen up. They were to share a small study with two tiny adjoining bedrooms, clean rooms which were very welcome indeed. Shortly after, they all went into dinner, followed by introductions to the many Chinese and English members of the mission who had come to meet them. Sister Edith was still grief-stricken over her sister's death, and neither Margaret nor Deaconess Sworder felt very bright. A sad impression, thought Margaret, with which to begin her life in China. Finally, they attended compline (evening service), led by Bishop Scott in the chapel. "It has been a long day since leaving our steamer at Taku [Dagu]," Margaret said. "How sleepy and bewildered we were, and so glad to get to bed."

The next morning began at six o'clock with a cup of tea, followed by matins in Chinese at seven-thirty. Chinese services took place every morning and evening, with three other services in English completing the daily routine. Margaret noted the children's great interest in the new arrivals, for they were well scrutinized as the youngsters trooped past.

Now it was a case of not wasting any time getting down to business. Margaret and Miss Sworder were put straight to work on their language lessons under two Chinese tutors, one young and the other elderly. Since the room was too small to accommodate both, they took turns. In those days, it was customary to throw a pupil in at the deep end, using the immersion method. Neither teacher knew a word of English. Instruction was by the Chinese method of repeating sounds and learning by rote. The two women virtually taught themselves with the help of C.W. Mateer's Mandarin primer in two large volumes, and the Chinese teachers' guidance on pronouncing the characters. Once Margaret felt she could recognize all the characters in one lesson, she would pass on to the next, though the teacher would remonstrate because she did not know it all by heart. She had learned to read and write both French and German at school but could speak neither, so she made up her mind to use her Chinese at once. From the first, she attended as many services in Chinese as possible and was able to pick out a word here and there as her vocabulary grew. In that way she felt that ear, eye and voice were all trained together. She somehow indicated to the tutor what was needed, and studied under him for two hours daily, supplemented by a further three hours of private study.

Margaret did not particularly relish her language studies. She considered Mandarin "terrible" and "awful," what with its 403 "sounds" (syllables), each with four different tones. In a letter home she described how it could be possible to tell a patient to drink a poisonous medicine when what she really meant was to apply it as a lotion. For the next six months her routine consisted mainly of language studies and medical work, although much of the day was taken up by the attendance of all five daily services held at the mission; indeed, a literal application of the First Commandment.

On her first afternoon there, Margaret was asked by Dr. Aspland, the resident mission doctor, to attend an operation on one of the schoolgirls, a leg amputation for tuberculosis of the bone. Margaret watched her condition under the anaesthetic, as the acting anaesthetist was untrained. Nurses were scarce, so when night came she sat up with the patient. Thus ended her first working day in China, which included attendance at several church services in Chinese.

The next day Dr. Aspland, who had arrived in China six months before Margaret and who was then building a small hospital, said he would give her charge of the women and children outpatients and the women's ward. So her mornings were spent studying Chinese, and her afternoons at the dispensary, where there were ten to twenty women and children outpatients every day. The pleasant ward had space for six women patients. Dr. Aspland kindly helped Margaret to gain experience.

When Margaret left England for China after completing her medical course, she had hoped that no one would guess how helpless and ignorant she felt, especially when she had to administer her first hypodermic or perform other procedures that had been assigned to nurses while she was a medical student. All the same, she felt her medical and surgical training there was as good as any. It was because of her inexperience that Margaret went first to Peking to work under Dr. Aspland for six months and visit the various mission hospitals there. Although she expected to be asked to help in those hospitals, among the four she visited she observed only one operation and administered the anaesthetic on a couple of other occasions. She usually travelled about the city alone by rickshaw, but if visiting a patient she went by mule cart, considered a more dignified mode for an important person like a doctor, accompanied by a Chinese duenna.

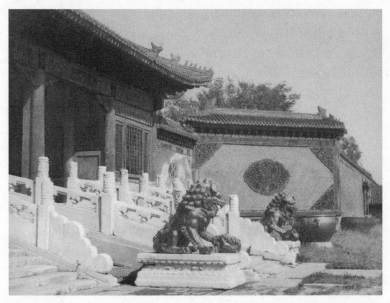

Two gilded lions guard an entrance inside the Forbidden City, the central quadrant of Peking. The left-hand lion has a cub under her paw while the male lion guards an orb.

♪❋

NOT UNTIL MARGARET SAW Peking's layout in daylight did she begin to understand the tortuous journey of that dreadful night of arrival. Her chief impression was a preponderance of mud combined with patches of wasteland and ruined buildings. There were but two main thoroughfares, on the east and west sides of the city, connecting with the north and south gates on either side of the Fore Gate. Each street had a raised portion down the middle with a section of macadamized paving reserved for the use of the springless, blue-hooded mule carts and the sedan chairs of the officials, while heavy goods carts had to keep to the mud tracks at the sides. Crossing the city west to east from the Anglican mission entailed heading south as far as the Fore Gate along Legation Street to Hatamen Street, or northwards to behind Coal Hill (also called Prospect Hill or *Jing Shan*), past the Forbidden City, before turning eastwards.

As the streets were unlit, everyone carried lanterns at night. Passing from one side of the city to the other necessitated going outside and around the Imperial City walls. The side-streets or lanes (*hutong*) were often impassable with oozing mud, with a view only of closed doorways let into high blank walls, for windows in a Chinese house never opened onto the street. No parks or palaces were open to the public in those days, and there was no thoroughfare across the Forbidden City from east to west. The appalling state of decay throughout the capital was a sad indication of the decline of the ruling dynasty. Margaret recalled Peking being described in a school geography book as having "a mean and dilapidated appearance"; now, she saw it as a city of ruins.

Rickshaws and sedan chairs, with outriders, often passed along the streets, but there were no carriages, much less motorcars. If a foreign woman walked in the street, she would be followed and her strange attire loudly commented on. Should a foreigner enter a shop, in no time the street became blocked by a crowd of spectators till the police came to clear them out. Every house kept a private mule cart, and since Margaret could not go to a patient in public view by rickshaw, she travelled under cover by cart with her chaperone.

The massive wall surrounding the Tartar City was twelve metres (40 feet) high, nineteen metres (62 feet) thick at the base and ten metres (34 feet) wide at the top, and paved and bordered with crenellated parapets. Westerners were granted special permission to take their daily exercise along the top of this wall in a southern section of the city. There they could walk freely and without a servant, as Chinese were not allowed on the wall. Margaret could stroll there in peace, enjoying the view of the countryside and Xi Shan (the Western Hills; also known as Badachu, meaning "Eight Great Places") in the distance, but she had to watch her step as the going was rough. Eventually she tired of the one walk, and once refused to venture onto "our prison Wall." On one occasion, the bishop received a letter from the British embassy stating that the empress dowager would be passing through the gate on that side of the city and foreigners were expected to abstain from walking on the wall for the next three days.

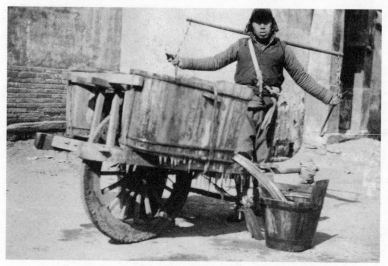

A water carrier and his cart. The two containers were rigged on either side of the main wheel, and would be filled from the top. The water would be stored in large earthenware jars—depending on the number of these in a residence—and the water carrier would deliver every other day.

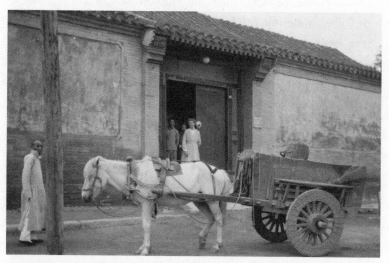

Not for passenger transportation, this photograph depicts the "honey-cart" used in Peking, c. 1918.

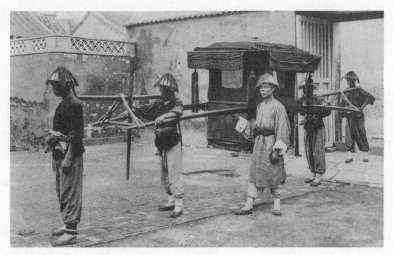

The Peking chair was one form of Chinese transportation in the early 20th century.

No electricity or telephones existed then, nor was there modern plumbing for running water. The water carrier with his squeaking wheelbarrow seemed to be ever at their gate. The wells were of two kinds: those with "sweet" water for drinking or cooking purposes, and those with "bitter" or alkaline water for washing; the latter, of course, being cheaper. Great care was needed to ensure that these two were not accidentally used for the wrong purpose.

The other wheelbarrow that appeared at the gate every night was the noxious honey cart. This crude but essential form of waste disposal was all that was available before any semblance of modern sewerage appeared years later. In a city of powerful guilds, two of the most powerful were the sanitation guild and, surprisingly, the beggars guild. These guilds served much the same purpose as unions do in the Western world.

♪✻

FROM NOVEMBER ON, the bulk of Margaret's routine consisted of medical work, caring for women in the mission hospital. There were but a few inpatients in the ward, and from 2:00 to 4:00 P.M. daily she saw the women and children outpatients, in disappointingly small numbers during the cold months. However, this gave her time to talk to the patients, which she greatly enjoyed. The first phrase she learned to use in her medical work was *"Shenchu ni shetou lai"* (Put out your tongue). Trying to understand the patients certainly helped her to get on more quickly with the language. A Chinese nurse, Miss Hong, aided Margaret by interpreting, putting the patients' remarks into easy words. The same words tended to be used often, so frequently only a few words were needed. By feeling the pulse and using her eyes and stethoscope, Margaret was generally able to determine the problem and prescribe accordingly.

Often diseases were due to uncleanliness and unsanitary conditions, and were at once self-evident. To further find out how medical work was performed in Peking, Margaret visited a number of hospitals of other missionary societies—the London Mission, American Presbyterian, American Board and the British Legation Native hospitals—since they all worked hand in hand. All were well equipped, but only occasionally did surgeons send for Dr. Margaret to assist with operations.

Margaret was still attending five church services daily, which tended to limit her Chinese studies. She concluded that if she had much more medical work, she would have to leave out either the lessons or the services. It would be impossible, she felt, for a doctor to live and work at St. Faith's. She enjoyed being there and had learned some useful lessons in Peking, but she admitted disappointment over the lack of medical work and felt her medical knowledge had suffered sadly. However, there was little time left for work anyway, and she was finding life quite strenuous. She was really trying hard to establish herself, and her efforts were taxing. She still felt shy and slightly ill at ease with some of her fellow missionaries, and as of yet did not know them very well. Her only recreations were invitations to tea with Dr. and Mrs. Aspland or with Rev. and Mrs. Benham-Brown, and hymn singing at Bishop Scott's every Sunday after supper. Otherwise the women sat in their small sitting-room and did a little needlework or knitting while Sister Edith read aloud. At nine o'clock they all went to compline in St. Faith's chapel, then to bed.

Occasionally Margaret and Sister Edith were taken to visit some of the Chinese Christians. For these events, the Chinese women all dressed in short coats and trousers, but when they went visiting, they wore richly embroidered satin or pleated silk skirts. The Manchu ladies always wore long silk coats, fuller at the bottom, embroidered in medallions or plain, with embroidered trimming and sleeve bands. Their faces were thickly painted and powdered, making them look devoid of expression, and they seemed hardly able to smile. Sometimes dirt showed through the powder. In Peking hot water was a luxury, and cold rooms were no inducement for ablutions.

One evening, as she was sitting with some colleagues in a nice warm room, Margaret was called out to attend to four schoolgirls who had been found unconscious from the effects of coal gas poisoning. Little coal-ball stoves were put under the brick beds (*kang*) to heat them for the night. Perhaps the girls had been put to bed too soon, before the gas had worked off, or the flue was defective; fortunately, someone happened to hear their moans during the first stages of unconsciousness, or they would all have died by morning.

Margaret snatched up a lightweight woollen jacket as that night was cold. The victims, brought out into the fresh air to recover, were well wrapped up in blankets, while Margaret was working out in the open for a half-hour, getting thoroughly chilled. It was then that some germ seized the chance to incubate in her lung, as ten days later she went down with pneumonia. This happened to be Christmas Eve, and as the weather that day was mild and bright, Dr. Aspland suggested taking a walk along the city wall to attend the British legation chapel, about half an hour away. Half a dozen of them went off together, and Margaret started off in the best of health, or so she thought. Before they arrived, however, she felt very tired, and had it not been for the service, she would have gone straight back. So on they went, and Margaret was enjoying the Christmas service when suddenly she began to shiver, feeling very ill. She stayed through the service, then got herself home in a rickshaw as fast as she could, putting herself to bed with a temperature of 101°F. When the rest of the group returned, Dr. Aspland went to see her and said she had appendicitis. "I may have," replied Margaret, for she had a pain in that region too, "but right now I have pneumonia."

The next day she was extremely ill, unable to think or move. Nor did she care to read her Christmas letters, which she had saved to read on Christmas Day, having arranged them all round the wainscotting in her bedroom. Afterwards, Margaret never kept anything back for Christmas, but opened each letter when it arrived. As it was Christmas, a priest came to give her Holy Communion, but she could not sit up and could hardly receive the sacrament.

There was an understood, if unexpressed, feeling in the mission that it was wrong to be ill. As Margaret felt dreadfully ashamed of giving trouble, she got up and tried to pretend that she was all right, but instead of getting better she got worse. On January 11, her thirtieth birthday, the Chinese assistant doctor was getting married, and all the missionaries had been invited. Margaret did not attend as she was not well enough to risk the cold in church. Just before the ceremony started, a woman patient arrived with a TB spine and a large psoas abscess, and Dr. Aspland asked Margaret if she could manage to drain it. She consented but felt desolate having limited and untrained help, and afterwards she was literally sick.

After a few more days with fever, she got up again but had no energy or appetite. There had recently been several of the germ-laden dust storms which frequent Peking and penetrate into every corner of the house. As consumption, or tuberculosis in all its forms, was exceedingly prevalent, it was not surprising that she had a relapse. She returned to her bed with a suspected invasion of the tubercle in her affected lung. Fortunately, this was only in a very early stage, and Dr. Aspland did all in his power to keep it in check. He advised her not to live in Peking any longer and to head to the country for open air treatment as soon as possible.

It was decided that she should go with Miss Bearder to recuperate in the mission rest-house, St. Hilary's, in the Western Hills, north-west of the city. The two undertook the journey separately with Miss Bearder in a sedan chair, as she was considered not strong enough to withstand the jolting of the cart in which Margaret travelled. Jolting along in a Peking mule cart along the rough camel and cart track, for no proper road existed then, was one of the most miserable experiences of Margaret's life. She felt faint with weakness, and all she could remember of that trip were strings of camels padding by and high dusty banks flanking the track. Her misery finally ended when the cart reached its destination in the village at the foot of the Hills and she was borne up the hillside in a sedan chair to the rest-house.

After the shut-in feeling of walled Peking, the wide vistas of the plain and the ranges of the hills were a sheer delight. The next six weeks were spent at first blissfully lazing in the sunshine, then taking longer and longer walks with Miss Bearder. It was very cold, however, and they had only a Chinese stove in the bedroom to dress by. The dining room also had just one small stove, which they needed to sit close to before feeling any warmth. Mission stoves were never allowed to show a red glow, for red-hot sides were a potential fire hazard. Margaret's condition developed into a bout of pleurisy.

Mrs. Aspland arrived for a week, and Dr. Aspland followed at the weekend. One day they hired four donkeys and rode to the Azure Cloud Temple (*Bi Yun Si*), a renowned spot several kilometres away. Dr. Aspland was immensely amused to overhear a Chinese passerby express admiration on his good fortune in having three wives. Despite all the fresh air, Margaret developed a troublesome cough and had little strength. Dr. Aspland was disappointed with his patient's progress and, suspecting some TB lung trouble, he considered sending her to the coast for a month or so until she was fully recovered.

∫✳

INWARDLY MARGARET SUSPECTED Peking had depressed her. Unwilling to trouble the others, she recorded her disillusionment in her diary:

I soon found that Missions and missionaries were not as ideal as I had thought, and the disillusionment nearly broke my heart as I had no preparation for the jealousies, the pettiness, or the quarrelling, for in fact I had never come across it to any extent before. Dr. Aspland was evidently born with a grouchy temperament and used to talk to me for half-hours at a time pouring out grievances and criticisms. He was older and more experienced (he had been many years in Dr. Grenfell's Mission in Labrador), but how was I to know he was extremely pessimistic and critical? It did seem as though there were but few Christians and not very earnest ones, that the services were mainly attended by servants who were lip-servers, and schoolchildren who were compelled to attend. No one told us about the many Christians who bravely died for their faith in the Boxer troubles five years before.

Still, I liked the old women who came to church, though I could only smile at them and let them hold my hand (which was something I have always disliked). These poor old women were very friendly, so smiles had to make up for rather limited chats. Their favourite questions concerned my age and family history, which interpreters often answered for me.

Then when my illness pulled me down I began to feel very depressed and supposed I was homesick, but I think that I was grieving for my lost ideals. Something was the matter with the Missions, or were we swamped by the evil around us? Certainly I received a very bad introduction, and was going to Shandong well on the lookout for something to criticize, aided by my nurse, Miss Bearder, who had thoroughly imbibed this spirit of criticism besides her natural gifts in that direction, for she had a wicked sense of humour which is not far removed. Perhaps our lives were too narrow. We each concentrated on our own work and became self-centred. For instance, Miss Sworder and I felt keenly the need of a little help with the language from those who already knew it, which would have made our task of directing our teachers much easier and we should have got on much faster, but everyone was too busy with their own work.

There had been little time for recreation or relaxation. No concerts, no clubs, no "at-homes," no movies, no sightseeing.

I was once invited to a dinner party at Mrs. Headland's in the Methodist mission across the city and as it would be too late to return home I spent the night there. It was my first experience of an American house and I was terribly shy. One thing that seemed strange and comfortless to me was that the rooms had no doors and all led into each other. The central heating was rather overpowering after the cold of the Mission. Several doctors, men and women, had been invited to meet me. I sat at Mrs. Headland's right and was served first, but I did not know what to do with all the little dishes around me but my hostess quietly put me straight. They did not realize that I had met hardly any Americans before and did not know how to make myself at home as I was expected to do. I was very gauche.

New Year's Day was an event in missionary circles, the day when the men paid calls on their friends in their own or other missions as they had been too busy (and self-engrossed) to do so during the year. I had several men callers, rather to the horror of the older missionaries, but I was in bed and could not "receive." Of course the Mission soon got less straitlaced and used to enjoy it themselves as the custom carried on.

Although her recovery was slow, Margaret was pining to take advantage of an urgent request from Bishop Iliff that she be transferred to his diocese. Dr. Aspland grudgingly agreed that a complete change might supply the answer. In February, with lifted spirits and Miss Bearder at her side, Margaret started off for a new way of life in a different sphere of activity.

In the shade of leafy lanes I long to wander
And breathe the rich scent of the good brown earth;
To pick the sprays of ivy from the mossy banks
And the flowers in season from the tall hedges:
First the hawthorn, then the wild rose or the clematis.
To gather the hazelnuts from the boughs above me
Or fill my basket with wild blackberries from their thorny sprays;
While the cows pass lazily by on their way homewards
Swishing the flies away with their whisk-like tails,
Rubbing their brown flanks along the hedgeside,
Enjoying the pleasant brushing of the branches and twigs;
Looking sedately at me with their large round mournful eyes
Or turning round to moo to a young calf.
Oh! The charm and quiet of English lanes!
Are they like this, I wonder, in England now?

(E. M. P.)

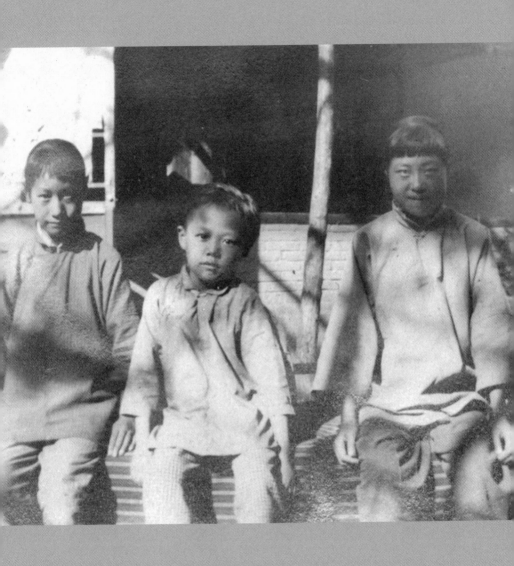

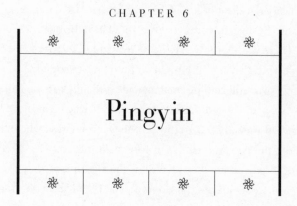

CHAPTER 6

Pingyin

ƒ* MARGARET BEGAN THE JOURNEY to her first mission station on February 28, 1906, thankful to be accompanied by Dorothy Bearder, who could speak some Chinese as she had already served in China for six months. Margaret was unable to speak the language adequately yet, having had no more than nine weeks of lessons before she had taken ill. Bishop Scott insisted the entourage should include a Chinese cook. Although Pingyin was scarcely 725 kilometres (450 miles) from Peking as the crow flies, Margaret and Dorothy travelled about 1,600 kilometres (1,000 miles) to reach their destination, first by train from Peking to Qinhuangdao (Chinhuangtao) on the coast, and then by sea to Qingdao (Tsingtao).

Their first stop was in Tianjin. The bishop had wired the Sedgewicks that the travellers would be arriving about six o'clock. It was their duty to send someone to meet them, as they received an allowance to cover expenses for hospitality, but when Margaret and Dorothy arrived, it was dark and no one awaited them. Porters burst onto the train and seized their bags, one grabbing Dorothy's handbag with the rest of her bags and dashing off. She rushed after him, as her handbag contained silver dollars for the journey. Margaret stayed behind to collect their luggage, then waited on the platform for Dorothy to return, but she had disappeared. Margaret did not know her way, but at last she managed to get herself and the luggage conveyed over the station bridge and outside the station. There was Dorothy, having recovered her handbag and bursting with impatience, saying, "I thought you were never coming."

Dorothy was still finding the language difficult, but she hailed some rickshaw men and stated their destination. They acted as if they understood, and off they went. Dorothy knew it was not far, so when they went on and on, the two women began to get alarmed. At last, after threatening not to pay unless they arrived at the right place, they drew up at the All Saints parsonage. The doors opened, and from the top of the steps, a voice called, "Why didn't you come this morning?"

"Why didn't you meet us?" Dorothy retorted. "Didn't you get Bishop Scott's telegram?"

There was no reply, so up the steps they went to shake hands with Mr. Sedgewick. In an offhand manner, he opened the door and invited the two inside. Margaret asked if it was safe to leave her handbag in the hall. "Why not?" said he.

"Because it contains silver for our journey," Margaret replied.

"Why do you carry so much silver?" he asked.

"Where is Mrs. Sedgewick?"

"In here," he replied, but she did not emerge to greet them. He was so obviously annoyed at having to take them in that Margaret picked up her bag and turned to Dorothy, saying, "Let's go to a hotel, Dorothy. We're not wanted here," whereupon Mrs. Sedgewick appeared from behind the door and asked them to come in. That first evening the husband and wife remained distinctly chilly, but the next day she was very kind and took the two travellers round the shops to buy their groceries and other necessities for their new life. Margaret had not realized that they needed to buy their own crockery and kitchenware, and that these had to be purchased in Tianjin to take with them.

This treaty port, as it was called, could provide a vastly better selection than Peking. In Peking missionaries received food and personal essentials, plus a salary of twenty pounds a year to cover incidentals such as stamps, shoe repairs, rickshaw fares and offertories. Bishop Iliff had advanced a quarter's salary to pay for their expenses, other than travelling, with the remainder to live on for six months. Margaret realized that meant very plain living indeed. Thankfully, the servants, including the cook, were on the mission payroll.

The next day the two women took a train to Qinhuangdao, where they boarded a German steamer for a day's journey down the coast to Qingdao. By now it was the beginning of March. The sea was rather rough so most passengers remained in their cabins. When Margaret sat down to eat, the captain complimented her on being a good sailor—an unfortunate remark, after which she had to retire promptly. Otherwise, she managed to enjoy the sumptuous meals and free wine. She noticed that the German passengers spoke to the Chinese stewards in English.

At Qingdao they were joined by two clergymen, the Reverends Burne and Perry, who were going to Pingyin for the consecration of a new church on March 11 and who would serve as escorts for the two women on the trip into the Interior. The latter was also going to release Mr. and Mrs. Mathews from the Pingyin mission for a new posting to the theological school for catechists, to be opened at Yantai. Before setting out, Margaret and Dorothy spent one night at the German hotel, where they shared a backroom, at the missionary rate.

Early the next morning they set off by train for Jinan (Chinan), the provincial capital of Shandong, where they were met by Wang San, a servant sent by Mr. Mathews to help them through the final stage of the journey. He took the group to a semi-foreign inn for the night, where the two women were chaperoned by an elderly Chinese woman. The city of Pingyin lies eighty kilometres (50 miles) south-west of the nearest railway terminus at Jinan. This meant a further two-day journey by wheelbarrow, the usual mode of travel, as the roads were too narrow and hilly for the mule carts so common in other parts of North China. It was also almost the same distance from Tai'an, the mission's cathedral city where Bishop Iliff was located. After an early breakfast they mounted their wheelbarrows for the final journey, which turned out to be the most harrowing part of the entire trip. Little did Margaret know then that she would travel by this means on many more occasions.

These vehicles were quite unlike the gardening wheelbarrows at home. There was a wide ledge on either side of a large iron-bound wheel about ninety centimetres (3 feet) in diameter and thirteen centimetres (5 inches) thick. The chassis provided handles for two men to propel the vehicle from the rear and the front. Each man had a wide leather strap attached to the handles which passed over his shoulders and took much of the strain from his hands. On the side ledges was set sufficient lighter luggage to balance the passenger. Heavier luggage was placed on another wheelbarrow. Finally a mattress was spread over the ledge in front of the luggage, thus providing a reasonably comfortable reclining seat. In the summer an awning mounted on poles would be stretched over the whole barrow, but that was hardly a requirement at this time of year.

Margaret served as ballast, balancing herself on one side with her luggage and medical equipment jostling to and fro on the other side as they made their way along the dirt roads, hardly more than tracks between the fields. She maintained her seat as best she could. These vehicles had no suspension, and the perpetual shrill screech emanating from the ungreased axle just below her was excruciating.

The two vicars led the way, balancing each other on opposite sides of one wheelbarrow, while the women had a wheelbarrow each. They trundled along the sandy road between high banks, sometimes getting off to walk up or down steep rocky paths over the hills. The most striking feature of the country was its bareness—it seemed one vast expanse of light brown earth. Though hilly, there were no mountains to relieve the monotony as they proceeded towards the great central plain of China. The trees were bare of leaves, and the fields, dotted with mounded graves. They passed through numerous villages, which were only clusters of mud huts with a few men, women and children standing about in the sun for warmth, their indigo clothing a striking contrast to the brown mud walls.

The travellers stopped for lunch at a village inn, where Wang San spread out the food he had brought for them. The *yang guizi* (foreign devils) were the objects of much curiosity. People simply swarmed into the inn, completely surrounding the group seated on benches at the table, wanting to see what and how they were eating, to examine their clothes and hairstyles, and to hear them speak. Closer and closer the crowd pressed until the travellers could no longer move their arms to eat. Wang San had considerable difficulty keeping the locals at a distance.

Taking to the road again, the travellers went on as fast as possible, but a couple of hours later they were horrified when the wheelbarrow men stopped for food and rest. Margaret and the others walked about to keep warm, but they were soon surrounded again and followed at every step, largely by inquisitive small children. In future, they quickly decided, they would take their meals when the porters chose to stop. Here was a lesson learned, for Wang San had been too polite to advise them. Having made too many stops the first day, they did not get as far as planned. That night was spent at a Presbyterian mission station, more pleasant than an inn, although none of them had ever before slept in a room with mud walls, dirt floors and a mud roof. Margaret had her own camp bed with mattress and sheets. Since Rev. Perry had none of these traveller's essentials, she loaned him the cot, while she spread her mattress on the Chinese brick *kang*. Needless to say, she found it difficult to adapt to such a strange bed.

They were off early next morning and this time had breakfast when the men stopped for their first meal, which was not until about ten o'clock. Here the crowd was even denser than the day before. Margaret suspected the country folk had never before seen foreign women.

♪❋

LATE IN THE AFTERNOON OF MARCH 9 they arrived in Pingyin, a small country city near the prefecture of Tai'an in the west part of Shandong Province. Pingyin stands on the edge of the Great Plain of northern China, surrounded on three sides, though not hemmed in, by gentle undulating hills practically bereft of vegetation, except where industrious peasants had built terraces to grow crops of corn and millet. To the west lay the winding Huang He (Yellow River), and beyond it a vast expanse of perfectly flat land, the Great Plain, dotted with innumerable villages, each within its small cluster of willow trees. To the east, north and south, as far as the eye could reach, rose range upon range of more hills. Above the highest hills emerged the peak of the sacred mountain Tai Shan, some eighty kilometres (50 miles) to the east.

Pingyin itself was an ordinary small Chinese city with narrow streets and mud houses, surrounded by a dilapidated battlemented wall with four gates facing the cardinal points of the compass. These were closed for security every night after dusk, after which they could not be opened without the specific permission of the magistrate, a Mandarin in absolute control of the city. As Pingyin lies on low ground about a kilometre and a half (1 mile) east of the Huang He, the land between the city and the river is usually flooded for most of the year. The floods sometimes surrounded or invaded the city, and the stagnant moat and numerous ditches harboured swarms of mosquitoes, rendering the place anything but a salubrious neighbourhood.

Despite that, the climate was generally pleasant and healthful, though marred by the fierce dust storms in the spring. Then the sky became the colour of the sand carried by the wind from the Gobi Desert. Over many millennia these winds have created the loess soil of these plains. Fine dust penetrates every crevice, even into the remotest corners of the houses, to the despair of any lover of cleanliness. The extremes of climate are marked, though possibly less so than in other parts of North China. The winter was milder, and the summer heat often tempered by clouds that frequently hung over the city. This gentle climate may account for the name of the city, which translates as "Tranquil Shade."

The houses in the city were one-storey, tentlike, flat-roofed buildings chiefly built of mud which tended to wash away in places every year during the heavy rains, necessitating annual repairs. Mud was cheap, and so was time to the Chinese, but the substantial advantages of a permanent homestead were becoming obvious and stone buildings were slowly increasing in numbers.

*∗

P INGYIN WAS OPENED for missionary work by the Society for the Propagation of the Gospel (SPG) in 1879 and permanently occupied as a mission centre in 1895. No other missions operated in the district, other than a small Roman Catholic church to the east of the city, under the control of German priests. Medical work evolved out of the bishop dispensing simple medication from a box he carried with him on his evangelical tours. Until 1900, the mission consisted of little more than a small church and a little old mud building which housed itinerant missionaries. Now it possessed a fine new church, a boys' boarding and day school, a girls' boarding school, several village mission churches and a few village schools preparatory to the Central School in Pingyin.

Mr. and Mrs. Mathews welcomed the travellers with tea. "It was wonderful to relax and feel that at last I had reached the goal for which my years of preparation had been spent," Margaret said. "I was at the beginning of my chosen life's work."

Bishop Iliff was in Pingyin for the consecration of the new church. Mr. Mathews had just completed its construction, which was of large blocks of grey stone after the pattern of an English church. At first it struck Margaret as looking somewhat incongruous in its Chinese surroundings; later she found that the Catholics also built their churches in the Western style. It was extremely well built and a monument to Mr. Mathews's energy and perseverance because he had only unskilled builders to work with. (Little did Margaret know that she too would proceed along similar lines in a couple of years' time constructing her hospital.)

The service of consecration was long, and Margaret could understand little of it. Chinese Christians came from all the surrounding districts, filling the church. The men sat on one side and the women on the other, but at least there was no partition down the middle of the church, as was deemed necessary in the early days of missionary work in China. Children wandered from side to side at will. It took Margaret a long time to get used to the late arrivals and the comings and goings during a service. This was rather in keeping with the people's only idea of a religious ceremony: simply a brief visit to burn incense. Only the priests stayed to worship. However, Margaret found the ceremony both impressive and interesting, and the church "absolutely simple and beautiful, so that on entering it one suddenly becomes conscious of a feeling of reverence, the feeling that a church ought to excite, but often does not." It had been erected in memory of the Reverend Sidney Brooke, the first missionary killed by the Boxers in 1900.

The bishop left soon after the consecration but not before speaking with Margaret about her future work, urging her specially to remember that she must be an evangelist as well as a doctor. She was instructed to see to it herself that evangelistic work was carried out in the dispensary, advice Margaret thought was uncalled for.

Margaret and Dorothy had rooms in the same courtyard as the Mathewses' two-storey building. The compound consisted of two parallel Chinese buildings facing south separated by the courtyard, with the kitchen and servants' quarters along the west side of the yard. Margaret's comfortable quarters were in front, and she enjoyed a small three-room suite with wooden floors. A bedroom and study bounded her tiny dining room. Dorothy's room at the back was more primitive, with brick floors and a flat roof. It was distinctly damp so Margaret changed over, as Dorothy was much troubled with rheumatism. (Later, after Dorothy had returned to Peking, Margaret changed back to the front room, and only a few days afterwards the whole of the back bedroom roof collapsed in the night. Margaret would have most certainly been killed.)

The courtyard was enclosed by a low wall to one side of the church compound with entry through a small gate. The Chinese were not supposed to enter the courtyard by that route, only through Mr. Mathews's study by another side door. Not knowing this, the two women annoyed Mrs. Mathews by constantly bringing Chinese people through this gate. Poor Mrs. Mathews was nervous in this lonely place and liked her privacy. Nevertheless, since Mr. and Mrs. Mathews were expecting to leave in due course, it was opportune that the two women came when they did, as it enabled them to achieve a degree of continuity.

For the first five weeks, Margaret worked primarily on her language studies since her small amount of Pekinese was of little use in the countryside, even though the Shandong dialect had the same Mandarin basis. On April 16, Easter Monday, she formally took charge of the medical work. She worked for the first month in the old mud building where Bishop Iliff had dispensed medicines several years previously. In the small, low building, only one patient could be seen at a time. The thick walls contained two small windows—or rather, holes—about sixty centimetres (2 feet) wide and forty-five centimetres (about 1½ feet) high. These did not open and were of little use in giving air or light. Most of the light entering the room came through the large cracks over and below the ill-fitting door, which had to be kept closed because a foreign woman doctor and nurse at work were objects of great interest and curiosity.

The crowd could not be kept from the doorway unless the door was kept shut; every patient wanted to be seen first. Closing the door was the only way of hearing what the patients said. Even then, a servant had to be posted near the windows to keep people from peering in and blocking out all the light. Occasionally the door had to be partially opened to allow a little more light, for the dried mud floor was uneven, causing frequent stumbling about in the half-light. In the rainy season it could be very damp, providing a most unsatisfactory situation for both doctor and patient.

Under such conditions, Margaret once had to do a major operation by the light of a small lamp. A man of seventy, in great pain, had been brought in, close to death from injuries received when a stone fell on his foot. His leg ought to have been amputated, but this was impossible, for the Boxers had carried off the necessary instruments. Margaret had the assistance of Dorothy and a medical attendant, Zhang Laoping, more familiarly known as Zhang Er (meaning Zhang the Second). With the help of chloroform, she did the best she could. To their great astonishment the old man recovered completely. Understandably, this case did much to enhance the regard of the local populace for the medical work now taking place.

There were also domestic problems to contend with. The cook from Peking proved unwilling to co-operate. Not only did they have to let him go, on Mr. Mathews's advice they paid his return fare to Peking. After that Margaret had a difficult time training a cook, for first she had to learn how to cook and bake bread in order to teach the new cook, although most Chinese men had a basic knowledge of how to prepare food. Eventually, order of a sort was restored.

Margaret and Dorothy got on well together, and they enjoyed many private jokes about the things that happened in the course of their work. Margaret felt certain that many patients came out of curiosity or to get medication for someone at home. Sometimes they seemed to find it difficult to remember their symptoms and to be so deeply interested in taking stock of the foreigners' appearance that they scarcely paid attention to what was being said to them. However, if another patient arrived, they would repeat to the newcomer what they had been told, as if to explain it and illustrate how well they understood the foreigners' language. Margaret believed they thought she was speaking English, which was not surprising, considering her poor accent. Foreigners were seldom credited with the ability to speak Chinese, and it often took a while for them to be understood, unless their speech was perfect. On the other hand, some Chinese people might compliment one out of the blue on how well one spoke the language. This was not really a compliment but a subtle way to put one at ease over an inadvertently badly spoken word or phrase. Margaret soon discovered the difference between the pronunciation of *soap* and *chair*, or *book* and *tree*, but she was often surprised to get sugar when she wanted soup, or vice versa.

Dorothy always saw the funny side of things. Finally Margaret refused to sit beside her in church, instead sitting behind, which was nearly as distracting when she saw her shoulders shaking. Occasionally Dorothy was given to bursting out laughing. Certainly it was funny seeing women throwing hassocks to their husbands across the aisle, or feeling a tug at her hat from behind when a woman wanted to know what it was made of. Sometimes there was a little lift of her skirt to see what she had on her legs; there was a great deal of doubt as to whether foreign women wore trousers.

In Shandong, all women wore short coats and trousers, and the men, ankle-length coats which looked like skirts. Embroidered skirts were seen only at weddings and ceremonial occasions. When the magistrate's wife called on Margaret, she wore a pleated skirt. Her feet were so tiny that she had to be supported on either side. All the women had bound feet, and it was marvellous how they managed to get about, even walking long distances to the market. They virtually walked on their big toes, supported by the other toes, which were turned under the instep towards the big toe. They toddled with a slightly swaying motion, though rather stiffly, as they could not bend their knees for fear of losing balance— hence arose the term "lily feet," as they were supposed to resemble the motion of lilies swaying in the breeze.

♪*

MR. AND MRS. MATHEWS remained at the mission. He was busy superintending alterations to the old dark dispensary, which was to become a sort of ward or temporary rest-house for men who had come a distance seeking medical attention. By then little of the old building was left standing, as the greater part had collapsed during the summer rains. For the women inpatients' temporary use, all Margaret had was one small room that could only accommodate two patients at a time. In this one room, they had to sleep, eat, smoke and see their friends.

Margaret had no great expectations as yet for results from inpatients work. So far her total number of inpatients was thirty-one, but these had been only the absolutely essential ones. She had purposely not encouraged any others, since she wanted to devote at least five hours a day to her language studies.

The old church, duly converted for use as a dispensary, was opened in grand style on Easter Monday. As damp conditions did not suit Dorothy, it was a relief to move into the new quarters. Although renovation had begun earlier in the year, directly after a pre-consecration conference with the bishop, progress seemed agonizingly slow. The wooden front on the south side of the church was removed and used to form screens which divided the building into three rooms. The south side was reconstructed of solid grey stone, with generous windows and a glazed door into the central room. The results were considered palatial by contrast.

The waiting room (*houzhen shi*) was the central room and larger than those on either side, but it soon failed to accommodate the influx of patients, becoming so crowded that people had to wait outdoors. Unfortunately, there was insufficient funding to provide a more adequate dispensary. To the east of the waiting room was the consulting room (*kanbing fang*), where patients were first seen by the doctor. After examination and treatment, Margaret would issue prescriptions when required. The patients would then proceed to the west room, the dispensary (*yaofang*, meaning "medicine room"), where Dorothy dispensed medication.

The waiting room was furnished with benches, a table and a chair— the seat of honour for the Chinese preacher, Mr. Xi. It was customary for him to address the waiting patients for at least an hour. His teaching was very much to the point; the people appeared interested and often asked questions. He seemed successful in getting them to understand that the missionaries loved Christ who loved all people; thus the missionaries wanted to emulate Christ and to help relieve suffering so that people might be happier. Margaret approved of Mr. Xi preaching in the waiting room, as she felt it was better to have a native speaker to address the group. Many Chinese had never heard foreigners speak their language, and foreigners speaking their own language would be just as incomprehensible.

One drawback was the lack of insulation against noise, the screens being made of open woodwork covered with paper. Unless the people in the waiting room were perfectly quiet, Margaret and her patient could not hear each other, and every word spoken in the consulting room was heard clearly by the whole assembly next door. The Chinese always imagined that, as the foreigners appeared to not fully comprehend their language, they must be deaf. As a rule they began by shouting at Margaret, hoping to help her better understand.

Margaret had mixed feelings over the new setting, but she adopted the philosophical attitude that work had to have a beginning, and she was most grateful and encouraged by the good start she was getting. However, she admitted to being insatiable: though this was satisfactory as a start, she would not be satisfied with it for long. Margaret's dreams, like a mirage, were constantly just out of reach and presented challenges she resolutely strained to meet.

It was hard to make an impression on the Chinese, and results were unlikely to be worthwhile in such work as this. Apart from the inability of the dispensary to handle more patients, the fleeting effect of clinical contact was inadequate to deal with substandard living conditions. The obstacles to be overcome were enormous: squalor, suspicion and bias on a general scale, all of which stood in the way of introducing foreign medical practices and converting patients to accept an alien religion. Nonetheless, Margaret felt that influence works secretly and is far-reaching. As long as she had the opportunities, she was happy to keep on working. She was aware that the local people dimly wondered why missionaries took so much trouble and were constantly willing to help out. For the time being, this was encouragement enough to persevere.

♪※

MARGARET FOUND IT DIFFICULT to give her consulting room the right ambiance. Her ingenuity was constantly challenged, but she went to work with a will. The main problem was its floor. She felt that floors in China generally presented a difficulty because of the way the bricks were laid. While bricks constituted a luxury as opposed to plain dirt, such floors were hard to keep clean, with the bricks or slabs set so far apart that there was always plenty of dirt to sweep up each day. Occasionally that room was used as a temporary operating theatre, and propping up the tables to make them steady on the uneven floor was tricky. One day,

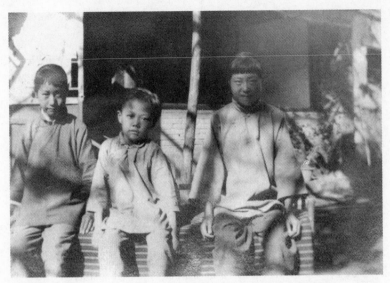

Many of Dr. Margaret's favourite patients in Pingyin were the local children.

when patients were few due to harvesting priorities, the floors were taken up and carefully relaid. The net result was quite rewarding, except for the need to prop up the instrument cupboard, and that proved to be the fault of the cupboard itself.

The next move was to put up mosquito netting over the windows and bamboo blinds over the doors. A colleague Margaret had met elsewhere in China had told her that he performed operations anywhere, even outdoors. She wondered how he kept the flies away, since a fly in the wrong place at a critical moment could be disastrous. Then she realized that being concerned over "a fly" was ridiculous. There was no such thing, as it would be invariably an entire swarm of flies. She hoped that the screens and blinds would be adequate to deal with any insect intrusions. Her next move was to paint the furniture black, and although she spoiled a good pair of overalls in the process, she finally began to feel more at home in her consulting room.

f^*

MARGARET FOUND MUCH SADNESS in her medical work, and she felt a tremendous compassion for the surrounding community. Much misery was borne stoically by her patients. It took a heroic effort on her part to reduce the suffering, since so much illness was due to ignorance and the sheer lack of education. To her, the Chinese methods of treatment seemed quite barbarous. If the people did try to emulate her treatment to any extent in their own wretched hovels, few had any chance of success, for they did not understand the purpose of their instructions or the need to carry them out. Thus, the educational work was important. Through outpatient work, mission workers could make known their aims and methods. Mission schools helped to create a friendly feeling in the district, but only through the inpatient work of a hospital was there any real hope of making Christians.

One cold day, a two-year-old boy in convulsions was brought in for treatment. After trying the usual remedies, the convulsions ceased and the boy at last passed into a peaceful sleep. There was no doubt that he was seriously ill, and Margaret begged his mother to let him remain with her to watch over him. This she was unwilling to do, and towards evening she took her son home. When she returned the next day as promised, her child seemed slightly better, but she was in a hurry to go elsewhere. Margaret gave her medicine and instructions, and off she went. But before leaving, she made a remark which Margaret, being still new to China, did not comprehend. Tapping the sleeping child on the head, the mother said, "He's really dead, isn't he? They all want me to throw him away."

"Indeed he is not!" Margaret replied indignantly, unaware that it was the custom for mothers to discard their sick children if they were thought likely to die. This was partly due to a fear of devils and partly because they had no idea what really caused convulsions or paroxysms, which they mistook for being possessed. Although she had no idea of the woman's true meaning, some instinct caused Margaret to make her promise to bring the boy back the next day—dead or alive—for her to see. The mother was most anxious to give her child to the doctor, and several times offered to do so. Margaret had to refuse, and tried to tell her, as best as her Chinese would permit, that she ought not to want to give him away.

The next day there was no sign of the woman or her son, which Margaret took to mean that the boy was better. But about nine o'clock that evening, Zhang Er rushed up in a state of suppressed excitement. He knew of Margaret's interest in the child, for she had been questioning him all day for news. The boy had been thrown outside the city walls to die, Zhang said, but he did have a little life left. Zhang had been buying tobacco outside the city gate when a man came by and said he had heard a baby crying on the bank of the moat surrounding the city wall. Zhang went to look and, recognizing her little patient, had immediately reported this to Margaret, since he feared to interfere himself.

She told him to fetch the baby at once. The responsibility now being hers, he quickly obeyed. A bundle of dirty rags was laid on the table. Inside was the unconscious little boy, only just alive and in dreadful convulsions again. He was dressed in his oldest and dirtiest clothes and was hardly recognizable. On his forehead, cheeks, nose and lips were streaks of black, and on the palms of his hands as well. Margaret could not understand the meaning of this, and then Zhang Er explained what he had not wished to tell her before. It seemed that the poor mother had been frightened by the convulsions. She no longer knew her child, and in her superstition believed that an evil spirit had possessed him. To her, he really was dead and she was afraid of him. Young children in China were seldom buried; their bodies were generally wrapped up in straw or rags and thrown over the city wall at night. Before daylight the dogs would have left no trace.

Since this boy was possessed of the devil, who would surely come to claim his own, the woman had daubed him all over with black paint and tied a piece of dog skin round each wrist. All this was a sign for the devil to claim him, so the child's appearance was truly ghastly. Margaret and Dorothy washed and tended him, and soon, under the influence of bromides, the convulsions were quietened and he slept. Zhang Er left to inform the mother and to beg her to return for her child. She arrived fearful and angry, giggling with nervousness, but she seemed pleased with what had been done and agreed to stay. Margaret knew that the child, who had meningitis, had not long to live, but the Chinese thought a wonderful thing had taken place. A report went round that she had brought a dead baby back to life, since they had declared the boy dead when he was thrown away.

Although his case was hopeless, especially after such treatment, Margaret aimed to show the poor woman how to treat a dying child and that there was no need for fear. She longed to be able to talk to the mother, but her Chinese remained woefully inadequate. The child seemed to improve so much that it was hard to feel there was no hope, but on the second day he suddenly worsened, and it was obvious he could not last much longer. With difficulty the mother was kept from running away again. Dorothy hardly left the boy's side, nursing him in her arms to show that there was nothing to fear. On the third day after he had been thrown out to die, he slept his life quietly away.

The mother showed no grief, though she did weep gently for a couple of minutes because she was frightened. She was made to promise to have her son buried, and Margaret sent Zhang to make sure it was done. Margaret was impressed with Zhang's conduct throughout. The mother in this tragic case subsequently became friendly and quite often returned to visit the dispensary.

♪✻

AN ASSESSMENT of how well the medical needs of the community were being served made it evident that a permanent hospital was needed to fulfill the mission's purpose, and Margaret had to determine the time needed for its erection. In the meantime, funds had to be found. Soon she found herself working virtually single-handedly. Dorothy was suffering from ill health, due to the crude and damp working conditions. While Margaret was undergoing identical hardships, at the age of thirty she was twelve years younger and stronger than her colleague.

Meanwhile, a change had been effected in the arrangements for the Mathewses, who, after many lonely years in Pingyin, were looking forward to going to the new school for catechists in Yantai. Unhappily, Rev. Perry, who had travelled with Margaret from Qingdao to replace Mr. Mathews, was found to be a heavy drinker. It was considered quite unsuitable to station him in Pingyin, where he could buy very cheaply the potent Chinese wine known as *mao tai,* which was almost pure spirit and highly intoxicating. The bishop had no one available to take his place other than a Mr. Jones, who was a bachelor, and this would be improper. In Margaret's opinion, it could hardly have been worse than the two women living in the same courtyard with Mr. Mathews as if they were his concubines.

There were obvious indications of friction between Mr. and Mrs. Mathews and Margaret and Dorothy, who on several occasions unthinkingly gave cause for resentment. While not intending to be aggressive, Margaret was eager to get on with her own agenda. Mr. Mathews's attitude suggested a grudge against Margaret; part of her trouble with him was her inability to accept having a man telling her what to do. After all his hard work in building a fine new church and then cleverly converting the old one into a dispensary, understandably he resented the turn of events. First was the irritation of having to surrender control of the dispensary and the first-aid work he had carried on for some time with the help of the Chinese dispenser. Rather belatedly, Margaret realized she could have been more tactful by discussing her intentions. Not only had she taken over the dispensary, which Mr. Mathews had started years before, to outward appearances she was asserting herself as if she was in authority. The Chinese would see this to mean demotion for her colleague with a resulting loss of face. Doubtless, Mr. Mathews was aware of this, while Margaret had been oblivious, not yet being entirely familiar with the protocol in Chinese culture.

More trouble arose from her zeal for evangelistic work. As there was no Sunday school, Dorothy and Margaret started one in the dispensary waiting room without consulting Mr. Mathews. After the Sunday morning service, they held a kind of reception for the Chinese women in the waiting room, followed once a month by an at-home in their own house. This meant bringing Chinese people onto the private grounds. Although Margaret considered the bishop's earlier injunctions as authority to do whatever she could on that score, eventually she realized that it was necessary to ask permission to do any kind of evangelistic work.

When Bishop Iliff had told Margaret that she should learn not to take things to heart too much, she had responded fervently, "I hope I never shall!" It now seemed to her that was just where the older missionaries were lacking; certainly they were deficient in charity for the younger ones and slow in offering a helping hand. Filled with the deepest contrition, she confided to her diary her fear of having failed in her line of duty.

♪❈

DOROTHY FOUND LIFE ALTOGETHER TOO HARD, and she frequently took to her bed for several days at a time, forcing Margaret to take care of her as well as all her other duties. Naturally this worried Dorothy, which made them both unhappy. Finally, it was decided that she should go to Yantai on the coast for the summer to escape the great heat. By the end of the year, Dorothy was feeling a little stronger. She took over the domestic duties but was unable to assist with the medical work. Whether she would stay in China remained to be seen. If she could, both the bishop and Margaret would be only too thankful, as Margaret could not live alone in Pingyin indefinitely. Dorothy was good about her limitations, but Margaret knew full well that she found it hard being forbidden from doing her desired work. In the end, a consultation between the two bishops revealed that there was a welcome awaiting her in Peking, where the climate had always suited her in the past. By springtime she was comfortably resettled up north.

In mid-December, Margaret's second in China, Bishop Iliff invited her to Tai'an to spend Christmas with his family, since she had not been away for a summer holiday. The invitation was gladly accepted, and Margaret at once prepared for the trip, engaging a wheelbarrow and packing in readiness to start the next day. Then Mr. Mathews arrived, telling her that she should not go, as bandits were massing in the district through which she was to travel and it was rumoured that they were threatening to take Pingyin. Margaret asked rather irritably what she considered a reasonable question: Why had he not told her earlier? He knew she would be afraid, he replied.

"That's a lie!" Margaret snapped, but she cancelled the wheelbarrow. A few days later Mr. Mathews said the governor of Shantung had sent down troops from Jinan, so the bandits had moved to the next province and now it would be quite safe for her to go. Off she went gladly.

At Tai'an, however, she felt impelled to tell the bishop how she felt, before taking her Christmas communion. That was the only time she confessed to a clergyman, though she did not regard it as a confession at the time. The bishop said she must apologize to Mr. Mathews and make allowances for his nervousness and concern. He had been alone in Pingyin when his friend the Reverend Sidney Brooke was cruelly killed by the Boxers, on the same lonely road on which Margaret travelled. Mr. Mathews had implored the bishop to write to the British consul at Jinan to ask protection for her, but this the bishop had declined to do. Finally, Mr. Mathews had written directly to the consul, who had reported it to the governor.

Margaret had a happy visit with Bishop and Mrs. Iliff and their small boys. There she met Mr. Cousins, a recent addition to the mission who was to teach in the boys' school. He lived in a tiny Chinese house in the church compound, and the bishop invited him several times to join them in the evening for games. Card games were generally discouraged for fear the servants might think that missionaries gambled. One evening, after the servants had retired, out came the cards for a round of bridge. Suddenly, a servant entered with a message. Someone hastily tried to put the cards out of sight, but the bishop stopped that, saying that they should not have been playing cards if they did not want the servants to know.

In due course, the Mathewses were reassigned to Pingyin as a result of the overall situation. Margaret made an honest attempt to bury the hatchet, and they all parted on good terms when the Mathewses departed for an extended break on the coast. They left behind a small oil stove, which was a boon to Margaret as she could then sterilize instruments and always have hot water on hand. Previously she had to send the gate-keeper out to buy a kettleful of hot water whenever necessary; naturally, this soon became tepid, while the waiting itself was simply a waste of time.

Between April 17 and June 17, Margaret attended to 2,300 men, women and children. Patients came from distances of 70 *li* (about 27 kilometres or 22 miles), which at walking pace took most of a day. On ordinary days she saw from 50 to 60 patients. The first harvest brought quieter days. For two weeks no one had time to have their ailments attended to; like-wise everyone stayed indoors for several days when it rained. Every fifth day was a market day, with no time to spare. Then Margaret had to cope with as many as 100 patients. Her record for a single day was 134. During those two months, it had been necessary for 15 patients to be accommo-dated intermittently in a private home or the old dispensary until such time the new dispensary was established.

After Bishop Iliff's injunction, Margaret believed that the responsi-bility for offering spiritual guidance was as much hers, being a missionary doctor, as the missionary staff's. She was confident that people would react more positively in a hospital environment than to the hasty occasional contact as outpatients. As well, with a patient in a hospital bed she could keep the person under observation and thereby carry out treatment of more substantial benefit than on a casual outpatient basis. Even a short stay could illustrate to the women how domestic conditions might be improved, if only by practising better hygiene. This, after all, would enable her to perform better medical practice and satisfy her professional duty.

She looked forward immensely to the completion of the ward, which would also enable her to save time for language study—devoting four to five hours daily was still essential—and serve as a stopgap until the hos-pital became a reality. She was still obliged to pay outside visits, for which she could ill afford the time, and she purposely avoided encouraging such patients. For the same reason, she had not yet started to visit the outlying villages. Although outside visits were being kept to a minimum, Margaret made seven trips in ten days to patients who were unable to be moved. She was frequently called upon to treat suicidal poisoning cases.

Often women took poison because of ill-treatment by relatives. Their purpose was to frighten their tormentors, as their death would bring the family into disgrace. Such patients were difficult to treat, as they had to be dosed with emetics or submit to a stomach pump against their will.

To realize her vision, Margaret had first to face the challenging task of building a hospital. This had been her ambition, even before leaving Peking for Pingyin, ever since she had seen how mission hospital work was carried out. For two long arduous years she had dealt with all the situations normally encountered in a general hospital. Without the backing of an organized hospital and trained staff to sustain her, she bore an enormous weight of personal responsibility. She had nobody to consult with over medical issues, all the while carrying out the roles of both physician and surgeon, and many times nurse as well.

Despite this, she never lost sight of that ambition to plan and erect a hospital, and still regularly found time to maintain a record of her work, her correspondence and observations of life around her. In her desire to encourage an active interest regarding missionary work in China, she compulsively wrote to friends and loyal supporters in England, thanking them for financial donations to her mission and describing in considerable detail various aspects of her work and where her needs lay heaviest— thus showing that their philanthropy was being well applied. Her friend Mrs. Mosse, who had staunchly backed her medical work from the beginning, wrote to tell Margaret that the SPG had started a medical needs supply department. She enquired about her needs, and Margaret quickly replied, "Wanted—A Hospital!"

"You shall have it," Mrs. Mosse replied with enthusiasm. She worked hard and long towards that goal. The two had a tremendous rapport, and Mrs. Mosse was well aware of Margaret's ambition. From this valiant effort, she later told Margaret, arose the SPG's medical mission department with Rev. Mosse as department secretary and Mrs. Mosse as head of supplies. Margaret was convinced that it was this interest and support that kept her going.

Thus October ended on a high note. Margaret had fixed up two contracts: one for the essential wall to surround the whole of the land bought for the medical quarters to the east of the city, and one for the new dispensary. The mission was anxious to recover use of the existing dispensary as a church room. After so many setbacks up to this point, one more would hardly seem to matter. At least things were starting to happen. Margaret was virtually quivering with excitement to have finally reached this stage.

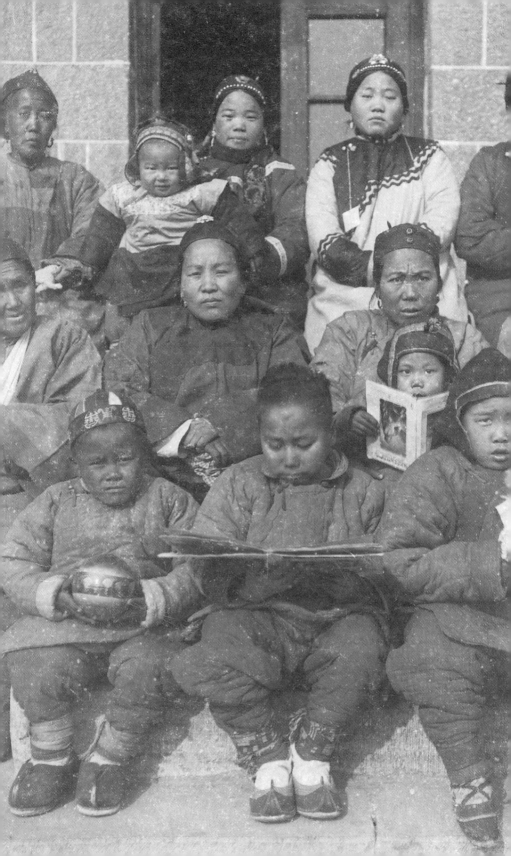

CHAPTER 7

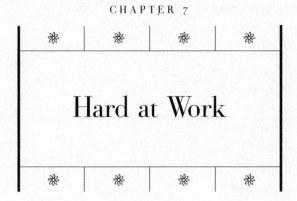

Hard at Work

♪* THOUGH PEOPLE WERE GENERALLY PLEASANT and friendly, Margaret found trying to treat their illnesses discouraging. She could give them only harmless medicines to take away, for if they liked the first dose, or the first dose relieved them, they would be likely to swallow the bottle's entire contents at once to hasten the cure. Medicines such as lotions for external use might be taken internally. Patients always enquired how the medicine should be prepared or what food should be avoided. The practice among Chinese doctors was to write a prescription for many ingredients which would be taken home in separate small packages, cooked together for an hour or more, then the whole draught taken at once.

To treat a patient who had taken opium and was slowly dying of the poison, typically the Chinese doctor would sit beside him, holding his pulse for about two hours. He would then order a remedy which required nearly half a day to prepare, by the time all the ingredients had been ground down into a powder:

2 oz. salted lizards, two male and two female

½ oz. Corea ginseng root [sic]

6 dried grasshoppers, three male and three female

1 oz. sweet potato stalks

1 oz. walnuts

½ oz. lotus leaves

¼ oz. tail of rattlesnake

2 oz. black dates

½ oz. elm tree bark

½ oz. devil-fish claw

½ oz. hartshorne

¼ oz. birds' claws

¼ oz. dried ginger

½ oz. old coffin nails

The whole to be mixed with two quarts of water, and boiled down to half the quantity. Then let the patient drink the mixture as quickly as possible.

Source: Honan Messenger

A traditional Chinese apothecary differed radically from a western pharmacist. To the Chinese, the foreign method of repeated doses seemed slow and strange. Margaret once gave a patient some worm powders, telling him to take one at night and one in the morning for two days, but before she had finished speaking he had swallowed all four powders, paper and all.

♪✳

OVER TIME Margaret's patients became accustomed to her speech, and she began to make friends. A new factor evolved in her activities. She was, in effect, helping to promote female emancipation by encouraging Chinese women to generally improve their lot. One branch of her work involved training nurses and other medical workers—a new concept for Chinese women, and difficult to achieve since the trainees expected to be paid. The ideal of service as a moral obligation had yet to take root. For one month she had a paid Chinese woman assistant, who was helpful and exceedingly quick. Margaret intended to teach her dispensing, but during the busy harvest time she left, and Margaret could not get her back for a very long time.

The two older schoolgirls who helped at the dispensary for an hour daily seemed to enjoy the work and to be taking to heart some of the lessons. One day one of their sisters brought her small and very dirty baby to see the doctor. The girls themselves suggested that the baby should be washed prior to coming before Margaret, then went on to get it done. This was truly a wonderful step forward because Chinese women never washed their babies and rarely washed themselves. Margaret was convinced that she was on the right track.

Another day a six-year-old with dysentery, in a state of collapse, was brought in by her mother. Having been ill for many days, she was practically starving, for if children were too ill to eat their ordinary food there was nothing else to give them. Margaret took the two into her small temporary ward for three days. Although the girl began to improve slightly, the mother constantly expressed her wish to leave, consenting to stay only after much persuasion. On the afternoon of the third day, just when the child had practically turned the corner and was safe, though still exceedingly weak, the mother made her getaway during Margaret's absence from the ward. The temporary ward was so situated that there was no way of controlling who came and went, and Margaret had no one to leave in charge. When she discovered their absence, she sent Zhang Er to beg the mother at least to let her give the child milk and medicine, but she refused.

A similar situation occurred not long afterwards, and that little girl died, also of dysentery, after a short stay in the ward. Again Margaret had only the unwilling mother to assist with the child's care. Had she been equipped with a hospital, Margaret might have been able to save such patients. She desperately needed nursing help, and although her reports were not intended to be complaining, she grieved over lost patients. At times she felt despondent. For the time being, lack of funds made the prospect of a hospital unlikely, and the loss of Miss Bearder meant she had to work alone indefinitely. With only the one small room to accommodate patients, she constantly had to turn sick people away. Once the ward was so overcrowded that two patients slept in Margaret's kitchen and one in her small dining room. She nursed all patients day and night with no servant to help with domestic duties. The amount of work was appalling, but the inability to accomplish much was more trying. Being so weary, she felt less and less likely to attract patients to the dispensary, where previously there had been a rush of patients during the "season."

Her greatest fear was that people were realizing how helpless she was, and doubtless spreading that impression. She also feared that the hospital might materialize too late, since Pingyin was liable to disaster. The nearby Huang He regularly flooded, occasionally to a disastrous level. Sometimes there were droughts, and either situation could easily drain Margaret's meagre resources.

One morning, just as she sat down to her Chinese examination, she was called out to attend a woman said to be dying of lockjaw. It was, in fact, an attempted suicide, and although the woman could swallow a little she resisted Margaret's efforts. Her friends and neighbours had gathered in large numbers to see her die. After spreading a straw mat on the ground to receive her, hanging red cloths on the bushes and lighting incense, they were waiting for Margaret to leave so that they might carry the woman outside. Chinese custom did not allow death to occur indoors. The Chinese believed that they may have more than one spirit, and their worst dread was lest one be left behind at home. For this reason, in the elegant funeral processions of affluent families, an empty sedan chair might preceed the coffin for the spirit to lead the way. This fear is also why the Chinese frequently moved house after a death in the family. For poor families, the best precaution was simply to move the dying person out of the house.

The day was bitterly cold, and Margaret heard afterwards that the woman did not die till three o'clock that afternoon. She had seemed to be enjoying being the object of so much attention and to fear Margaret might deprive her of that. Her friends appeared to be of the same mind, so it was difficult to see why they had sent for Margaret. She concluded that it was of no use to try to find an explanation. As time went on, she did achieve a deeper understanding of the Chinese culture and morality, and their effects on the people.

♪*

BY YEAR-END Margaret had passed her first-year language examination. One paper was on the Chinese grammar and exercise book by C. W. Mateer, another on Chinese characters and radicals, and another on St. John's Gospel and the prayer book (matins, evensong, litany and the Holy Communion). This examination was the same as that taken by priests and deacons. She had asked to be allowed to take St. John's Gospel instead of S. Wells Williams's *Middle Kingdom*, the subject normally assigned to an unordained missionary.

After several futile attempts at a holiday, Margaret visited Tai Shan, the most sacred and oldest of the five sacred mountains of the Daoist religion. Located some eighty-four kilometres (52 miles) south of Jinan, it is, at 1,545 metres (5,070 feet), the highest peak on the Shandong Peninsula. An elderly Chinese duenna accompanied her as chaperone, and a servant took care of the cooking. Meals were somewhat monotonous, with everything boiled over a primitive Chinese stove, giving a smoky flavour to food and water alike.

Most of the time it rained heavily, but Margaret took advantage of breaks in the weather to chase the clouds up the mountainside with her Brownie box camera. Since there was no colour film then, she could not capture the lovely greens, browns and purples of the tree trunks, or the many hues of the shining wet rock. She tried to portray the filmy wool-white cloudy mist filling the valleys with the rock barely peeping through, then to imagine the whole as one sparkling mass of raindrops. She later wrote: "I have never seen so many raindrops before. It is a feast of the beautiful. 'The Idea of the Beautiful,' which is God."

Words cannot describe the glory of the setting sun;
Art cannot portray its radiancy;
Too gorgeous are the colours and swift the changes;
We gaze enthralled.
How exquisite is the sunset glow
Spreading streaks across the pale sky,
Lighting up the dark green of the trees and the brown branches;
Softening the hard lines of daylight
And drawing a blaze of reflected light from some window.
The sunset is a parable of the end of life's day;
How will it be with you and me in the evening of life?
Shall we catch the reflected glow of Heaven
Or pass over in storm clouds dark and grey?

(E. M. P.)

Margaret took many long walks on the mountain, but she did not attempt the ascent in the traditional manner of climbing the six thousand steps to the summit, which rose steeply to just over fifteen hundred metres (5,000 feet) above the plain. She did what most foreigners do, and many Chinese too, and ascended by sedan chair. The way up, with its many flights of steps and wayside temples, was beautiful. Cypress trees of all ages cast a delightful cooling shade over the path. Picturesque bridges led across deep ravines packed closely with huge boulders, loosened and brought down from the mountainsides by the bitter frosts of winter and the heavy rains of summer, concealing the flow of water far below. Beggars' huts abounded on the sides of the roadway, adding to rather than detracting from the scene. The smallest space seemed to suffice; every conveniently overhanging rock was utilized as a dwelling chamber, the sides roughly built with the loose stones lying abundantly about. The beggars relied on the passing sightseers and pilgrims to provide for their support.

This was the coldest time of year and also the time of the Spring Festival, commonly referred to as the Chinese New Year, when the Chinese had virtually no other occupation, as frost prevented both the cultivation of soil and the repair of the usually broken-down houses. The steps were thronged with people, ascending and descending, in chairs or on foot. People came from all parts of China to make the sacred ascent, and all were besieged with the clamours of the crippled, maimed and disfigured, who laying waiting for them to pass.

Often these pilgrims were representatives of their various villages, chosen and sent off by joint subscription to do good by proxy for those unable to leave home. Pity the poor women toiling up those steep and narrow steps on their pinched and distorted "lily" feet. At the sides of the last and steepest flight of steps, chains were provided by which people would drag themselves up to the Gate of Heaven, the archway at the top of the last flight of steps. Wonderful were their powers of endurance, and their reward was ensured, for they were honoured and respected by their neighbours for the rest of their lives. Fear of one's neighbours' opinions was probably an even bigger god in China than elsewhere in the world.

The Analects of Confucius stress that conscientiousness about funeral rites for parents and worship of ancestors will increase the family's standing. Such is one way to "gain face" in one's neighbourhood, and such is the weight it carries that no effort is spared to gain face wherever possible. The corollary is, of course, not to "lose face"—this, to the Chinese, is tantamount at times to losing one's honour. Several foreign pseudonyms amount to the Chinese conception of *face*: prestige, reputation, honour, public standing, self-respect. Anything said or done, intentionally or not, that may harm this can cause a loss of face. Remarks likely to diminish someone's ego must be avoided, as well as anything suggesting sarcasm, or criticism in public. On such an occasion a Chinese may put it down to foreign ignorance and overlook the gaffe. In a circumstances where a foreigner might fire back a pointed retort, a Chinese would remain silent. For the hurt given, he would rather get even than get mad.

Margaret's "pilgrimage"—regardless of motivation—certainly gave her face, because it indicated a respect for Chinese culture, thus gaining face for the Chinese too. Passing through the Gate of Heaven leads to an astonishing space on the summit of the mountain, with numerous temples and even a colony of small dwellings, though mainly deserted. Only one temple was in any state of repair; the rest, in various stages of decay. The chief Confucian temple had recently undergone a process of renovation lasting almost three years. The main shrine was reasonably well maintained, and the broken-down roofs had been renewed and were ablaze with yellow tiles. Bright yellow flowers sprang from cracks between the tiles, making the beautiful roof more beautiful still but numbering its days. The Chinese never seemed to think of removing those destructive weeds or of renewing any missing tiles. Consequently, ruin was a certainty and quite rapid. Nor did they appear to repair their temples without an imperial decree. The magistrates of the district came and went every two or three years to be promoted or degraded, as the case may be. Unless His Imperial Majesty so ordained, rather than repair temples for their successors to enjoy, they kept to themselves all the money they could levy from the people.

♪⁂

THAT YEAR, patient numbers diminished to only 80 a day. Margaret began visiting two village stations once a month, each involving three to four hours of travel by sedan chair. She longed to set up a base so that her patients could come to her. Too much valuable time was lost taking doctor to patient. In one day she would have seen anywhere from 98 to a maximum, once, of 139 patients. Among so many people she often recognized potential candidates as inpatients. She wanted so much to be able to do something more for them, both physically and spiritually, than could be achieved in one necessarily hasty examination.

A scourge of Shandong Province was trachoma, an infection of the eyelids due to flies, dirt, dust, poor food and bad air in the mud huts in which the country folk lived. This widespread infectious disease, which often led to blindness, existed in all levels of society from the Mandarin of the city on down to the peasants. The eye cases were usually hopeless by the time the patients came for help, and often they refused to attend enough to gain much benefit. "I have been here four times," one patient complained on her final visit, "and yet my eyes are not cured."

Another patient used her written prescription as an application to her eyes; yet another drank her eye-drops in water. Nonetheless, Margaret did her best under the circumstances, and the extra attendances she had made at the eye hospital in Manchester were paying off. A great many patients were eye cases although they might be attending the dispensary for other reasons, such as skin diseases, all of which arose from poor hygiene. Years later, after Margaret had achieved her dream of building a hospital in Pingyin, Bishop Iliff commented, "If this hospital has done nothing else, it has justified its presence by the enormous amount of suffering and pain relieved in these poor sightless eyes, suffering from and through the effects of this dreadful disease—Trachoma."

Often medical work at this level of squalor called for a strong stomach, and Margaret usually wore a mask while working in the dispensary, to protect against contagion but also as a barrier against the stench. The smells of the patients were largely due to being unwashed but occasionally exacerbated by putrefaction, depending on the nature of the injury or its prior treatment by some herbalist or local charlatan. It did not take long to become inured to these noisome conditions, though sometimes Margaret's eyes watered behind her spectacles.

Some native medicines were extremely repulsive. Margaret was reluctant to use tar ointments for skin diseases in case this treatment encouraged the use of a native medicament of similar colour. She was always careful to use clean-looking ointments and, whenever possible, to cleanse with hot water.

Happily though, many patients recovered beyond all expectation. One patient, near death, had arrived with a spinal abscess; in ten days' time he walked from the room without assistance.

Unsurprisingly, the Chinese faith in their own doctors was beginning to pall, but it was to take some time before experience taught the people to trust Western medical practice. With serious illnesses, a foreign doctor was seldom called in until too late and only after the sufferer had given up the various Chinese doctors. In such cases Margaret took the line that she could hardly make matters worse, and there was a faint hope that the "foreign devil" doctor might work a miraculous cure.

The lepers had found out at last about Margaret, and several came to her, some from considerable distances. Here again she could render little help since leprosy was so contagious. It was impossible, on account of the other patients, to receive lepers into the compound. At first the Chinese attendants would not admit them even into the dispensary. She managed to overcome their prejudices eventually by reminding them of the main essence of their calling, which was to serve all patients without discrimination.

The local people were extremely poor, and during the early springtime the tender shoots and leaves of almost every kind of tree or wayside weed formed a staple portion of their diet. Margaret often treated injuries caused by falling from trees, and sometimes gangrene of the face and hands sustained by eating poisonous plants.

A man arrived with a severely lacerated hand, the result of a bite from his brother during a violent quarrel. Thanks to the liberal application for many days of some particularly revolting Chinese medication, his whole arm was in a state of intense inflammation. Ten maggots were extracted from the wounds, and a simple treatment with an arm bath worked marvels. Yet the man complained about the slow rate of recovery and left before the cure was complete. This behaviour was rather frequent and, understandably, imposed a considerable strain on Margaret's patience.

Although recovery was the rule, she was seldom allowed to see the result of her labours. She did not ascribe this to ingratitude but rather to her patients being unaccustomed to continuing for long with any one line of treatment.

In August, with the encouragement of Bishop Iliff, Margaret took a furlough to Japan. Her health had deteriorated, likely due to her burden of work; again she had haemoptysis. She expected to be away for at least a month, but in the end she was not back on the job until mid-October.

In England there had long been concern over Margaret's being on her own in Pingyin since Dorothy's departure. She pleaded with the bishop not to move her elsewhere, stoutly assuring him how strongly she felt about the medical work where she was and stressing the unlikelihood of finding another candidate for her position, in which case her medical work would be closed down. Any hopes for a hospital after that might then have to be abandoned, a fate too sad to contemplate.

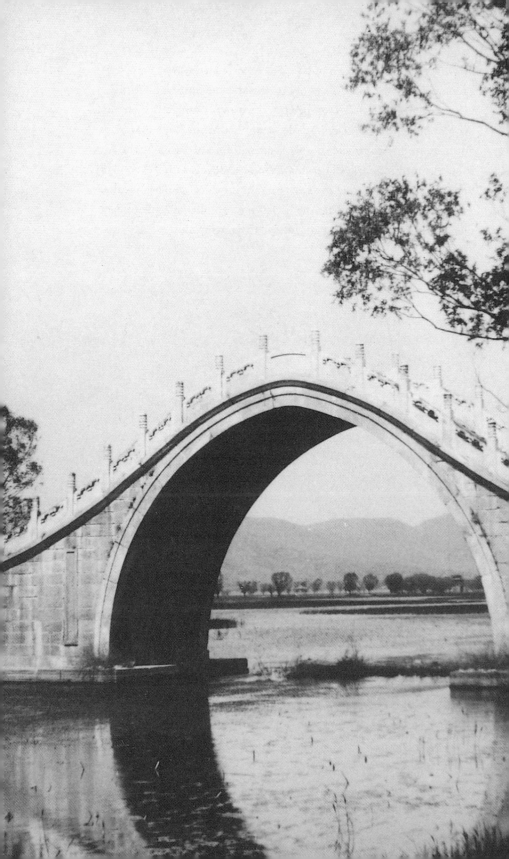

CHAPTER 8

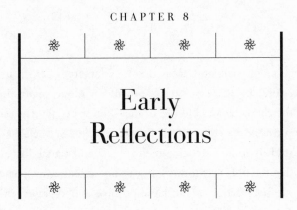

Early
Reflections

✿ PROGRESS TOWARDS THE REALITY of a hospital
was excruciatingly slow, but the mission had purchased a piece of land
for the site—unfortunately, at some distance from the compound housing
the church and other mission buildings. This disadvantage, in Margaret's
opinion, was more than compensated for by its location on rising ground
well above the city, outside its east suburb opposite a Roman Catholic
church. It was a healthy site with a good rock foundation, in contrast to
the mission compound's location in one of the most unhealthy positions of the city. Neighbouring land, which the mission had originally
tried to purchase, was not only expensive but low-lying and inconvenient
for medical work, being cut off by floodwaters on practically all sides
during most of the year.

The new compound was always accessible, and Margaret expected its
healthy location to be an advantage for the workers and sick alike. The
first action would be to build a good strong wall right round the land,
always a necessity in China. Mr. Mathews had calculated that this alone
would cost about one hundred pounds, a sum beyond their existing

budget. Nonetheless, Margaret felt that the acquisition of this land was a positive first step towards achieving her heart's desire.

∫✴

A FEW YEARS had now elapsed since Margaret's arrival in China. Medical work, by its very nature, provided unique opportunities to observe the character and lifestyle of the Chinese people. The essence of this was most intimately revealed at times of sickness, when the Chinese were least likely to be practicing their so-called inscrutability. She soon learned that the only way to work in this unfamiliar atmosphere was to sweep aside first reactions as quickly as possible, and to preserve a "mental mobility." As time passed, she generally found she was more inclined to trust those people who initially had impressed her less than favourably.

Margaret came to China with many of the preconceptions about the Chinese people common to the times. She soon saw the error in the popular notion that the Chinese nature was too complex for Westerners to understand. Overall, the people were intelligent, but their childhood environment offered little scope, the educational system seeming to develop the memory at the expense of intellect. The Chinese were taught to revere the written word, hence becoming credulous and ready to believe anything they saw in print. Margaret believed this explained why the purveyors of native medicine did such a good trade.

Although the Chinese were reputed to be a peace-loving people, heated arguments were frequent in the family, between neighbours or with shop-keepers and other businessmen. Teachers, officials and servants were constantly at variance, their noisy quarrels as good as a play to the onlookers crowded round. Much acting went into a properly conducted altercation, which could become so realistic and emotional that someone in a fit of rage might actually commit suicide to bring disaster to the opponent. Then came the opportunity for the peacemaker, who was usually successful, whereupon custom required the opponents to seal the peace with a banquet.

In daily situations, people tried to respond in speech and demeanor in the way they thought Margaret might expect, while controlling their own feelings, if necessary. This habit partly accounted for their reputation of inscrutability, but it was untrue that they hid their feelings. They could be highly emotional, and those living amongst them always knew whether they were pleased or angry—largely a case of being familiar with their body language. Many digestive ailments were caused by fits of hysteria and emotional outbursts.

Although the Chinese were often stigmatized for dishonesty, Margaret found that most people spoke the truth even when it appeared detrimental to them. What seemed to be lies were usually figures of speech, a form of acting, which they well understood but Westerners took too literally. Time was when a Chinese man's word was his bond. No contract was necessary, and he would fulfill an agreement even at his own loss. Bargaining was a game, and shopkeeping lost much of its zest when fixed prices became established. Curio dealers still expect to bargain, which is conducted in a most friendly fashion.

Gambling games, resembling a form of Stone, Paper, Scissors, were quite usual at a feast, with the object of getting the opposition drunk, since the forfeit each time was another drink for the loser. The Chinese seemed to be born gamblers, and good losers. Scheming was the spice of life to these people, giving them the reputation of being crafty.

Despite their reputation for industry, Margaret found that, although the people were certainly capable of long hours of work, they took frequent rests; paid workers seldom put in much more than the equivalent of half a day. Their meagre diet was partly to blame; legitimate holidays were few, but family obligations and other excuses frequently interrupted work. "Those who do not work do not eat" was their principal work ethic. Margaret was impressed by the people's powers of endurance and ability to bear cold, pain, hunger and general discomfort without making much effort to alleviate their condition. They could sleep anywhere at any time, with only a brick or a piece of wood for a pillow. Apprentices were constantly seen sleeping on their handcarts by the roadside.

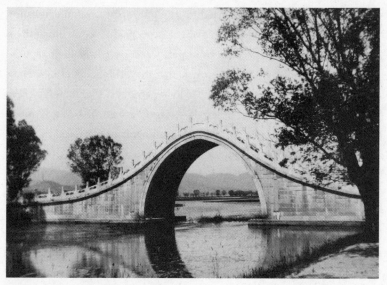

A camelback bridge designed to reflect as a full moon when the water in the pool is placid.

A tendency to live in the present on the traditions of the past seemed, Margaret thought, to result in a lack of foresight. Many people seemed chary of embarking on large enterprises, leaving the future welfare of the family and country to the care of their descendants. Overall she found people to be kind and hospitable, willing to assist anyone in misfortune, although often they expected a return of benefit. In her writings, she characterized the Chinese people as imaginative, keenly observant, naturally artistic and fond of poetry, literature and music. They liked to give presents, and enjoyed entertaining and being entertained. Among her Chinese neighbours, she found faithful friends and grateful patients, who never forgot a benefit conferred.

∫*

MARGARET HAD MUCH TO LEARN about her neighbours' habits, all of which were strange to her. Apart from what was the right or wrong way of doing things, she became increasingly aware that the Chinese way, under the circumstances, was far more important. Her first great missionary concept lay in zeal, but she soon realized that, though needful, this had to be exercised sparingly. Excessive enthusiasm would fail entirely with the tranquil Chinese; sympathy was far more essential. She had often noticed its effect in the dispensary, to the extent that she most longed for the strength to persevere with the essential efforts to give each patient an individual share of sympathy. The high numbers of patients necessitated that her consultations were brief, which in itself was a strange proceeding to the Chinese, who would have preferred to stay and chat for at least half an hour as they would have done when visiting native doctors. Margaret learned that even ten patients in one day would be considered a great many, so naturally Chinese doctors had the time to contribute to each patient.

When she explained that she had other patients to see, her patients were compliant. When she showed them out with a kind word at the doorway, invariably there were many backward smiles. When she became irritable, it was because patients had disobeyed instructions. Margaret did not take kindly to what she considered to be a lack of discipline, and she could behave sternly on such occasions. She knew this was not conducive to the most persuasive bedside manner, and she was at pains to refrain from showing her disapproval. All this more than made up for her inability to speak Chinese fluently.

Once in a letter to a friend Margaret categorically debunked the myth of what superb results Chinese washerwomen produced. Perhaps, she said, this might have been so in Europe or America, where facilities and competition combined to derive the best results at Chinese hands, but the same exigency definitely did not apply locally. The usual method was to take laundry down to a dirty stagnant pool to soak. Margaret doubted if there were any really clean pools in all of Shandong, for she had seen many women washing in greenish black water. After soaking the clothes, they would beat and belabour them with a rolling pin upon a stone by the waterside. She had even seen a small child dip a cup into the foul water and drink it with great relish, with his mother at his side washing clothes in the same water.

Under such rough treatment, the mission's white blankets soon ended up looking old and shabby. Margaret would have liked to wash her own clothes, to get them truly clean as well as to preserve them, for their lives in China were comparatively short. However, doing all things herself was impossible, and she knew it would be a bad policy to even try. This largely accounted for her constant requests for bandages, cloth or flannel, or flannelette and cotton materials of sober colours suitable for women's clothing. She was grateful for old sheets to cover the operating table but hoped also for coloured blankets or even patchwork quilts.

Margaret soon discovered that, while Chinese could not wash clothes to her liking, they did cook well. No self-respecting Chinese person could fail to know the rudiments of basic cooking, such as boiling rice and other staples. This, in effect, gave the Chinese cook a head start in her foreign kitchen. Yu Zhi quickly picked up the ability to cook an English meal—manifestly different from what he cooked ordinarily, yet in a short while he produced dishes and flavours to Margaret's tastes. Not once, however, did she see him sampling his work. Yu simply followed instructions as assiduously as possible and waited for reactions from the dining room—a normal procedure for most Chinese cooks in foreign households. Food was unlikely to be overdone, as Chinese cuisine generally required quick cooking, over great heat, for the most economical use of precious fuel, and conforming with the Daoist culture, which called for lightly cooked food.

♪✳

Margaret's correspondents often asked what China was like when she arrived. China was then an empire, she told them, with the Empress Dowager Tzu Hsi (Zixi) acting as a self-appointed regent for her nephew, Kuang Hsu (Guangxu), who was detained in a palace on a tiny island in the centre of Peking. The despotic regent had declared him mentally unstable, thus unfit to rule this mighty nation of eighteen provinces and the enormous tributary states of Tibet, Turkestan and Mongolia.

Actually, the emperor's ideas on reform were too progressive for the times, and the dowager lady feared that they might cause the downfall of the Manchu dynasty—which did, in fact, occur barely six years after Margaret's arrival.

This situation was one of the main topics of conversation at that time. The empress dowager had to acknowledge that China was overdue for a measure of reform, which she promised would occur gradually over the next decade. She decreed immediate changes to the educational system, the consequence of the Western education being taught in the mission schools and the intercourse with Westerners due to the spread of international trade following the treaties made with the Allies after the Boxer Uprising. That incident was another common topic, and none too cheering for the newcomer. However, mission schools were reviving, and new buildings were replacing the damaged ones.

∫*

THE CHINESE did many things opposite to what Margaret was used to. For some time after her arrival, she would fumble at a door, expecting it to open the "usual" way only to find she had turned the knob the "wrong" way; at first she was certain the lock had been installed upside down. Chinese men wore long gowns, like skirts, down to the ankles, while women's costumes, at least at home, consisted of short jackets and trousers, but outdoors they wore long gowns following the Manchu style. While a foreign gentleman removed his hat upon entering a house, a Chinese continued to wear his indoors. Women did not usually wear hats, although old people wore warm ones in the winter. When putting on a jacket or overcoat, instead of thrusting the arm down into a sleeve, the Chinese usually thrust the arm upwards into the garment, which was then lowered down onto the body with a kind of flourish.

During her language lessons, she was amused to learn that a number of figures of speech combined opposite meanings. For example, the Chinese equivalent of "size" was da-xiao (big/ little), while the term for "height" was gao-ai (high/low). In those days it was customary for Chinese calligraphy to start at the right side of the page, written downwards instead of across the page. The paintbrush was held in an upright position with the hand not touching the paper, so as not to smudge the writing. A book began at what she considered the back, but she soon became used to opening a book from the other end. Nowadays books are produced in the universal manner, but when encountering a banner strung across the street or against a wall, it remains necessary to check both the right and left ends to make sense of the message.

Whereas in England cars festooned with white bows and ribbons outside a church indicated a wedding, in China the same would indicate a funeral, for white is the color for death and mourning. Red signifies happiness and good luck, and weddings were termed "red affairs." In China the bride always wore red, with a red veil over her head, and she walked upon a red carpet to reach her red carriage or sedan chair. When she alighted, red carpeting led to the place of the wedding ceremony. Margaret wondered if it was for good luck that in England red carpeting was used to welcome the participants of balls or banquets.

Chinese hand gestures also differed considerably. Beckoning was done with an outstretched right-hand palm down, energetically waving the fingers or whole hand downwards towards oneself to invite someone to approach. Never would a crooked finger be used for the purpose, nor on any account would snapping the fingers be tolerated. One clap of the hands, at most, would suffice to attract attention. Applauding by clapping was usually achieved by holding the left hand still with the palm upwards and moving the right hand up and down to create the sound. When offering something—anything from a cup of tea to a gift or visiting card—to another person, the Chinese would present it with both hands; to do otherwise was considered slovenly and ill-mannered. The recipient would reciprocate in like manner.

Rarely did the Chinese refer to left or right when giving directions, using instead the cardinal points of the compass. A driver, for example, would be directed to turn west or to take the third road to the east. Similarly, one would refer to the north wall rather than the back wall of a room, likewise to the south side instead of the front of the room (always supposing the house faced south, as was usually the case). The Chinese refer to compass points in a different sequence, beginning with the east where the sun rises, then south, west, north. The seat of honour for a guest was on the east side. Politeness required that one should at first decline the honour proffered, but after a little gentle pressure it would be appropriate to accept the courtesy. Tea was always served directly when a guest walked into a Chinese house, but only after the host raised his cup as an invitation to drink was it polite to imbibe at will.

Margaret found that the weather was not necessarily a suitable opening gambit for conversation, which sometimes left her at a loss for a topic, knowing that it was considered brusque to go straight to the point. Politeness demanded that business wait until she and whoever she was with had dealt with the normal opening courtesies. Though the Chinese language lends itself admirably to the art of punning, it was all too easy for a foreigner to mispronounce or inflect a word to give it an altogether different meaning, often humorous and sometimes vulgar. The weather could lend itself to the occasional rude meaning, which Margaret took care to avoid.

While Western manners caused foreigners to be shy about asking personal questions, there was no need to be shy about answering such questions in China. No embarrassment was intended by asking one's age; the foreigner's objection to providing this information was considered odd, for in China, the older the person the greater the esteem. It was perfectly acceptable to ask the host his age, his birthplace (often his ancestral home), the number of children in the family, their ages and educational standing, as well as the health of his parents and his wife, who was referred to as the "mother of his children." Invariably it was taken for granted that Margaret was married, since nearly every man and woman in China had wed.

Margaret also learned to avoid the usual foreign practice of leaving after completing the business in hand. This the Chinese regarded as rude and abrupt, so she would appear reluctant to make her departure. There was little danger of outstaying her welcome, for eventually the host would order some fresh tea to be made, which was the signal to depart.

The reason why her Chinese callers seemed to linger, she found, was that they were waiting for a cue to permit them to leave. Paradoxically, when a banquet at a restaurant was over, it was quite in order to leave at will, "to eat and run," as it were. This may be why speeches were often dealt with before the feast was served, in contrast to the usual foreign practice.

A gracious host would accompany his guest not only from the room but also across the courtyard and even to the gate, where he would bow and see the visitor into a vehicle. If this was a first-time call, the host would return the call within a few days or even the next day. Margaret made it a point not to delay her return visit to a first call. Contrary to the old English custom of calling on the host to express pleasure for a delightful evening, it was customary for a Chinese host to call on all guests a day or two later to thank them for their presence at his party, and to express the hope that they had not been wearied by their journey.

Chinese women were clever at needlework and embroidery, but to Margaret, they seemed to do their sewing upside down and backwards. They wore their thimbles like a ring round the first joint of the middle finger instead of a metal cap on the tip of a finger. It was considered impolite to wear spectacles in the presence of a superior, but in Margaret's view this was too bad since she was blind as a bat without her bifocals. This rule was slowly relaxed, but dark glasses were expected to be removed on entering the house.

Margaret noted for future reference that when erecting a building, the roof is usually finished first, which has the virtue of protecting the interior against the weather at an early stage of development. Soon after she first arrived in Peking, Margaret witnessed the Fore Gate (*Qian Men*) being rebuilt after the ravages of the Boxer Uprising. It seemed strange to see the roof standing without any walls, but later she found out that the roof of a building rests upon its pillars and the walls are filled in afterwards. The Chinese have always been clever at the art of scaffolding. The tower was a mass of intricately interlaced poles with daylight showing through, and the solid tiled roof on top.

♪

IN TIME Margaret came to understand certain Chinese facial expressions and body language. The latter was the hardest to recognize, but she soon realized the significance of various looks. One most familiar, and the first to be encountered, was the bland expression which conveyed virtually nothing—precisely what was intended. The Chinese were inclined to adopt this countenance when being at their most difficult, and when they had no intention of revealing feelings, but Margaret learned how to get round that one. This could lead to considerable discomfiture for the person whose bland shield had been penetrated, which then called for a good deal of tact on her part.

The Chinese were considered to be cheerful people, which, generally speaking, was perfectly true. There is, however, a marked difference between a talkative, pleasant throng and a group of people with fixed grins upon their faces. Margaret realized this expression served mainly to cover up embarrassment but also indicated no intention of revealing true feelings or answering an embarrassing question, especially if the answer was to cause a loss of face. If a Chinese could not give an appropriate answer to a question, rather than incur an adverse reaction, it was considered best to say nothing at all. She soon appreciated the significance of the fixed grin and either changed the subject or tried a more subtle approach, knowing that to show her impatience or disapproval would only add to the embarrassment of the situation. On the other hand, the Chinese had an almost implacable attitude towards foreigners, and until it was patently clear that foreigners could be trusted, they frequently and deliberately avoided any collaboration. Margaret, as a physician, was in a good position to break down such barriers, but this was not to be accomplished in a trice. She set about getting to know the Chinese people as quickly as possible, making a persistent effort to quickly assimilate enough of the language to enable her to communicate.

Over the years Margaret's doctrines became an amalgam of two powerful cultures. One aspect that never varied or faltered was her determination to do whatever it was that she felt God wanted her to do.

Frail though she might have appeared to be physically, and poor though her health was from time to time, nothing could divert her from her convictions regarding her faith and the power of her mind. Rarely did she waver from what she saw as her duty, despite the hardships and misunderstandings that beset her day. She grew to love the people around her. Despite their differences, China was where she felt she belonged.

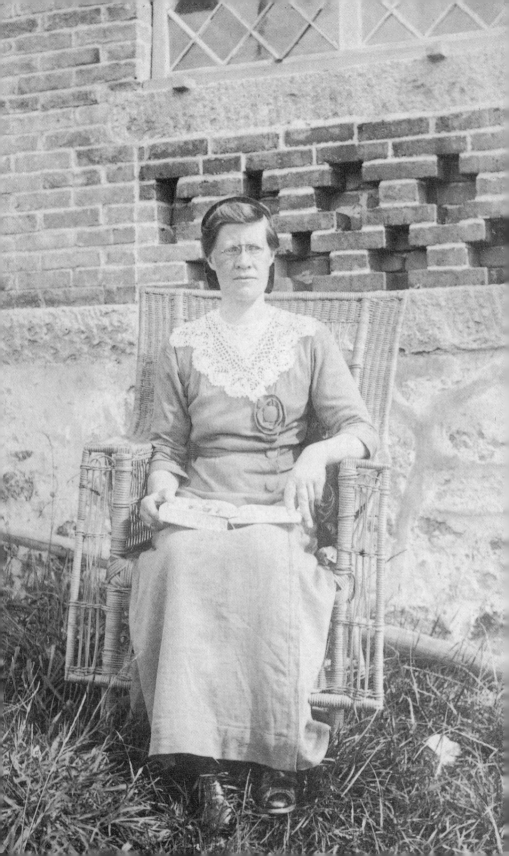

CHAPTER 9

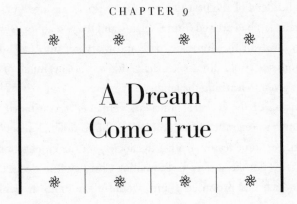

A Dream
Come True

🌸 FINALLY, the dream Margaret had harboured for so long began to take shape. She had been agonizing over the budget for this great project, which could run the mission into debt. Thanks to an unexpected windfall from a pan-Anglican fund-raiser and other sources, sufficient funds had accumulated for Bishop Illif to grant his permission to begin building St. Agatha's Hospital. In a letter dated February 3, 1908, an ecstatic Margaret wrote:

> Today I have news…of the splendid results of your energetic efforts…
> I am so greedy for my hospital that almost my happiest moments
> are those which bring me news of the thoughts and prayers, and
> keen practical interest of the helpers at home. I have never had the
> slightest tendency to insomnia, but…I cannot sleep for joy. I think
> the happiness lies both in the thought of the helping force and
> sympathy behind one, and the work to be done in the future…I
> shall not feel that we have begun our medical work until the hos-
> pital is opened. These are but the preliminary stages.

Margaret's spirits had now improved considerably. The break from her work during the holiday in Japan had done her the world of good, and her burdens of the past two years were finally easing: an assistant, Miss Sarah Gay, had arrived from England, and the two got on well. Sarah assumed much of the domestic load, and Margaret now had someone with whom she could discuss her daily affairs. Initially, much of Sarah's time was given to learning the language.

Financing of the construction work remained a constant concern. While funds were gradually accumulating, the complete budget had yet to be met. For some reason, neither the Society for the Propagation of the Gospel (SPG) nor the Society for Promoting Christian Knowledge (SPCK), both of which had promised grants, would make funds available until the building was completed. Margaret was at a loss as to how she could avoid running into debt with the Chinese—to her, quite the wrong principle to exemplify. Moreover, if she were to try to borrow, she doubted if anyone could lend the amount required. If it came to the worst, she might be obliged to run into debt at the local bank since prices had started to soar, being double already to what they were two years ago when she arrived. If she were to wait too long, the cost could treble, and the wish for a hospital might become hopeless.

Nevertheless, she remained optimistic, and in preparation for construction, she recruited the services of her old tutor and cook, Yu Chih (Yu Zhi), for his expertise in the delicate intricacies of the art of bargaining. Undoubtedly, with the advent of the impending work, he had already been discussing the matter at some length in the neighbourhood. Instructed to find a suitable contractor for the job, Yu quickly produced one to furnish the lime.

The use of cementitious materials goes as far back as the building of China's Great Wall, and even in Margaret's time, lime rather than cement was used for making mortar. Rope was shredded to provide hemp for improving the mortar's tensile strength, as necessary when laying heavy blocks of stone. Yu apparently had a figure in mind, but certain formalities had to be followed before reaching an agreement. A solemn conclave took place in Margaret's small dining room. She was utterly at sea as to the price of lime or the quantity required, but Yu glossed over her ignorance as far as possible. Bargaining began over several small cups of wine, eventually reaching a price which she suspected had been fixed beforehand. The two men then sealed the deal with more wine and drew up a written contract for the required amount. The same day a builder arrived, offering to build the wall that would surround the compound. His price was easily brought down to a remarkably low figure, and a contract signed. The next morning Yu ushered in two other contractors who wished to be partners in the construction of the dispensary and other buildings.

By now, Margaret was rapidly adding new words to her Chinese vocabulary. At the same time she realized how small that vocabulary was, to say nothing of her ignorance of the affairs of construction. She had initially been given to understand that the Chinese must not be hurried over such matters, yet three days after her return to Pingyin two contracts had been drawn up and signed, ratified by the usual ritual of wine drinking.

Unfortunately, Yu then suffered a paralytic stroke. Sarah, who turned out to be an excellent cook, assumed his culinary duties, but as yet no replacement had been found as building manager. Having lost the full use of his right arm and much of his speaking ability, Yu seemed to have made up his mind to die rather than live on as a helpless burden. He refused food and medication for a while; Margaret had to administer the dosage herself or send in the dispensary attendant three times a day, otherwise he would not take it. Eventually his spirits improved and he agreed to allow his wife to work for Margaret, doing light housework and sewing. She was a Christian, although he was not, so Margaret intended to teach her how to read. This would enable her to be a Bible-woman in due course in the new hospital.

For two reasons, work did not start until October 28. First, the workmen had to be assembled from the surrounding villages, and secondly for the more important consideration of *feng shui* (meaning "wind and water"), the practice of geomancy. According to Chinese custom, it was essential to select a propitious day for undertaking building operations so as not to offend the aura of the neighbourhood. This meant construction was delayed until early spring. Margaret utilized the respite to study the basics of building and architecture; her early training in art proved useful in drawing up simple layout plans. She learned how windows, doors and doorways should be constructed, and discovered the intricacies of staircases, something rarely seen in Chinese buildings, most being a single storey.

On Good Friday—a date not yet observed as a holiday in China—the first barrow-loads of stone arrived, deposited in heaps in readiness for the stonemasons, who set to work the next day, chiselling the attractive grey stones into rectangular blocks with a level outer face. To speed the process, two builders would work simultaneously on different parts of the site, one masonry group contracted for the construction of the buildings, gatehouse, men's wards and intervening wall, and the other for building the "great" and—in China—indispensable wall around the whole compound, no less than 2.7 metres (9 feet) high and 325 metres (1,060 feet) long.[1] The builders subcontracted other workers to provide and transport the stone by cart from the nearby quarry, and to dress and lay the blocks received from the stonemasons.

It was an experiment in building procedure to have two separate crews of labourers at work together on one site. As it turned out, the two crews were a spur to each other, and the work progressed speedily and harmoniously. Margaret's eagerness for the hospital seemed infectious. An undertaking of this importance was also not without a degree of prestige for the community.

The provision of other materials—lime, sand, rope and scaffolding—necessitated continuous bargaining. The workmen were paid per cubic foot of completed wall, and the sum of one hundred Chinese dollars was advanced to each contractor. The building, once started, was immediately ahead of the money paid. It was Margaret's object to keep it so—theirs being, of course, to keep the payment as near as possible to the work accomplished. For the roofing, plastering, painting and carpentry, labour was hired and paid for at a daily rate, necessitating strict quality control to ensure an appropriate standard. The men were allowed to keep their own registers of work, but these required close scrutiny. One man claimed 368 days' attendance in one year, including absences for Sundays and during bad weather and winter frosts when all work came to a standstill!

Margaret visited the work site twice daily to ensure the work was done properly, as the contractors were unaccustomed to the foreign style of construction and needed ongoing instruction. Most of the area housing was of adobe, whereas the principal building material for the hospital was stone. For the woodwork, Margaret had to arrange piecemeal agreements with the carpenter and provide him with the timber. An American variety available in Qingdao was brought up the Huang He from Jinan in small junks, hauled by a long line of men tracking along the riverbank. It entailed about two weeks to bring the load upstream, although the return downstream journey took only a day. Margaret anticipated that, all going well, the wall and the dispensary building could be completed in April.

The next phase of development involved erecting the hospital building and dwelling simultaneously. Funds did not allow for a large hospital but rather what Margaret called a "cottage hospital," with room for about twenty-five patients or "thirty at a pinch." The site's size allowed for future development with additional buildings and extensions, and Margaret was optimistic of forthcoming funds, heartened to know that money was arriving from her parish and personal contacts, above any SPG grant. She was aware that claims from India, Africa and Canada were so strong that agency grants to China might well be less than the immensity of her needs, the size of the land and the remaining amount of work. The only reason she was developing such a small hospital, she emphasized, was that there was no prospect of adequate funds for one larger—certainly not because a small one might suffice for the needs of the two and a half million people in her district.

The ongoing suspense and inequality over funding distribution was somewhat exasperating. During her recent trip to the coast to meet Sarah, Margaret had encountered an English Baptist missionary who asked about the probable cost of her new hospital. She told him she anticipated erecting the hospital, dispensary and a residence for about six hundred pounds, building costs then being cheap. She worried that, at the present rate of progress, her costs could increase to as much as one thousand pounds, as a widespread prolonged rate of inflation was developing during the declining years of the Qing dynasty, due to the uncertain political situation. He responded that his mission doctor was about to build a hospital costing four thousand pounds, implying that funds were already to hand. Without wanting to appear covetous, Margaret wished that the people connected with her English mission were giving in the same wholehearted fashion as other missions seemed to enjoy.

Perhaps, Margaret thought, other missions were connected to more enthusiastic supporters at home. In whatever time she had to spare, she strove to maintain contact with her friends and her colleagues in Manchester; doubtless this did much to encourage the supply of funds. Another source of support materialized in the Birch Missionary Association. Under her heavy financial cloud, Margaret always emphasized that the hospital was designed as far as possible towards economy and utility rather than convenience or appearance.

It had troubled Margaret greatly that there would be no private wards. It was difficult to reach the women of the Chinese upper classes, and she felt certain they would not leave the privacy of their homes to go into a public ward. With the latest donation, she planned to set up a special fund for constructing a block of a few small private wards, one to be named in memory of Miss Anne Vaudrey, a keen fund-raiser and truly a Lady Bountiful to the mission field in general. Margaret felt honoured that her hospital project had enjoyed Miss Vaudrey's patronage.

The hospital compound was divided into three sections. The single-storey hospital, in the middle section and occupying the greater area, had no communication with the outside world except through the other two sections—the doctors' quarters and the outpatients' building—thus ensuring the privacy and seclusion essential for a women's hospital in China. The house intended for the doctors' quarters had plans for an upper storey, unusual in those parts. The other buildings conformed more closely to the conventional style of Chinese architecture, with certain modern modifications. In the traditional style, the roof of any substantial building is supported by heavy horizontal beams on thick pillars. Those roofs were extremely heavy, having tiled ornamentation along the ridge. Without wishing to detract too much from native art, in the interests of economy such embellishments were kept to a minimum and the roofs modified to be lighter. The outer walls between the pillars, designed primarily to contain the doors and windows, would be load-bearing and sixty centimetres (2 feet) thick to provide good insulation.

In due time foreign-style doors and windows were fitted. Each room would have a ceiling rather than a bare roof overhead, further improving insulation and considerably reducing heating costs in winter. All floors were tiled. Maximum cleanliness would be far more easily maintained under these improvements.

As she kept a close eye on the progress of the construction, Margaret discovered that the unexpected task of building was fascinating. Her imagination feasted on what she expected to achieve within those new walls. It seemed almost too good to be true that, after three weary years of waiting, the hospital was becoming a fact. However, she pointed out that no one ought ever to imagine that construction work in China was performed as simply as in England.

For a start, every kind of material had to be bargained for, since that was the Chinese method of purchase. Only small quantities could be bought at a time, partly because the source of supply was soon exhausted and partly because the building funds were usually in a similar condition. Materials almost invariably cost more than expected. Wondering whether she was an unwitting dupe for the wily Chinese merchants who con-trolled the supplies caused Margaret much anxiety, but she admitted to receiving such wonderful answers to prayer—and not only to her prayers—just at the times of dire need, that she resolved to try to put that kind of anxiety aside forever.

The builders were uneducated; not one could read or write. Plans were quite unintelligible to them at first, and elevations even more so. Margaret measured the foundations herself, with frequent corrections until the walls were well underway; being inexperienced herself, she made a point of keeping well abreast of the situation through assiduous studies. She took pleasure in how the verandahs were paved with large slabs of stone—fine examples of the degree of smoothness achieved by the manual skill of the stonemasons—and in the attractive dog-toothed edging of stone under the eaves. The verandah is an essential feature in Chinese house design, as it is constructed deep enough to ban the hot rays of the sun during summer and lofty enough to admit the lower sun's rays into the rooms during winter.

The hospital's main entrance was up a flight of steps to the gateway in the encircling wall, at the south-west corner leading into the outpatients' compound. In this section were the dispensary buildings with a waiting room to the left and the gatekeeper's lodge to the right, as well as the manager's cottage and two wards for the boys and men patients. A deep well under a shed would supply the whole compound unfailingly with excellent water for all purposes. It was cut through almost solid rock by two men working daily for nearly twelve months. The shed was large enough to be used for open air treatment and to store the wheelbarrows and sedan chair. Hanging from a roofed stand near the manager's cottage was a bell, specially commissioned by Bishop Iliff and cast in Tai'an. When struck with a heavy wooden club, it would announce the short prayer services to be held daily, morning and evening, in the hospital chapel and attended by everyone in the compound, including servants, visitors and all patients not bedridden.

Two gates in this compound led into the hospital compound proper, which was for women and children only. No men were allowed to enter except for chapel services, and the gates were usually kept locked. Men-servants had to enter at fixed times and generally under supervision. Most of the work in the hospital would be done by women. In the main building were the wards, three large and public, two smaller and private, named after Anne Vaudrey, Fanny Fernside, Helen Stephen, Bethany Leslie and John Leslie, all hardworking fund-raisers. Also within this building were the operating theatre and anterooms, the dining rooms, the chapel (St. Agatha's) and the nurses' room. Behind the hospital were the bathrooms, kitchens and laundries.

In the third section of the compound was the doctors' quarters with kitchens and outhouses, and a flourishing garden. Trees were planted in all three compounds, initially providing little shade, though already forming an attractive setting for the new buildings.

The work was not without a few near mishaps. More than once Margaret proved, to the workers' dismay, that defects existed. Many times the workmen altered the lines to suit their own purposes or the particular blocks of stone they were trying to fit. On several occasions, she pushed over with her bare hands what she rightly suspected was a poorly laid wall, which on no account could be expected to bear a heavy load. Her eyes widened in disbelief when she found a wooden beam set across a chimney. On this occasion her Chinese oratory rose to new heights to make quite certain that such irregularities did not occur again.

The contractors became very much aware that here was a person who knew what she wanted. After the buildings were finished and the walls were being measured for payment, the men completely lost their way indoors, for paint and plaster had quite altered the appearance of the walls they themselves had erected. Margaret got on well with the head carpenter, a white-haired man of more than seventy years, who wore spectacles almost the size of small saucers. She was fascinated with the beautiful designs he had drawn and carved on some of the larger door panels.

Rapid progress was made during the two months before frosts intervened. As soon as weather conditions permitted, the work continued, with the hospital completed for all practical purposes to allow an official opening, most appropriately, on February 5, St. Agatha's Day. The new dispensary was put to use that very day. Remaining details were soon completed, and the formal dedication ceremony was held on May 1, 1909. According to the official report of the occasion:

[I]n 1905 Bishop Illif made an urgent appeal for six doctors to come and carry on the medical work in the diocese…Dr. Margaret Phillips alone came in answer to that call in 1906.

…[In] the mission field…we must be prepared to put our hand to anything, but many of us fail to realize what that may mean…

One of the first things Dr. Phillips had to do was to build a hospital. The site chosen for it was on a hill opposite the Roman

Catholic Church. It commands a delightful view of hills in the background, and gives one a sense of space in front.

... [I]magine you are deaf and dumb (a true state of affairs when you are ignorant of the language)...trained to look after people's bodies, but have little or no technical knowledge of other professions, and you are suddenly confronted with a problem such as building or architecture (and Dr. Phillips was confronted with both)...[A]ll your orders must be conveyed by mysterious signs which constantly will be misinterpreted. If you can imagine all this...you will understand a little of what St. Agatha's Hospital owes to her pioneer doctor...[who at the same time] was carrying on dispensary work in the old Church (instead of the damp mud building which had been used since 1896).

...

The whole of the medical work, with nursing in addition, now rested entirely on Dr. Phillips, for in the coming year our only assistant nurse was obliged through ill health to return to Peking. We also added to her responsibilities by opening two outstations for the sake of the women in the more distant villages, who were unable to travel far over the bad roads.[2]

St. Agatha's was the first SPG hospital built in the diocese of Shandong, and naturally its opening was a big event in the history of the mission. Workers from all parts of the diocese attended the impressive services held that day in Pingyin, including Bishop Illif (who took the dedication service), Rev. and Mrs. Mawson, the Reverend I. Stoker, Dorothy Bearder, Sarah Gay, Dr. F. M. Cunningham and, of course, Dr. E. M. Phillips. It was a great day, with hopefulness as the predominant note.

The opening ceremony began at seven-thirty in the morning with an English celebration and a short address by Bishop Illif in the private oratory. The bishop drew his text from John 14, verse 12: "He that believeth on me, the works that I do shall he do also; and greater works than these shall he do; because I go unto my Father." He explained what to many people must have seemed an incredible saying: that they could indeed do greater works than Christ himself, and that no difficulties need be too great to overcome, even in this most difficult of lands, if they believed in him.[3]

The Chinese ceremonies followed with a short service in the dispensary waiting room including an address by the bishop. Nearly one hundred Chinese Christians attended. Only Christians had been invited to attend; this prevented people from coming out of curiosity, which otherwise they would surely have done in large numbers. The congregation formed a procession and filed out to the hospital, reciting psalms along the way, and pausing in each of the three principal wards and the operating theatre for prayers or hymns. They then headed into the doctors' house in the third courtyard, where prayers, still in Chinese, were read on the verandah, and in the dining room, the hall and upper landing. Bishop Illif prayed for blessings on all who might sleep and rest there.

The service concluded with a dedication prayer back in the oratory, the singing of the hymn "Oh God, Our Help in Ages Past" and the blessing. After the company had dispersed, the inevitable feasting took place— but exclusively for the Chinese women guests, for whom the occasion of opening the first women's hospital in the district was of particular significance.

♪❋

ACCORDING TO CHINESE PROCEDURE, the completion of such a project as constructing a hospital deserved nothing less than a banquet, and on that occasion Margaret earned her Chinese surname. The highlight of the evening was when the head contractor presented his erstwhile employer with the bill—not only for the final payment for the work discharged but also for the cost of the feast. This was perfectly in order, since it acknowledged the prestige of the hostess, thus giving her much face, as well as serving as a gratuity for all concerned.

After formally acknowledging receipt of the document, Margaret made a special request. In front of the assembled company—which included a number of patients, especially the Chinese Christians, as well as the

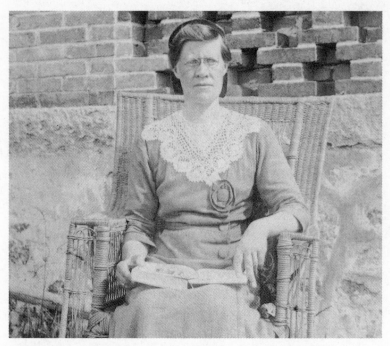

The Lady Named Thunder, c. 1909.

labour force—she told the contractor that she would deem it a favour if he would be so kind as to confer on her a proper Chinese surname. It has always been the custom for Chinese to put the family name first, and it usually consists of only one syllable. So far Margaret's surname had been pronounced with the phonetic rendering of "Fayleepusser." She knew that there was a Chinese character pronounced "Fei," which was a surname. But since several families of that name lived in a village not far down the road, she rather doubted the suitability of the name Fei for her, as it could be considered presumptuous for a blonde female foreigner to assume their name, implying a family relationship.

The contractor responded magnificently. Considering the number of tongue lashings he had received from his employer over the past year, his reply was the essence of tact. He assured Margaret that he understood her sentiments perfectly, for they had collaborated closely for a long time. Since the name Fei seemed inappropriate, he suggested a not dissimilar sounding surname: Lei. For a brief moment there was a hush in the room, followed by a burst of laughter, led by Margaret herself. She took the point directly, as did everyone else: *Lei* meant "thunder." No doubt the thought going through Margaret's mind just then was *"Touché."*

Not long afterwards, Bishop Iliff heard of this, and he told Margaret that he felt she deserved more than simply a Chinese surname. She being fair, he was inspired to attach Baiju, thus making an authentic-sounding Chinese name: Lei Baiju. The characters for *Baiju* mean "white chrysanthemum," which seemed a pleasing compliment to pay her. It can only be supposed that neither realized, at least not at the time, that it was customary for ladies of the night to be known by such flowery names— not that it would have made any difference to Margaret.

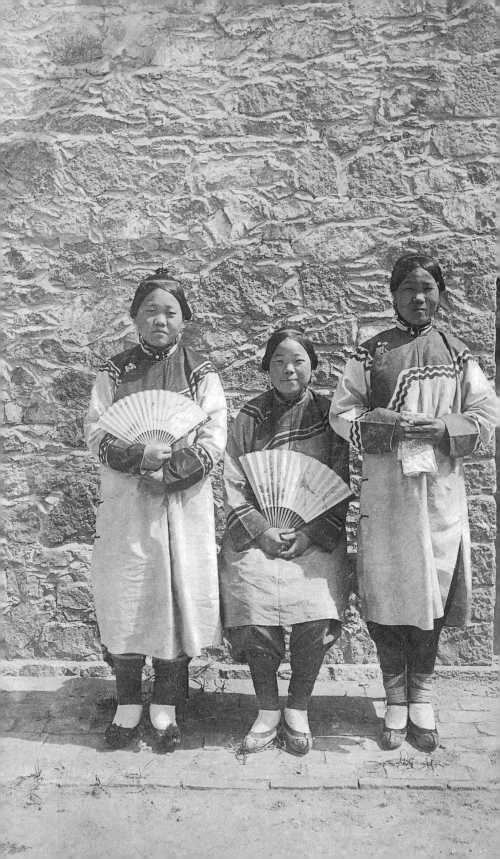

CHAPTER 10

St. Agatha's Hospital

♪* THE NEXT TWO MONTHS were spent tying up loose ends as quickly as possible, for patients could not be admitted while workmen were still about. A separate block, housing the kitchen and bathroom area, had been left until the main building was complete. By then funds were used up, and the bishop ordered a stop to further building. Since some kind of a kitchen was essential, all leftover materials were used to build a temporary room until funds became available again. That would have to do for now, though Margaret considered the kitchen inadequate and the bathroom area "shameful." The contents of the old dispensary were removed by hand, the drugs carried openly in baskets slung from a long flexible pole supported on the shoulders of two men, who supported the lot so steadily that not a single bottle was lost.

Except for a few minor deficiencies, the buildings proved comfortable and convenient, a result of Margaret's plans and preparation. She was much relieved to welcome Dr. Frances M. Cunningham to assist in running the hospital, and Liu Shengming, a Chinese Christian from the mission who had experience from running the dispensary, to manage the hos-

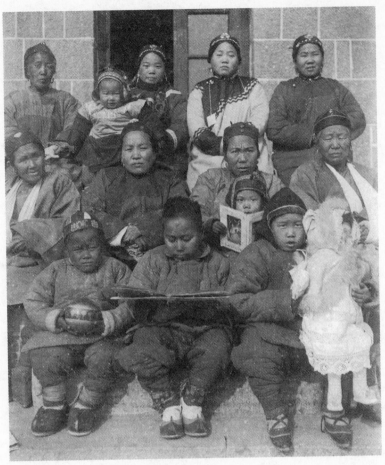

A group of patients at St. Agatha's Hospital, Pingyin.

pital compound. As they had no fully trained foreign nurse, Sarah returned
to England for training.

By the autumn harvest, St. Agatha's Hospital was in full swing. The first
patients were admitted on November 15—not the most favourable time
to open, since patients were always fewer in winter, but illness had prevented an earlier start. The first inpatients were Mr. Liu's wife and their
young daughter, Faith, Margaret's godchild.

Faith had been ailing for several months, so Margaret was getting
anxious about her, as well as Mrs. Liu, who had been a constant attendant

at the dispensary. Two months' stay in hospital did for them what years of outpatient treatment had failed to accomplish, and afterwards both remained in good health. Mr. Liu was so delighted that when he received his January salary, he donated it all to hospital funds. Margaret graciously accepted his donation, even though it was obvious that he could ill afford it, especially on the eve of the Chinese New Year.

The hospital's chief expenses were the maintenance of the doctors and nurse, and the wages of servants and hospital attendants. Winter brought the added cost of fuel, usually coal. Drugs and instruments were expensive, as they were purchased from England, entailing added shipping costs. Hospital fees were a problem at first, due to the poverty of the district. Margaret did not want to deter people from coming, since it was for her convenience and to their advantage if they were admitted. Since feeding patients was inexpensive, thanks to the low cost of living, she decided to provide food at no cost, to ensure an appropriate diet. The common Chinese diet consisted principally of rice or flour and other kinds of grain and vegetables. People rarely ate meat, which they could seldom afford. The hospital food was rather better than what people were accustomed to, and probably more necessary for them than the medicines.

There was no fear of patients coming solely for free food, for they were admitted only if it was thought they would benefit from treatment. Each patient paid a fee on admission, the equivalent of about one shilling, and on leaving a subscription towards hospital upkeep was requested according to their means. Should patients wish to leave before treatment was complete, they had to repay in full the cost of their food during their stay. That plan seemed to be the answer.

∫*

THE EXTENT OF THE UNCLEANLINESS in rural China was appalling, and one reason for hospitalization was to provide the hygienic conditions needed for satisfactory medical treatment. Though Margaret's constant endeavour, now and for years to come, was to retain the style of living familiar to her Chinese patients—which was why, for example, she had chosen to have wooden beds hand-built in the Chinese style rather than standard hospital beds—some radical changes were needed. Hers was a radically different standard of hygiene and not easy for patients to emulate once they returned home, even if they tried to.

She primarily wanted to break away from the custom, prevalent in most hospitals, of allowing patients to bring in their own bedding. The country folk did not undress at night but would wrap themselves up in a *beiwo*—a coverlet thickly padded with cotton wool or flock stitched inside. It was never washed. They did not sleep between sheets and blankets, so she concluded that the only alternative was to supply each patient with sets of night and day garments, which would be washable and reusable, and with warm yet washable quilts, all of which would remain the property of the hospital. In this way the patients would be happy to continue with the type of bedclothes they were accustomed to, and the hospital could maintain a good standard of cleanliness. The day and night clothing could easily be bought locally, but the quilts would need to be specially made. Margaret's design for a washable quilt was similar to a modern duvet. In place of cotton wool she used woollen blankets as the filler, with a detachable cotton cover which could be removed for frequent laundering.

She had some pretty lengths of cloth made into housecoats, which could be loaned to patients, since they had no change of clothing. Another item on her wish list was some overalls or aprons of a particular type, measuring 130 centimetres (50 inches) from neck to bottom hem, to be used for daily work in the dispensary. Dark blue was preferred; white, being the colour of mourning, would shock the Chinese.

Wound healing was difficult if the patients continued to live in filthy clothes. A change of clean laundry was essential. Unfortunately, the missionary societies in England did not readily appreciate this, nor could they see any justification for that expense. It was hard enough to raise money for the purchase of the necessary drugs and instruments; stretching funds to buy clothing and bedding seemed unthinkable. Margaret was constantly at pains to explain how this was a matter where help was particularly needed. She wrote a letter to her alma mater, pleading with the

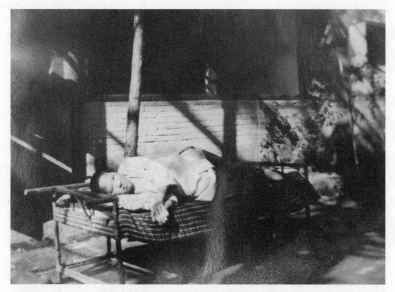

Margaret implemented a number of her own health measures in an attempt to assist in the care of sanatorium patients. Patients were given clean bedding and were moved outside during the day to the courtyard.

Ashburnian Society for anything that could be done towards meeting this requirement on a regular annual basis.

What a great comfort it was knowing that people at home in England were supplying the mission not only with practical support but also with their prayers. When Margaret received financial contributions as well, she thought humbly that it was these people rather than she who really did the missionary work. Certainly they were the ones who made it possible for her to perform her duties.

♪✳

ON DECEMBER 27, 1909, the first infant was born in the hospital. He was christened John, and when last seen six months later was a chubby and sturdy baby. Many of the patients were children, and it was a great pleasure to see them getting fat while in hospital. As a rule they responded readily to treatment, being much easier to handle than their elders.

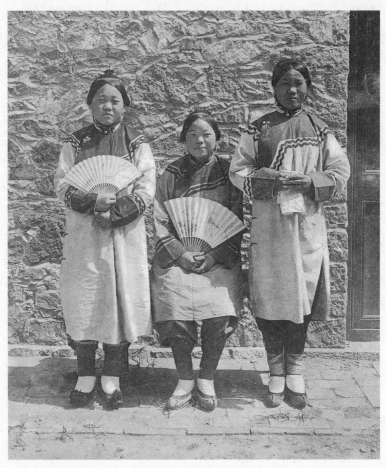

Early nurse probationers outside of St. Agatha's Hospital, c. 1910.

Women patients, on the other hand, provided little encouragement. Usually chronic cases of several years' duration, after a month or two of treatment, just as the doctors hoped that they were at last gaining some ground, they would beg to go home. They credited the hospital with the power to do most wonderful and impossible things, yet were unable to trust themselves completely to the doctors. Margaret hoped, nevertheless, to slowly gain their confidence. She was aware that the district people were in awe of foreign methods, so she should tread warily.

From just one nurse probationer at the start, by the end of the year the hospital had four. Eunice, the eldest and most useful, had no wish to get married, so the doctors hoped she would long remain on the staff. Minnie, the second one hired, was one of the Pingyin schoolgirls and the bishop's protégée; it was probable that she would leave one day to get wed. The third was a new arrival, lately a schoolgirl in Tai'an, while the fourth and youngest had never been to school and was there only temporarily, as the girls' school was full and she could not be admitted. While waiting for a place, she took daily lessons at the hospital with Minnie. Her mother and her brother, a schoolboy who had been baptized on Whit Sunday, were both inpatients during the winter. While there, the mother, one of Margaret's former inpatients at the old compound, began learning the catechism of preparation for baptism, something she had little time or opportunity to do in her non-Christian husband's home.

Margaret regretted that so little evangelistic work was being done. A woman from the American Presbyterian mission had recently visited St. Agatha's. Her delightful accompanying Chinese Bible-woman—someone Margaret felt she could easily befriend, and whose keenness and missionary zeal far exceeded her own—spent three days at the hospital, preaching and talking nearly all the time. She much lamented that there was no Bible-woman in a place where she too felt the need was great. The young nurses were not ready to preach to the women, nor was it expected of them.

Someone was needed who could devote her time to preaching and comforting patients, though the staff did their best as occasion and strength permitted. Regular morning and evening prayers in the small chapel were attended by all in the compound who were able. A simple hymn and a prayer, borrowed from Methodist friends in China who provided many helpful lessons, were much enjoyed. Nearly all the patients managed to learn the words, which were the epitome of the gospel message in simple Chinese.

In the outpatients' compound, the few rooms available for men were constantly filled. The catechist from the church compound came daily to preach, and every fifth day he took a class for the men patients and servants but did not seem to inspire them. Either he was a poor preacher or his heart was not in his work. The best evangelist was the gatekeeper, for his voluntary preaching, the outcome of his passion, was remarkable for an illiterate person. While the catechist had but a short time to spend with the men, the gatekeeper preached at all hours to anyone who came, though he had never been asked to do so. He had the best interests of the compound at heart and maintained the rules with rigid severity, even where Margaret would have relaxed them.

♪﹡

WHEN TIME PERMITTED, Margaret continued to visit outlying villages to attend to those who could not make it to the hospital, encouraging all who could possibly be carried to be brought in for examination. Now she was able to share that duty with Dr. Cunningham, and between the two of them they visited four villages within a day's journey of Pingyin. Often, itinerating was disappointing from the medical point of view, though valuable as a means of evangelization and useful in attracting the sick to come to the hospital. In the intervals between the doctors' visits, patients who experienced real benefit from the medicines sometimes found their way to the central dispensary at Pingyin. Others resorted to Chinese drugs and treatment, thus neutralizing the possible benefit from the foreign treatment before the next visit to the village was due. Margaret was convinced that inpatient work was the most hopeful from every point of view, and the only means of giving real medical relief. After a few days, most patients became accustomed to the foreigners' manner of speech and were generally willing to listen to the story of the gospel and to attend hospital prayers or church services.

Dr. Cunningham, an experienced horsewoman, often rode a pony on her travels through the countryside, escorted by her assistant, who walked or rode a donkey if the distance was far. A comment on this "romantic" way to go about the countryside led to Dr. Cunningham retorting that there was nothing romantic about waving off flies, mosquitoes and other winged pests hour after hour throughout a hot and dusty summer's day. In no way did it resemble a comfortable hour's hack or canter along English country lanes.

A typical trip to a country station took place one October to a village named Shuilipu. At eight o'clock that morning Margaret began her preparations for the journey. Following an early lunch she attended the afternoon dispensary, where patients were few, due partly to weather conditions. After seeing to all patients, Margaret set off by sedan chair, accompanied by Zhang Er, who was in charge of travelling arrangements. Bedding and medicines were carried on a donkey, and with four bearers to carry the sedan—two at a time—the six of them made up quite a procession. The twenty-five-kilometre (15 mile) journey would take four hours, and longer in bad weather. Margaret used the opportunity to read. At dusk the group arrived at the hut serving as the village mission building, where she had her evening meal. Margaret always took her own food and crockery with her, and hot water was readily obtainable. Zhang Er fixed up her camp bed, then he and the bearers went off to an inn for the night, as there was no provision for them in the tiny hut.

The native Christian in charge and his wife arrived to chat, immediately describing their ailments, expecting that Margaret would diagnose and prescribe on the spot, but the candlelight was insufficient and their cases were not urgent enough to justify such prompt attention. She persuaded them to wait till the next day. While noisily drinking tea, they asked her age and why she was not married, to which she responded: how could she have time to come to China to see patients if she were married? Next they asked how much money she received for her work. She replied that she had sufficient for her food, pointing out that missionaries did not come to China to make money, or to earn a living, but rather to help the Chinese. They seemed to find that hard to believe, so they went on to ask whether she liked England or China better; she confessed a preference for her own country, realizing that this reply could be considered rude, but at least it was honest and helped to drive home the fact that it was not for China, nor pecuniary advantages, that she had left home.

Maintaining a lengthy running conversation with her limited vocabulary was rather tiring, so she was not sorry when after about an hour and a half the company politely suggested she might wish to rest. She admitted she did, whereupon the woman said she would stay with her till she was asleep. Margaret did not relish that prospect, and warned her she might have to wait a long time. As tactfully as possible, she indicated she preferred to be left alone.

Margaret hoped to one day, when she had sufficiently improved her powers of Chinese rhetoric, be able to get a few village women together for an evening for a little teaching, although generally she did not feel up to work immediately after arrival. People tended to come late and stay late, and in the summer she started work early each morning.

Very early the following morning a young man arrived, requesting that Margaret attend to his sick mother. He presented her with the fee for home visits—five hundred cash, equalling about sixpence—then escorted her to a nearby neighbouring village. The way lay through many beautiful neat gardens of cabbages, carrots and onions. Margaret often wished that the Chinese would keep their houses as tidy as their gardens. They had yet to learn that they too, like their cabbages, would be healthier if they did so.

Margaret could not spend long with the woman, as other patients were waiting. She left her with specific instructions but had little expectation of having them followed. On her way out, she remonstrated with the neighbours who had trooped in, filling the doorway and blocking out all light and air, there being no window in the room. The sick woman's son accompanied her back to the mission, then took the prescribed medicines home to his mother.

By then most patients had arrived. The mission had no catechist for that village, so there could be no preaching. Each patient paid gate money of twenty cash, the equivalent of one farthing. There was no charge for medication, since the villagers could not possibly afford to pay the full value; also it was better that they not think the mission was making a business of it. That day Margaret saw seventy-two patients, a relative few compared with some summer clinics. She could not help wondering how she had once managed to see to more than twice that many during a visit to that village in the hottest weather. It may have been that the amount of work was the same, for when the patients were fewer their complaints were generally longer.

Her last patient was a suicidal young girl who had eaten lead and phosphorus about a month earlier and who, naturally, was feeling extremely ill. She was unlikely to recover. Then another patient returned, saying that he had been showing his pills to another man, who had picked up two to taste and accidentally swallowed them—so could she please let him have two more? She heard him out with some scepticism but acceded with a caution. At last she packed up her medicine chests, got into her sedan chair and set off for home, arriving just before dusk. Thankfully, there were no inpatients requiring her attention, and no emergency cases awaiting her return, as would have been the situation in summer.

♪❋

ONE OF MARGARET'S SADDEST PATIENTS was a friendless, homeless nine-year-old orphan named Meihua (Plum Blossom). A kind Catholic priest heard of her circumstances and found her a home amongst his parishioners, whom he paid for her support. Meihua soon proved very helpful, gathering sticks for fuel, minding the baby and helping to cook. One day, while dishing up porridge for breakfast and carrying the large heavy pot to the table, she stumbled and spilled the hot stuff, badly scalding her leg. A mixture of oil and mud was rubbed over the burn, and her leg was then bound up in rags. In great pain, she lay moaning in bed, unable to sleep or eat. After several days she became very ill. Fearing for her life, her foster mother brought her to the dispensary. Margaret told her at once that the child must remain as an inpatient. The woman consented and agreed to remain to look after her, as there was no nurse.

Meihua's leg was in such terrible condition that she had to be given chloroform while it was attended to. Margaret initially feared she might not recover, but in a few days' time she began to mend. Her foster mother, however, was tiring of nursing her and, feeling bored in a strange place, went home to fetch her two-year-old, who was fretful without her. She provided and cooked food for the two of them, while Meihua's meals were provided by the hospital. Because Meihua needed nourishment, Margaret often supplemented her supplied meals with extra dainties, only to find that these were often taken from her and given to the toddler. Meihua was not getting enough to eat, thus was making slow progress. A week later, the mother again wanted to take her home. As Margaret knew that Meihua would certainly die if she left at this point, she told the woman that she could leave but not take the patient, then found another woman to take charge of Meihua. She also notified the priest of what she had done. He thoroughly approved and said the child was to stay as long as Margaret wished, and that he would pay for everything that was required. Meihua was fed the most nourishing food and she mended rapidly.

Once she could walk about, Meihua was free to come in and out of Margaret's house and prattle to her when she was not busy. Margaret was living alone and she enjoyed the child's company. Meihua grew to be strong and merry, and Margaret longed to keep her, but she knew that was not to be. One day, when she had quite recovered, the priest sent an escort to take her away, and little Meihua left, sobbing bitterly. However, Margaret felt easier about her, knowing she was getting a new foster mother and not returning to the former neglectful one.

A year later Margaret heard that Meihua had suddenly taken ill, a few months after leaving, and died. Apparently no one had realized the severity of her ailment in time to send for a doctor.

♪❋

ONE SUNDAY MORNING Margaret awoke to the tolling of a church bell, a rather dismal sound in China. She realized that she had slept in, having been up late the night before dealing with a case of attempted suicide by opium poisoning. It was too late for the morning service, so she began her day with breakfast.

Immediately afterwards she headed off to see a patient who was dying of heart disease. Wang Chengfu was about twenty, a Christian and former mission schoolboy, at a time prior to Margaret's arrival in China, though she had been told his story. His parents were extremely poor, but they wanted him to have a good education, so they had allowed him to attend the mission school as a day scholar, as did his cousin Qingfu, whose father was a Christian. Every morning and evening the two attended church services, but Qingfu sat among the Christians near the front of the church, while Chengfu had to sit behind. However, this had its advantages as he could escape attention at the back, and since he had entered school comparatively late, he had much to make up for. He got through quite a lot of study during those half-hours in church.

Chengfu was clever and gradually made his way to the top of the school. When he knew his Bible and his catechisms thoroughly, he was baptized and confirmed, and allowed to sit in front among the Christians in church. Then began the first trouble of his life. His parents, thinking him old enough to be married and needing someone to help with the housework, allowed an engagement to be arranged for him in the usual way. A friend was asked to find him a wife, and one of his friends had an available girl. With no direct communicating, the two families allowed these middlemen to fix up the engagement. Both families were poor and could not expect to make a very good match. The girl's parents paid the middlemen heavily for getting their daughter married and taken off their hands. It occurred to no one that the couple might not be suitable life companions, or more importantly, that the girl might not get on well with her new mother-in-law—for a person of that status reigned supreme in the Chinese household. The two most deeply concerned had no share in the arrangement at all.

Chengfu would have preferred to marry a Christian, but Christian girls were scarce and the middlemen did not know any. Nevertheless, he was resolved to have a Christian marriage in his own home late at night. The groom, with a complete set of new clothes, had never before been dressed so well. The bride was, of course, clothed entirely in red, her head and face covered with a large red veil. She was escorted down the aisle by two friends, for she could not see to walk, and deposited at Chengfu's side. They had never met or even seen one another before, and still he could not see her face.

The service began, but when asked if she would take Chengfu as her husband, the girl refused, saying, "I won't be a Christian." Her friends whispered angrily at her to be quiet, and the clergyman tried to soothe her into saying the necessary words. For some time she refused, still calling out that she would not be a Christian. At last she felt assured that she was not binding herself to be a Christian, and as the clergyman understood she was not objecting to the marriage itself, the ceremony continued. Thus poor Chengfu was married to a girl older than himself who was actively opposed to Christianity.

She led him a most unhappy life, jeering and mocking his faith, and quarrelling with him incessantly. Fortunately, he escaped a great deal of misery as he still went to school daily. But hard study, poor food and overall stress so undermined his strength that a few months after his marriage, he became very ill and had to take to his bed. The one-room mud cottage, which he shared with his parents, wife and younger brother, was partially divided by a screen, and dark and dirty. The door, a straw mat in a light wooden frame, was usually open during the day, but the small square openings which served as windows had been completely blocked up to keep the wind off him. He lay in a dark corner, where no fresh air or light could reach him.

The walls and roof consisted of thick straw plastered with mud. The hard mud-brick bed, a *kang*, was hollow and heated by a meagre fire of straw below, coal being unaffordable; it filled nearly the whole room. Chengfu lay there, semiconscious and delirious, for two months or longer, rolled up in a thick wadded quilt, without washing and with no change of clothing. Small wonder he felt little inclination for food and that his fever gained on him.

When he first became ill, his mother went to a medicine shop and brought home a bundle of dried herbs and roots to be boiled for an hour in a litre (2 pints) of water. The thick brown fluid was then ladled into a bowl, which he drained in one draught. The next morning there was no improvement, so another mixture was bought from a different medicine shop, and that was given a trial. Many remedies were tried and the fire lit many times in the hope that the heat would drive out his disease, but it only weakened him. Meanwhile, Chengfu could not eat any ordinary food. As his family was too poor to procure better food, he became thinner than ever and grew steadily worse. Then money was borrowed and Chinese doctors were called in. One after another they came, prescribed for the patient and left. According to custom they paid just one visit; there was no chance of seeing the effects of their medicines, or of being blamed if the result was not good.

Finally, Chengfu became delirious and his condition so serious that the current Chinese doctor proclaimed nothing could be done. The neighbours declared that he was dying, so word was sent to the English priest, which was when Margaret came into the picture. When she saw him, his state was even worse, and he had been without food for about six days. His parents were not willing for her to try to feed him. She headed back to the dispensary for medication, then returned to administer it. The family did seem grateful that she had taken the trouble to make a double journey, and they asked her to pray for them, which she did, then departed.

When she got home, she found her little Sunday school class of three awaiting. They were learning to read St. John's Gospel and getting on very quickly, especially the oldest girl, who had learned almost four chapters since she began barely five months previously, accomplishing this despite having only the one weekly lesson. The reading lesson was followed by a short discussion. Margaret felt the children would begin to understand better when they knew more Chinese characters. After the lesson the children went home to mind babies while their mothers attended church. Meanwhile, Margaret was called to the dispensary—which normally remained closed on Sunday except for urgent cases—to dress the wounds of a burned child. The usual sixteen women were in church that day, a number considered quite good. Few could read, and a number of them would fall asleep, or play with their babies, or inspect another missionary lady's hat and clothes—Margaret's, of course, they were quite familiar with. Still, so far as she could tell, the women were benefitting by their church attendances.

After the service the women went into the dispensary for tea and a little social conversation. There was no suggestion of making this a class. It was simply a means of keeping in touch, and all seemed to enjoy the friendliness of it, being much given to hospitality and social intercourse amongst themselves. Margaret hoped that this type of ladies' meeting, *taitai hui,* could have the makings of an auxiliary group in due course. After an hour's chat, the women politely invited her to go for lunch, which she was quite glad to do as it was then half past one.

As to how Margaret spent her time between lunch and tea, she preferred to draw the curtains on the subject, which is what she did in reality. During her teatime a message arrived that the suicidal patient of the previous night had come to see her. He complained of not feeling very "comfortable"—a natural state after the quantity of fresh opium he had taken, but on the whole he seemed well and quite grateful. He had only taken it in a moment of rage and was glad to find himself still alive.

Accompanied by Sarah, Margaret then returned to see Chengfu, but his condition was quite hopeless. His parents had asked her not to give him any further medication, and she yielded to their wishes. Sarah washed Chengfu's hands and face so that he "looked" more comfortable, and that seemed to be all that could be done. By then it was time for evensong; the rest of the evening passed quietly, and Margaret's day ended early. Two days later news of Chengfu's passing reached her. Due to his impoverished state, the mission provided a Christian burial.

∫✳

LIKE MANY HIGHLY PRINCIPLED PEOPLE, Margaret had always been her own harshest critic. Filled with the deepest contrition, she once confided to her diary her fear of having failed in her line of duty:

I fear that I let God down often by sheer overwork and neglect of prayer, which was too great a strain on my health and temper.

[Sometimes feeling as if I were working] without human aid, I studied Chinese, built a hospital (only those who have done it can have any idea of what it meant, and a dim idea of what it meant for a woman), I saw patients daily, paid outside calls, nursed patients and wrote begging letters to get money for the building. I see now that it was all wrong, for I had tried to do impossibilities.

She had always been concerned over how few patients returned for follow-up visits after her assessments, though she knew this expectation was foreign to them. In one instance, however, she derived considerable satisfaction. The previous autumn a little girl with an extreme contraction of the knee joint following a burn had been admitted for a lengthy stay in hospital. Straightening the leg proved an easy matter, though no local Chinese doctor could have done so. The mother, who was very poor, had been sorely distressed at the thought of her daughter being a helpless cripple. Never would she be able to find a mother-in-law for her, a state of affairs too terrible to contemplate. When she saw two straight little limbs instead of only one, she wept for joy, becoming so hysterical in her expressions of gratitude that Margaret felt quite alarmed. To further express her gratitude, the mother insisted on her being given some sewing to do. She worked at this without a moment's rest except when Margaret compelled her to stop.

That year many of the hospital's patients included workers from some nearby government quarries and stonemasons working on a new Roman Catholic church a few kilometres away. Working safety standards were primitive, and industrial accidents occurred frequently. However, from an evangelical aspect, the victims' spiritual welfare was attended to at least as well as their medical needs.

♪❊

MEANWHILE, an enormous political change was occurring in China. Margaret felt the situation was aptly described in the book *My Father in China* by James Burke:

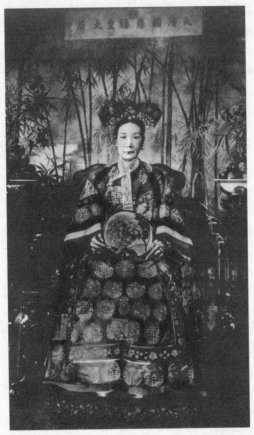

The Empress Dowager Zixi (Tzu Hsi) played an important and controversial role at the end of the Manchu Dynasty.

In 1906, the Empress-Dowager, had reluctantly signed an Edict preparing for constitutional government. Provincial assemblies met in 1909, and in 1910 a provisional national assembly was convened. However, this progress towards democracy was too slow for China's countless revolutionary societies which smouldered behind the doors of their secret meeting rooms throughout the country. Constitutional government meant nothing to the masses…[but they] were only too well aware…that the existing Imperial régime was over-burdensome with taxes…[which]…in itself, was sufficient…to warrant an overthrow.

…[T]he Revolution of 1911 [began with]…the explosion of a bomb in a Chinese house in the Russian quarter of Hankow (Hankou), on October 9th. Raking around in the wreckage, the police found a quantity of unexploded bombs…a huge supply of revolutionary flags and badges, as well as documentary evidence revealing plans for a major outbreak…the following April.

…Viceroy Rui Cheng (Rui Zheng) in Wuchang across the Yangtse from Hankow, spent October 10th executing and otherwise incapacitating radicals. The revolutionaries…hastily marshalled their forces. Fires broke out in Wuchang that night and Imperial troops mutinied. The leading mutineer, Li Yuan-Hung,…helped [the viceroy] to escape, then proclaimed his intention of overthrowing the Manchus. Within a few days the three combined cities (Wuchang, Hankow and Hanyang) were in the hands of the People's Army.

In a panic over the initial successes of the insurgents, the throne was driven to the humiliating recourse of recalling Yuan Shi-Kai… the former military chieftain who had been sent into retirement by the Empress-Dowager three years earlier. A cabinet was formed and Yuan was made premier…Li Yuan-Hung proclaimed the establishment of a Republic in Wuchang, with himself as President… [T]he fever of revolt was spreading rapidly, picked up by the secret societies all over the land.

In Shanghai, the revolutionaries…set up a republic under… veteran diplomat, Wu Ding-Fang, independently of the rising in Wuchang. Then a campaign was launched to capture Nanking, but the commander there, General Chang Hsün (Zhang Xun)… of a sterner breed than most Imperialists…fought savagely for three weeks before he was compelled to withdraw northwards on December 1st. However, the Old Tiger, as Zhang Xun was called, was not gone for good.

China was now effectively split into three camps…republics at Wuchang, Nanking and Beijing, the latter…under the dictatorship

of Yuan Shi-Kai...[F]ighting [had given]...way to the more typically Chinese method of talk-banquets...[when]...the elusive
Tongmenghui hero, Dr. Sun Yat-Sen...reached Shanghai on Christmas
Eve...[He was] inaugurated provisional president of the Nanking
junta on January 1st.

After more fighting between the Imperialists and the revolutionaries north of Hankow, the self-appointed Field Marshal Yuan
Shi-Kai engineered a nonresistance ultimatum to the throne from
the forty-six Imperial commanders in the field...[forcing] the
throne's abdication...on February 12th, 1912. So ended finally and
ignominiously the rule of the Manchus in China after two hundred and sixty-eight years.

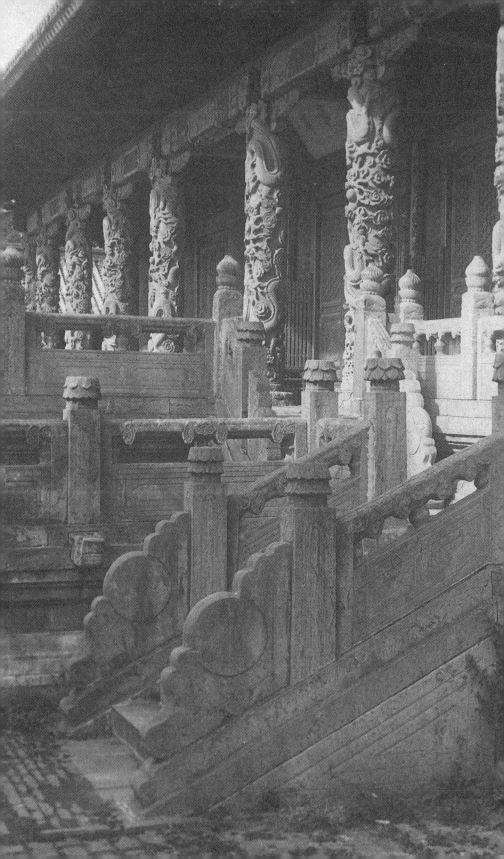

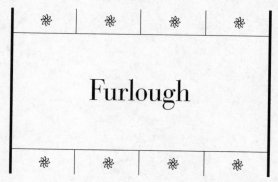

Furlough

ƒ✴ MARGARET WAS OVERDUE for some dental work, so she seized the opportunity to have a short holiday and departed for Qingdao, which entailed the misery of a day-and-a-half-long wheelbarrow journey to the railway station at Jinan. The rest of the trip, a far greater distance by rail to the coast, took the same amount of time. At Qingdao, by pre-arrangement she met a nurse, Miss Abbott, who had just arrived from England. Before leaving for Pingyin, the two briefly visited Qufu, where Confucius was born about 551 B.C.

The Kong family were still in residence there after seventy-seven generations. Qufu had acquired the status of a holy place because of its worthy son, Confucius; the direct descendants, being still present, were considered its guardians. Sightseeing of this compact town could be accomplished on foot in a day. Thanks to its fine imperial architecture, most of which dated back to the Ming dynasty, the place was an oasis of culture and elegance. The Temple of Confucius is large; its grounds contain over one thousand stone steles with inscriptions dating from Han to Qing times, as well as profuse clusters of cypresses and twisted pines. Another note-

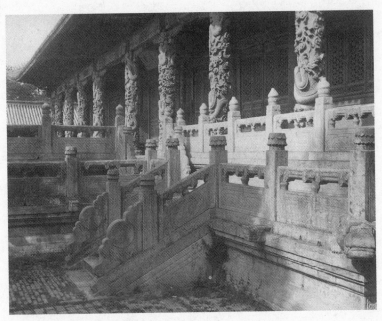

CHAPTER 11

The Temple of Confucius in Qufu.

worthy spot was *Kong Lin*, the Confucian Forest, containing the burial place of the sage and his many descendants.

Miss Abbott's arrival was timely for two reasons. Margaret was due to go home on furlough, but she refused to depart until the Society for the Propagation of the Gospel (SPG) sent out a nurse. With the hospital fully functional and Sarah still away, she was not prepared to leave Dr. Cunningham alone to bear the load she previously had to endure. The second reason was that it had become essential for her to take leave. She was haemorrhaging again and obviously needed an extended period away to recuperate. She made arrangements to return to England, travelling via the United States to see her sister Mamie, visiting Hawaii en route. Unable to complete her arrangements on the spot, she set off with some concerns on her mind and with hope in her heart—a situation that was nothing new.

♪

AFTER ANOTHER ARDUOUS WHEELBARROW JOURNEY to Jinan, this time in the blazing heat of the summer, and a train journey to Qingdao, Margaret boarded a coastal steamer for three uneventful days, arriving in Shanghai on Saturday, July 1. To her dismay, the banks there were closed for three days to balance their half-yearly accounts. She was due to sail on Monday. How was she to draw funds to pay for her sea passage to the States? Luckily, the administrator of the missionary home where she was staying agreed to cash her cheque, albeit at a fairly high rate of commission. Nonetheless, she was grateful.

The SPG travel allowance covered only second-class fare, but for the sake of her health, Margaret preferred to go first class. She booked her passage through a Japanese shipping company and, for an additional sixty pounds, negotiated her ticket to London at the missionary rate, which included first-class rail fare across America but no meals.

Appropriately, on the Fourth of July, Margaret sailed for America. The *Chyo Maru* was oil-burning and clean, and served good food. She was pleased to find that she knew a number of people onboard, including Deaconess Hart from Hankow and two other missionaries from the American Episcopalian mission, who invited her to join their party. They went ashore together at Honolulu, where they watched the surfers and visited the museum and the aquarium with its brilliantly coloured fish. At the end of a beautiful day, the satisfied passengers sailed away, decked out in their leis.

THE SEA HATH HER MOODS

How soothing is the sleepy sea with scarce a ripple on her face—
Yet how dull!
How pleasing in her playful mood as she lightly tosses feathery crests
Here and there!

How menacing is the sullen sea when she's a heaving mass of
    grey-green billows
Everywhere!

How awesome is the angry sea as she moulds the restless waves
Into mountainous ridges!
How beautiful is the sea when the sun shines again after rain,
And the white-capped waves are tumbling about in joyous confusion!

Azure-blue, ultramarine, silver-grey, jade-green,
Turquoise and milky-blue—
Many are the colours of the sea.

I love to see the silver fish sporting through the rainbows in the spray
As they fly in crowds above the waves, then plunge into the
    dark blue sea.
I love to see the dolphins gambolling in the waves,
Leaping in graceful curves from crest to crest
As they race each other through the sea.

(E. M. P.)

In San Francisco they booked a hotel for the night, then amused themselves touring round Chinatown. The following morning the group travelled on a new line, the Southern Pacific, indulging in a drawing room for two nights.

As they approached the Rockies, Margaret witnessed her first forest fire, so near to the track that she could see flames crawling from tree to tree, smell the reeking smoke and hear the crackling flames and crashing trees. While waiting to change trains at Denver, they viewed a western film of the most sensational kind. The next stopover was at Salt Lake City for two nights at a big hotel where, according to Deaconess Hart, the American president stayed whenever he visited the city. Bathing in the lake was amusing. People bobbed about on the water like corks and had to hold their heads up to keep from turning upside down. When they emerged, their bodies shone with crystals of salt. The next day, being Sunday, the group attended a morning church service, and an afternoon service in the Mormon Tabernacle, a huge building with a circular seating arrangement thronged with thousands. Leaving Salt Lake City, the train passed over miles of dazzling white salt—to Margaret's mind, a world supply.

In Chicago, the party went to Marshall Field's and rode the elevators up the fifteen storeys of the tallest skyscraper. There they parted ways, with Margaret going on alone to Toronto. Her trunk was bonded on to New York, and her hand luggage examined during the night as she crossed the border. On reaching Toronto, one item was missing. She was told that it was in the customs room and that she would not get it till the afternoon. In the six-hour break, she wandered about the streets of Toronto, going into the Eaton's department store and venturing up and down a "moving stairway"—an escalator—several times, purely for the novelty. Later, back at the station, she was still unable to retrieve her suitcase, as the customs official had not arrived. Margaret was in despair. If she missed her train, where was she to spend the night? In a flood of tears, she stormed, "If this is the way you do things in Canada, give me China!" The case was restored, and the man hastily put a chalk mark on it to let her take it away. Of course, she had to carry her own luggage—so different from China!

Margaret proceeded to Bowmanville, near Toronto, where Marion Service was staying with missionary friends from Japan and where she would be married to Rev. Kettlewell. The wedding quietly took place the following day in the local church, and Margaret then went to Niagara Falls for an overnight visit. She had been told to be sure to go to the cave on the Canadian side, where one looked through part of the waterfall from behind, but she searched for this in vain. Presently she spotted a sign which read THIS WAY TO THE CAVE OF THE WINDS. Assuming her original instructions were faulty, Margaret concluded that "some people are wrong even when they are most positive."

"Come and put on a bathing suit," she was told. "There's a party getting ready to go down now."

"A bathing suit" sounded strange, for her friend had said a mackintosh, and "going down" was not right either, but she did what she was told. They mustered together a group of eight with a guide in front, though Margaret thought there should have been one behind too. Down they went on a spiral staircase, down, down, down till they were nearly at the bottom of the Falls. Then they turned and began to climb stairways made of slippery wooden planks with one handrail and nothing to prevent one from slipping through or over the side. Up and down they went, blinded with spray and deafened by the thunder of the waterfall. Margaret could only see two or three people ahead of her, when the person directly in front turned round and, holding out her left hand, shouted, "Hold hands and go sideways."

She turned round and held out her hand to the woman behind her, the last in line, shouting the same message. Her reply almost petrified Margaret: "I can't!" Margaret yelled back, "You must!" Grabbing her hand, she pulled for dear life. She had no intention of letting go. Finally, they stopped along a narrow plank bridge. As they were holding each other's hands, they could not grasp onto any support. Then it seemed as if tons of water were falling on their heads, for they were actually passing under a small detached bit of the Falls. Suddenly, they were at the spiral staircase again and back to safety. She was never to know whether that woman realized it, but Margaret was quite certain she had saved her life.

Back in Toronto, Margaret took a boat cruise on Lake Ontario. She had a day's visit in Ottawa, where she visited the parliament buildings. Despite feeling a cold coming on, she boarded another steamer and sailed down the St. Lawrence River, passing through the Thousand Isles en route to Montreal, where she spent the night. Her hotel room was on the sixth floor. How thankful she was when morning came, for she had a morbid dread of fire in high buildings.

Margaret's ticket allowed her to travel down the Hudson River, which would have taken an additional twelve hours. Her cold was getting worse, and she thought as she had already done pretty well by way of sightseeing, she had better take care of her health by not going. She regretted that decision but considered it wise. She did manage to catch glimpses of the river as she travelled on the train to New York. Margaret had found it pleasant to be with a small group of American missionaries, although they were expensive to travel with as they had a sightseeing allowance and invariably went first class. She acknowledged that sightseeing had widened her experience, but she arrived in New York virtually penniless.

At New York Central, Margaret was disappointed to see no one on the platform. She walked up the long platform and there, behind some railings, she found Mamie and her husband, Owen, anxiously looking around for her. Margaret spotted them first despite the intervening eleven years. Her lingering memory of her first evening was eating supper with four pairs of young eyes gazing at their "China Auntie."

Margaret liked New York very much. She was quite surprised to find that the architecture was not at all monotonous, and she admired the Singer Tower, which a few years earlier had been promoted as the world's tallest building. The department stores fascinated her with their displays of desirable goods of every description, and she spent an entire day going from floor to floor, resting in the lounges and having lunch or tea in the restaurants. The Metropolitan Museum of Art had a wonderful collection of Chinese treasures on display, and she was enchanted with Central Park with its zoo and the squirrels, so tame they took peanuts from her hand. When her cold worsened, she knew she had made the right decision over not taking the river trip. She felt rather panicky, fearing a haemorrhage might recur.

Mamie took her to see the lot of land she and Owen had bought on which to build their new house, then simply a grassy field with a few trees. They were not far from Brighton Beach with its crowds of bathers in bathing suits of ample proportions, wearing long stockings and even gloves to avoid an unfashionable suntan.

One day cousin Winifred came for a visit, and they went to Coney Island. The tricks were hilarious. When a bench collapsed under them, Margaret caught sight of a man on a nearby gallery, who had obviously pulled a lever. As they walked along Margaret's dress blew upwards and off came her glasses—her only pair as she had already lost a pair into the water during a sudden squall on a ferry crossing. In the thick crowd, she spotted a man in the act of picking them up. Dashing forward, she seized them, just as he was about to pocket them, saying, "Mine, I think," and rushed away.

From Mamie's, Margaret went to Providence to stay with her cousins Edith and Winifred and Aunt Mattie for ten days. One day she was out walking and noticed a man across the street, putting up a large signboard while standing on the railing of a balcony. He appeared to take a step backwards to look at the sign, then fell, crashing down onto the pavement. Horrified, Margaret ran across the wide street, but it was hopeless. Some men had rushed out of the shop and were lifting him into a sitting position. "Put him down," Margaret ordered, and they obeyed, but he was dead. The incident haunted her for a long time afterwards.

♪✳

IN OCTOBER, Margaret crossed the Atlantic onboard the *St. Paul.* For two days the ship was in thick fog. The booming of the foghorn day and night made her nervous, especially on the second day when another foghorn repeatedly answered theirs. Eventually, the fog lifted and the other ship was sighted. It was the *Caronia,* heading in the same direction, but she felt it was somewhat too close for comfort.

When Margaret left England seven years previously, her brother Frank had promised he would be there to meet her on her return. However, at Plymouth she received a letter saying that as the ship was late he could not be at Southampton due to pressing business, so he would meet her in London instead. Margaret was tempted to disembark at Plymouth and catch the through train to London; on the other hand, since she had left England from Southampton she fancied landing there, so she remained onboard overnight while the ship slipped across the English Channel to Cherbourg and back. As they were docking at Southampton, Margaret sat on deck chatting with some shipboard acquaintances, when a steward asked if anybody was going ashore. She quickly got up and rushed down the gangway, straight into the arms of Frank—much to her surprise. He had been waiting anxiously in view of his letter about meeting in London, and had even tried to force his way onboard without success. It was a wonderful reunion, and they made their way back to Birmingham together with much happiness in their hearts.

When she landed, Margaret was in good health. Three rather hectic weeks later, she was instructed to present herself to the SPG doctor in London for a report on her condition. She stayed with Rev. and Mrs. Mosse, the two kind friends who had been unfailingly supportive. Mrs. Mosse had collected most of the money for the building of St. Agatha's Hospital. Dr. Pulteney reported that Margaret was underweight, which was true, and the society ordered her to go to a sanatorium for three months. This she was very willing to do.

She was dispatched to a sanatorium at Peppard Common, a delightful place, ten kilometres (6 miles) from Reading and six kilometres (4 miles) from Henley. The kind and capable superintendent, Dr. Esther Carling, originally ran a private sanatorium for women, Kingwood, for which she had recently obtained official county recognition. She was granted a subsidy, so that Maitland, a sanatorium for men, and Kindercot, for children, were all combined in her charge under the title of the Berkshire and Buckinghamshire Joint Sanatorium, more commonly known as the Berks and Bucks Sanatorium. The food was excellent, and at every meal Margaret enjoyed a glass of rich milk from the sanatorium cows. She lived in a wooden hut in the garden and sat in a shelter during the hours of rest. She made great progress and was soon allowed to take long walks or bicycle rides. She much preferred walking and often covered sixteen kilometres (10 miles) in a morning, for the country was pleasant with lovely beech woods nearby. There was a good deal of rain, but that was to be expected in wintertime.

THE GLEANERS

Early this morning the sparrows had a meeting
On a branch of an old tree near my balcony—
All sitting in a row like good children at school—
Turning their little chests towards the warm sun.

At some word of command down together they flew
Like little brown leaves falling from the tree,
And fluttered like butterflies over the ripe grass
Then busily pecked at the scattered seeds.

Till something disturbed them when up they rose
And flew swiftly back to the bough.

Now they are twittering and chirping around me
Giving praise and thanks for their new day,
For the fresh moist air and the joy of living
And their good fare.

(E. M. P.)

Three months later, Margaret had put on two stone (i.e., averaging almost a kilogram or 2 pounds a week). She bounced into the SPG doctor's office, declaring, "You won't find anything wrong with me now."

"I hope not," Dr. Pulteney answered, rather chillily. She listened to Margaret's breath, comparing one side with the other, then said, "I'm sorry to say that it has spread to the other side."

Dumbfounded, Margaret managed to blurt, "How could that be when I'm so well?" There was no response. She then asked, "Can I go back to China?" To this came the grim reply, "It would be better for you to stay in England near your people, in case anything happens."

Margaret returned to the sanatorium, feeling almost as ill as the doctor had told her she was. "Stuff and nonsense about spreading to the other side," Dr. Carling said. "Of course you feel ill. It's enough to give you pneumonia. We'll go and see what Sir William Osler has to say."

Sir William Osler was then in Oxford, so Mr. Carling got the car out and drove them there. After listening carefully to Margaret's chest, Sir William said, "I can hear nothing at all. I see no reason why Dr. Phillips should not go back to China, or anywhere else she likes."

Nonetheless, Margaret was not surprised to receive a letter from the SPG saying that they would be unable to send her back to China, but they could send her to Africa, which would be better for her health. A letter from Bishop Iliff followed, expressing his regret that she would not be returning to Shandong, and saying that she was entitled to the half-rate salary of six months' furlough. As more than six months had already elapsed, Margaret was furious. She had stayed in the field a year beyond her agreement, she replied, and felt entitled to a year's furlough; certainly she required six months' notice.

The SPG eventually accepted her argument and she received the year's furlough allowance, then was left on her own, supposedly broken down in health and without any enquiry into her financial situation. Her relatives were in no position to help, and she would not live on them. She had no "call" to go to Africa; after all, she spoke Chinese. She believed she was needed in China, where the climate generally was as good as in Africa, and that she would keep well if she had reasonable help. She sent Sir William Osler's letter to the SPG, who replied that they were glad to know she had received such a good report, but they felt bound to abide by their own doctor's decision.

Dr. Carling was a wonderful friend. She had already offered Margaret the position of assistant medical officer at the close of Dr. Sollan's term, which she accepted. Now, at least, she was temporarily earning her own living, since Dr. Carling paid her an honorarium. Soon after she was installed in Dr. Sollan's rooms, Dr. Carling asked if she would carry on alone while she took a much needed vacation in Italy. Margaret felt most gratified by this sign of confidence.

She was kept fairly busy, spending three to four hours every morning examining patients' chests. Dr. Carling asked her to administer pneumothorax injections—a rather new method—and TB injections. On her advice, Margaret also gave herself a course of TB injections, to which she really attributed her own cure. The capable sister at Maitland was kind and helpful to Margaret, so in return she was glad to help out by carving the meat at the men's luncheon. One of the patients kept the carving knives well sharpened, and she proceeded to cut up three large legs of mutton in record time. Appetites were good, and some of the men went back for second, and even third, helpings.

Dr. Carling believed in occupational therapy, graduated rest and exercise, and the psychological factor was not overlooked. Various amusements were arranged, including playing bridge with the doctor, her husband and other staff members.

⁂

REGRETFULLY, Margaret had to leave in June, as she had promised to help the SPG with a big missionary exhibition in Westminster. Again she stayed with the Mosses. She had been asked to take charge of the medical side of the exhibition, and for that she brought a complete scale model of the St. Agatha's Hospital compound, a number of scrolls and other interesting objects. The model was displayed on a table in the centre of the exhibit, with compartments set up on both sides of the hall to represent a room in a Chinese house, a ward in her hospital, and the consulting room and dispensary with people dressed up to represent nurses and patients.

As Her Majesty Queen Mary was to open the exhibition, the ladies practised the curtsey required on being introduced to her. Margaret bought herself a nice dress with a smart new hat from Dickins and Jones—one of the better department stores—specially for the occasion. The exhibition was to open at three o'clock. Margaret arrived early and, to her horror, was told she was required to speak at five o'clock about her medical work in China. She went up into the gallery for a half-hour to marshal her thoughts.

The Queen was first taken around the main hall, where she saw exhibits from missionary stations in different parts of the world. Then a small procession, consisting of Queen Mary, the young Princess Mary, the Archbishop of Canterbury, Bishop Montgomery (general secretary) and Dr. Robertson (medical secretary), all came into the medical hall, which was devoted to China. Margaret, on being presented to Her Majesty, performed her curtsey and kissed her hand, then took the Queen round and explained various items to her. The Queen inspected keenly and asked many questions. When she had looked at the model of the hospital, she turned round, eyed Margaret up and down, and said, "Good 'eavens, did you do that all yourself?"

Immediately afterwards, Margaret was called upon for her talk. As there was no podium, she was asked to stand on a chair; barely one and a half metres (5 feet) tall, she would be difficult to see otherwise. She launched forth and found that the going was not too hard, once she had taken the plunge. An assistant dressed in Chinese clothes, the "patient," climbed into a large wicker basket slung from a pole and was carried by two stalwart "Chinese" to the dispensary for treatment, then to the ward. When she got down from her chair, she found three fellow missionaries from Shandong had been listening. Margaret wondered what sort of impression she had made. She was gratified when Mrs. Mosse later showed her a most complimentary report in the *Guardian*.

This performance was repeated several times daily for ten days. Margaret attended the exhibition each day from 2:00 to 11:00 P.M., but she cried off attending at 11:00 A.M., when schools were shown round. She felt that would be taking too much risk with her lungs.

♪✳

AT THE CLOSE OF THE EXHIBITION, Margaret left her kind friends in London to make her way to Manchester. There she attended a degree ceremony to receive her delayed M.Sc. and participated in a college reunion. She stayed at the hall of residence, now removed to a new building in Fallowfield. Jess, Marion and Ethel Carpenter were there with a number of other fellow students; they celebrated with a cocoa party. After leaving Manchester, Margaret went to Liverpool to see her sister Annie. They had last seen each other in London, where Annie was taking nursing training in a nursing home. Later she had gone to a cottage hospital in Kent, and now she was in Liverpool, though no one knew why. Margaret was anxious about her and went purposely to see if she needed help. Annie did not tell her anything, nor did she let Margaret see where she lived; they met only in the street. Margaret was unhappy, but she could do nothing for Annie against her will. The family was aware only that there was a man in her life. Once, when she wrote to Margaret, she signed herself "A. Hill."

Ethel Lomas had advised Margaret to stay at the Adelphi, but she found it too grand and expensive, so she decided to push on to Bristol to stay with Jess, now Mrs. Skemp. The trip took over four hours although she went by express, London to Bristol direct. En route, somewhere in Shropshire, the steam pressure in the engine ran out, bringing the train to a standstill in the midst of beautiful country, with no sign of a house anywhere. Apparently someone had to walk to the nearest telephone to explain the predicament. It was a lovely day, so the passengers got off the train and strolled around the fields until another engine came to the rescue. Nearer Bristol, the train passed through the Severn Tunnel, the longest Margaret had ever been through.

Jess's husband, Arthur, was away, so Margaret never saw him. Their daughter, Margaret—her namesake—was a dainty child of five. Jess had a nice semi-detached home in Clifton, and Margaret anticipated a happy visit. But on the third day as she stooped over her trunk, she felt a ghastly little bubbling in her throat: the beginning of haemoptysis. She told Jess, who made her lie down. She hardly dared breathe, and certainly not to cough. Only those who have experienced it can know the panic that an attack of haemoptysis can cause. She shook the bed with trembling, unable to stop. It was heartbreaking after her long stay at the sanatorium, where she had been so fit. Margaret suspected the long stuffy hours at the exhibition had something to do with it, plus the fatigue and anxiety in Liverpool over Annie. The haemorrhage was mercifully slight, but it would not clear up. A nurse came to attend to Margaret and she had absolute rest, distressed to be such a trouble and disappointment to Jess, whom she never saw again after that episode.

♪

DR. CARLING INVITED Margaret to return to Peppard Common. Dr. Lily accompanied her on the cross-country journey. How comforting it was to have such a good escort, and how indescribably kind of her. A strong bond existed between many of the women doctors in those days.

To Margaret, reaching the sanatorium felt like coming home. After a few days' rest she was up and about again. Then she suffered a bigger haemorrhage than she had ever experienced before. However, she was in good hands and was probably all the better for it, so she said, since it stopped completely. At that time, earwigs were rather plentiful, crawling along the cracks of the wooden ceiling of her shack and sometimes falling, *plop,* onto her bed. Margaret had a great dislike for earwigs, and as she was afraid to move suddenly, she persuaded the sister to poke all along the cracks each night before she turned the light off. Only then did she feel she could sleep peacefully.

For months, Margaret stayed with Dr. Carling, who said that things always went well when she was around. She already had an assistant medical officer so there was not much for Margaret to do, but she helped with secretarial work, enabling the secretary to take a holiday, and assisted with occupational therapy. She learned embroidery from Sybil Welch, an old friend of Ethel Lomas's who, for health reasons, had been held up in the middle of her medical course and was resting at Kingwood. They taught the men embroidery. One man had been run over by a train; he lost both legs and an arm, yet learned to do beautiful embroidery with a frame clamped to a table. Later Sybil sent Margaret a nightdress case of cross-stitch which he had worked. Many of her designs were copied from the South Kensington Museum. Margaret gave Dr. Carling her first piece of work, which she had framed and hung in her cottage.

♪

AT LAST, in March 1913, Margaret felt well enough to return to China. She considered the climate there better for her than the perpetual

English rain. She wrote to Bishop Roots in Hankow and offered her services, as Deaconess Hart had urged her to do; he replied that Hankow or anywhere in the Yangzi River valley would be too risky. She toyed with the idea of serving in Fuzhou, but climatic considerations and the thought of having to learn a new dialect changed her mind. Then she remembered what Dr. Aspland had said about the Canadian Church Mission in Henan (Honan) Province, so she wrote to Bishop William White in Kaifeng, telling him about her health problems and Dr. William Osler's opinion. As she posted the letter she had a feeling of irrevocability, yet she wondered if she had done the right thing. She had little confidence as to the outcome. Certainly she never expected such a prompt and definite answer: "ACCEPTED GLADLY. PROCEED IMMEDIATELY VIA SIBERIA." That was indeed a day to remember.

Margaret met Sir William Osler one day when he was visiting Dr. Carling, and she told him about her bad turn of events, but he said, "Never mind. I shall not change my opinion."

She had been invited by Bishop and Mrs. Burroughs to spend a few days with them in Brighton. He was president of the North China and Shantung Mission. There she met Miss Wyatt Smith, who promised to pay Margaret's passage to China whenever she was ready, and gave her one hundred pounds for her fare and expenses. During the next three weeks, as she prepared to return to where she felt she really belonged, Margaret wrote:

I was told, "Go back to your old China; you'll never be happy till you do." I'm afraid I must have been a bore. To tell the truth, my impression was that English people were not interested in China. They would ask me to tell them about China, but as soon as I began I saw they were already thinking of something else. The person who seemed most interested and asked the most questions was Professor Withers, the Professor of History in Manchester whom I met when I went there for my M.Sc.

One Saturday night Mrs. Burroughs invited Margaret to hear a talk on Africa given to the girls of the Girls' Friendly Society by a returned missionary, and she asked if Margaret would care to say an impromptu few words about China. The meeting was held in an upstairs room of the church house, and they were asked to be quiet as there was some kind of service going on below. They were certainly quiet, for the speaker's talk was dry, merely a chronicle of church work which could have been done for any part of the world. Then came Margaret's turn.

The girls must have been feeling bottled up, for they laughed at everything she said. She told them about Chinese customs being the opposite to the English, and the native ways of treatment, and about the patient who swallowed four powders while she told him how to take them, another who drank his liniment, and one putting the powders on his leg. They laughed and laughed, till Margaret got quite nervous about the noise. She sat down as soon as she could. Although Mrs. Burroughs might not have approved of her talk, she was certain the girls had enjoyed it.

Margaret spent a day with her father to say goodbye once more, and before they parted, he presented her with one of his most treasured possessions: a handsome travelling clock in its own case, which he had received from his father on his twenty-first birthday. This clock was to remain with her until she died. Margaret's final stay was with Frank and his wife, Frances. During a farewell visit to a local friend, Margaret had a severe attack of nausea, and Frank was called to fetch her home in a cab. Exhausted with her preparations and farewells, she had developed yet another cold, which turned into bronchitis.

In London, Margaret again stayed with the best of her friends, the Mosses. Mrs. Mosse was quite distressed and urged Margaret to postpone her journey. But Margaret dared not forfeit her ticket, so Mrs. Mosse saw her off at Charing Cross. The channel crossing from Dover to Ostend was uneventful. Margaret took this to be a happy augury as she set out for China. Once there, she realized, she would have circled the globe.

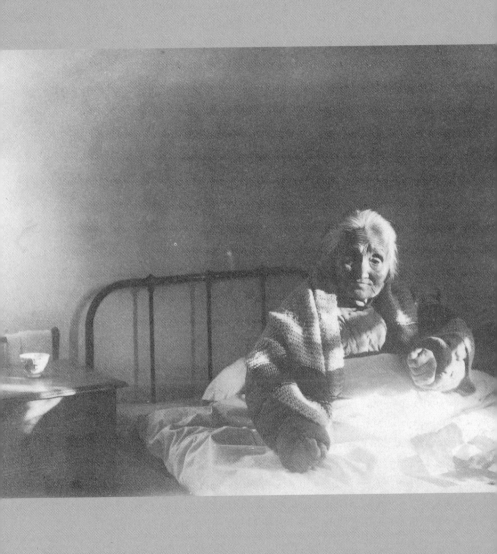

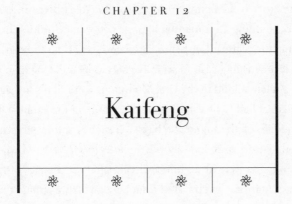

CHAPTER 12

Kaifeng

♪❋ MARGARET PLACED FAR GREATER IMPORTANCE
on her arrival in China than on the journey there. At Ostend she boarded
the Nord Express to Moscow, again travelling first class for her health's sake.
The carriage was overheated and the windows locked shut, but happily, it
cured her cold, for it was gone in one day. Although it was springtime,
the scenery was uninteresting. All she saw of Berlin from the train were
the ugly warehouses and rail sidings on the outskirts.

At the Russian border town of Alexandrovitch, all passengers had to
leave the train and go into a waiting room, where their passports were
collected and taken into a side room for examination. After a long anxious wait, the railway official re-emerged. As he knew no English, the
passengers crowded round him to claim their documents as they came
into view. He made no attempt to establish whether or not they had the
right ones. Margaret was greatly relieved when she spotted her name and
hurriedly repossessed her passport.

In Moscow she changed trains for the Trans-Siberian Express, which
was quite straightforward. All she had to do was to get off her train and
walk forward along the platform to board the train in front. Now there

were to be three passengers in the compartment instead of two as before, but they were quite comfortable. The food in the dining car was excellent. The train crossed the famous bridge over the Volga River and travelled on slowly, stopping at numerous stations with opportunities for a brisk walk along the platform. A bell rang when it was time to return to the train, with an ensuing rush to scramble back onboard. One man was too late and got left behind in the Ural Mountains without his luggage.

All luggage had to be examined at Manchuli on the Chinese frontier. In the middle of the night, the bags were taken into a large hall and placed on platforms. Everybody was anxious to get back to bed, but the customs officials were in no hurry. Finally, after six changes of trains in twelve days, Margaret had travelled from London halfway round the world, across the whole of Europe and Asia. She arrived in Peking just in time to spend a happy Easter at the mission before completing her journey by travelling down the Peking-Hankow line to Kaifeng. Even this leg involved changing trains at Zhengzhou (Chengchow), the current capital of the province of Henan.

Mr. and Mrs. Herring of the American Southern Baptist mission kindly offered Margaret their hospitality while she awaited her final change of trains. Mrs. Herring told her there were rather sore feelings in the China Inland Mission (CIM) in Kaifeng, as Bishop White of the Canadian Church Mission planned to build a hospital in a compound adjoining the American Southern Baptist mission, where a hospital already existed.

Kaifeng was a medium-sized walled city, too close for its own good to the Huang He—a waterway often referred to as China's Sorrow. Kaifeng had little to show for its two one-time distinguishing features. Prior to 1127 A.D., the Northern Song dynasty had established itself with Kaifeng as its thriving imperial capital. The Mongol invasion from the north drove them to re-establish themselves in Hangzhou in Zhejiang Province for the period known as the Southern Song dynasty. The second and possibly more remarkable feature was the Jewish community that could trace its ancestry at least as far back as the Ming dynasty (1368–1644). An emperor had conferred upon the residents seven surnames by which they could be distinguished, such as Shi, meaning "Stone," and Jin, meaning "Silver," both common surnames among western Jews today. Chinese Jews boast one of the most amazing histories in the Diaspora. Evidence points to their presence in China as early as the eighth century; they are believed to have travelled from Persia to China, in all probability along the Silk Road.

By Margaret's time, few traces of their synagogue remained, but it transpired that Bishop White had conducted considerable research on this subject, and published his findings. Margaret stayed with Bishop and Mrs. White in Kaifeng for a few days. When she questioned him about duplicating hospital facilities virtually in the same location, he informed her that only a rather primitive men's hospital existed. After he took her to see it the next day, she agreed that there was indeed room for his hospital, which was to be for women and children only.

Bishop White presided over a new diocese of the Anglican mission (*Sheng Gong Hui*), and the new Canadian Church Mission was supported and staffed by the Episcopal church in Canada. The various Canadian Protestant missions were autonomous; while each acknowledged the other's work, there was virtually no liaison between them, instead an acrimonious degree of rivalry. Bishop White had previously worked in Fujian (Fukien) Province, and was currently in the process of learning Mandarin. The rest of the missionaries were young and new. Margaret was the senior missionary, as she was on her second term and could speak the language; consequently, Bishop White put her in charge of the women's work. He also ordered her to supervise the boys' orphanage and the construction of his new hospital.

The plans for the hospital had been drawn up by architects in Canada. It was to be a three-storey building with a basement, a construction twenty-five metres (80 feet) long with verandahs on the east and west sides. The east wing was to be the residence for a foreign doctor and nurse. The foundations had already been excavated, and to Margaret's horror, they were full of water where the builders were driving in strong piles. Margaret's hospital in Pingyin was built on rock. She was so shocked to see the water that she went to ask the bishop if he knew. All the foundations were like that, he said, and she need not be concerned. This area was near the Huang He, which was higher than the surrounding land. To offset the situation there was a system of levees beyond the banks.

It gradually became apparent that the bishop intended to establish this hospital as his key project to mark his authority and influence. His presence was invariably apparent due to his vainglorious manner as well as the unmistakable noise of his motorcycle—his usual form of transportation around the diocese.

Although the work on the building progressed apace, Margaret was far from satisfied with the workmanship. She began by having the miserable door and window frames taken down, saying that no frame was to go up without her signature. The workmen complained to the bishop that they could not work to Margaret's standard for the agreed price. It amused him to quote their comment: "She wants too good work." For all that, it had to be her way or no way, which suited the bishop well enough.

Suddenly there began a spate of serious illnesses in the mission. The nurse, Miss Holland, was sent to Hankow for an appendectomy; the Reverend A. J. Williams developed a type of typhoid that lasted, with relapses, for twelve weeks; Mrs. Beatrice Jones, who was doing evangelistic work in the city, came down with smallpox. The CIM was not willing for their newly arrived nurse to help and there was no nurse available from Hankow, so Margaret moved into the city, where she and Miss Bessie Benbow nursed Mrs. Jones. She called in a CIM doctor for a consultation, as she thought Mrs. Jones might not survive. She was completely covered with spots, and twice daily Margaret wrapped her in wet sheets saturated with mercurochrome. She eventually recovered without a blemish.

When the women were out of quarantine, Mrs. Jones was sent to Jigong Shan (Chikung Shan) to join Miss Holland for convalescence. Then Margaret had to look after Mr. Williams, until she contracted typhus fever herself. By this time almost everyone in the mission had gone to Jigong Shan for the summer vacation.

Henan and the neighbouring provinces were in a state of famine during the summer of 1913. Although Margaret had warned the bishop prior to her arrival that she needed to be careful of her health, he added yet another duty to her busy schedule: to provide medical assistance in a famine camp nearby. The camp, some distance outside the city, was reached by mule cart. The magistrate in charge took the relief group round, and Margaret admired the way the camp was organized. The people came from all over the countryside, an extremely desolate region. Only women and children, forty thousand in all, were admitted. The men had to fend for themselves. They were housed in long mat sheds with half-open fronts; there was no fear of rain in summer. Their millet porridge—the main food—was cooked in great cauldrons. Of course, the mission group attracted attention, and the people crowded round. When the crowd obstructed progress, the attendants in front flicked their whips and the crowds fell back, people sometimes tumbling over like ninepins, causing great amusement and shouts of laughter.

The magistrate authorized a large tent to be erected as a dispensary, part of which would be a waiting room, with a consulting room partitioned off at one side. This was situated in a small yard enclosed by a mat fence to keep the crowds at bay. One or two women warders ushered in the patients and kept order. Margaret took a Bible-woman with her, but she had no other helper. One long tent made of matting served as an infirmary, with a separate one for cases of smallpox, which was very prevalent. The Chinese have many superstitions about smallpox, known as *tianhua* (heavenly flowers), and they were none too willing for Margaret to even visit that tent. "It's only smallpox," they would say. Actually, there was nothing she could do, for there was no possibility of nursing. She doubted if her efforts would have been any more than a gesture. Smallpox had long been endemic in China, and fatalities were relatively rare.

At last the spring rains came, the land began to look green and the camp could be disbanded. People were as anxious to leave as they had been to be admitted, but all was carried out in an orderly manner. Some people trekked back to their homes; others had too far to go or were too weak. They wandered about the Kaifeng streets to beg, and many died where they collapsed.

Bishop White, seeing further need, suggested making a mat shelter on a piece of mission land behind the new hospital. The CIM doctors had their own work and were disinclined to give assistance. The bishop again turned to Margaret to care for the refugees, and she agreed. Then the CIM doctors advised that typhus was rampant, so he should not let her undertake it. The bishop consulted Margaret, telling her that she must stop if there were any typhus patients. She had never seen a case of typhus, but she answered that she would not give the work up once she had begun. This he well knew would be the case.

Margaret's shelter, a long tent of matting spread over bamboo scaffolding, could hold one hundred patients. It was soon filled. Her helpers were some of the women refugees, and the Bible-woman with her son. He assisted with dressings, and acted as her orderly. They were no beds or equipment, so the sick women lay upon straw on the ground. Margaret visited them twice daily, first seeing to new patients, then going round the "beds." She had seen lice before—but never in such profusion. With each new patient, one of the helpers took a stiff broom and brushed off the lice, which were thick on the outside of every ragged blue coat. There was no sterilizer, but they did their best to wash the clothes.

After her rounds, Margaret headed straight home to bathe and disinfect herself, followed by a complete change of clothing. However, there was plenty of time for her to get bitten while in the tent. One day she felt shivery and feverish, so she took quinine and felt better for it. On the third night her temperature rose to 104°F. Dr. Guinness had invited her to dinner with the Reverend and Mrs. George Simmons, but she could not go. When he called round early the next morning, Margaret told him she had been "fitting her head into triangles all night."

Both doctors were well aware that this was typhus fever. He called her spots "mosquito bites," but she knew it was the work of lice. Dr. Guinness was most concerned, and he wired to Hankow for a nurse. Margaret took an intense dislike to the Hankow nurse and would not let her do anything for her; consequently, she left. Margaret had no recollection of this. Miss Holland was called back from Jigong Shan, and she nursed the recalcitrant invalid most efficiently and patiently back to health, but it took quite a while.

The day after Margaret took to her bed, Mrs. Simmons brought her a blank cheque to sign. This was a sensible thing to have done, for had she died the mission would have been without funds to carry on the women's work. Margaret thought to herself, "They think I'm going to die, but I won't." Her resolve helped her to recover, although at times she wondered if she really could pull through. When the ends of her fingers had swollen almost into knobs, she cried, "Look at my hands! It's no use trying any more."

From time to time she suffered hallucinations, including children being swept out from under her bed, and patients waiting in the next room for her heart—and that being many decades before the first heart transplant took place. She also became almost blind and very deaf. Her orderly, the Bible-woman's son, died of typhus and was buried in a plot across the road. The others were afraid Margaret might hear the funeral music and ask questions, but she heard nothing, not even the loud claps of a passing thunderstorm.

After the crisis, Margaret was so weak that she could not turn her head for Miss Holland to do her hair. When she tried to read all the words were blurred, but gradually both sight and hearing returned to normal. One night there was a terrific explosion. When Miss Holland checked if it had alarmed her patient, Margaret said quite calmly, "Oh, that was only an explosion."

Then she had a copious haemorrhage from the lung. When she saw the anxious face of the nurse holding out a kidney basin for her, she announced serenely, "It's all right. I often do that." Strangely, this event seemed to set her mind at ease. The great thing was that it was her last haemorrhage.

Margaret attributed her persistent vomiting to weakness. She never refused a glass of milk, though she would say, "It will all come back, but I will drink it anyway." One day she begged Miss Holland to let her have some English cabbage, as she knew there was some growing in the bishop's garden. Miss Holland was apprehensive but yielded to Margaret's pleas. She could not eat much, but she kept it down. A few days later she craved sardines and managed to consume a couple. At last she was well enough for Miss Holland to leave her for a while. One day Margaret demanded to see how the hospital construction was progressing, and she was carried round in a chair, but still she found it exhausting.

Once again, almost everyone had gone to Jigong Shan for a respite from the summer heat. Dr. and Mrs. Guinness had been waiting till Margaret was strong enough to join them. Though barely recovered, she made them believe she felt fine. She was carried to the train in a chair and along the platform, only to find she could not climb the step. At Jigong Shan most people walked from the station up the hill, but she had to be carried. It was wonderful to arrive safely at last and join the other missionaries in a substantial stone building belonging to the mission.

At first she could barely walk, falling down readily for no apparent reason. All the same, she applied herself assiduously to fostering her recovery. She had always enjoyed walking, so despite her stumbles she concentrated on both exercise and physiotherapy, reverting to needlework to keep her hands busy. Margaret was an avid knitter and keen on crochet. She designed and created a simple yet beautiful embroidered piece of red silk thread on linen, using every known stitch to embellish her work. It remains a treasured heirloom in her family.

With dismay Margaret heard Mrs. Jones, her smallpox patient, coughing frequently. She was horrified at the condition of her lungs, which showed signs of advanced TB. Mrs. Jones realized that nothing could be done about her condition. She told Margaret that her fiancé had gone to Canada and she had followed to marry him; after he had failed to meet her, she found him in hospital, dying of consumption. She asked that they be married, and she nursed him to the end. Afterwards, she took some missionary training and was accepted for Henan, as there was no evidence of her having acquired the disease.

The smallpox was too heavy a strain on her system, so the seeds flourished. Bishop White had gone to England several weeks previously, and when he returned in October 1914, he insisted that Mrs. Jones go to

Switzerland, refusing to listen to Margaret's opinion that she was too weak to travel. Obliged to carry out his orders, with a heavy heart Margaret accompanied Mrs. Jones as far as Hankow and saw her safely onto a river steamer. After Mrs. Jones arrived in Switzerland, Margaret received an irate letter from her Swiss doctor, expressing disapproval of her subjecting a patient in such poor condition to an arduous journey. Though this served to confirm Margaret's opinion which had been dismissed so cavalierly by Bishop White, the damage was done. Mrs. Jones was sent home to England, where she died a few months later.

♪⁂

MEANWHILE, China was undergoing a considerable amount of political turmoil which, fortunately, had little impact on Kaifeng. Although Margaret had been too busy or too ill to be aware of political happenings, she did hear a related explosion while recovering from typhus. The situation consisted mainly of rumours and ill-informed discussions. Yuan Shikai, first president of the Republic of China, was really a monarchist at heart. He had been a prominent figure in the Manchu court, but later court intrigues brought him into disfavour. When the final revolt against the Manchus took place, Yuan threw in his lot with the rebels led by Li Yuanhong. Dr. Sun Yat-sen was initially acclaimed as the leader of the Republic, but he passed on the honour to Yuan, a popular, more experienced statesman.

Margaret returned to Kaifeng after convalescing from June 3 to August 22, the dates inscribed on the flyleaf of her well-worn, leather-bound Chinese copy of the New Testament. Even this long recuperation was not adequate, but she wanted to relieve Rev. Simmons, who had been overseeing all the construction work on the hospital as well as the orphanage, now being transferred to a new building in the boys' main compound.

By the time Bishop White returned to Kaifeng, considerable progress had been made. With some pride Margaret showed him around the building, but to her chagrin, he uttered not a single word of approval, instead pointing out a number of minor defects. By now, Margaret was beginning to understand the full measure of Bishop White's character. While she respected him as being capable, she saw him as hypercritical and arrogant. She was hurt by his chauvinistic attitude and told him so. His imperious attitude had not been conducive to a happy state of affairs throughout the mission for a considerable time.

Before the end of the summer, the hospital was completed within and without, and was well-equipped. The former boys' orphanage was consigned for use as an isolation hospital, for both Bishop and Mrs. White were morbidly nervous about infection. The bishop was interested in help for the lepers from his time in Fujian, and he enquired whether Margaret would care to specialize in leprosy. She responded that as far as she knew there was no leprosy in Henan. He then insisted that she not take any more tubercular patients. Disregarding his advice, she continued to isolate and treat all cases of TB that came her way, viewing his counteraction as unacceptable, for he was unaware that many people had it in their systems already. Without question, she would keep all recognizable cases separate in the annex.

The fine operating theatre had good north light, and the floor was of the best Ningpo lacquer. Although only a two-storey building, it had the advantage that its roof could be used as a drying area. Rainwater from a large cistern, connected to pipes from the roof, was pumped to a cistern above the operating theatre so as to ensure a constant supply of cold water upstairs. There was a separate laundry, which Margaret supervised personally, due to her low regard for Chinese laundry abilities.

Bishop White planned a public ceremonial opening of the hospital. He had a silver key made, intending to ask the governor to unlock the main door and declare the hospital open. It all sounded very fine. Then he wrote to Margaret to inform her that he had decided to be the president of the hospital.

After all her trials and tribulations, Margaret could not face the perpetual interference that would undoubtedly ensue, so she promptly wrote back, saying in that case she would have to resign. She sent her resignation to Canada, returning in the meantime to Jigong Shan for a holiday.

She was there on August 14, when the Great War broke out, so she expected to return to England to do her bit. Instead she received a cablegram from Canada saying, "RESIGNATION NOT ACCEPTED; AWAIT LETTER."

A call for medical assistance arrived from a mission station at Jiujiang in Jiangxi Province, downstream of Hankow on the south bank of the Yangzi River. The American Baptist mission asked Margaret to come to their aid, as Dr. Mary Stone was down with typhoid. She wired Bishop White for permission, then proceeded to Hankow to await his consent. While permission was granted, the bishop made his displeasure clear by first stating his disapproval.

Margaret took a river steamer down to Jiujiang, where she received a warm welcome. The fine hospital had a good staff of Chinese nurses, including one of her faithful trainees from Pingyin. She also found herself in charge of Dr. Stone's eight adopted children of various ages. The hospital ran smoothly and she did several operations. She was once called to a case of a difficult labour. The usual crowd surrounded the house, blocking the light from the window. After the baby was safely delivered, as Margaret stepped into a sedan chair, almost under her feet came a great burst of fireworks—a sign of rejoicing and felicitation.

Two or three nurses came down with typhoid, and suspicion fell on one of the hospital wells. Then Miss Woodruffe, with whom Margaret was living, went to Guling, a nearby mountain resort, for a weekend, and whilst there, she too developed the disease. At last Dr. Perkins, who had been looking after Dr. Stone, came down from the mountain resort, and Margaret was asked to go up and take care of Miss Woodruffe, who was still seriously ill. By then Guling was practically deserted, all the summer visitors having left. Margaret had a lonely two weeks with only two Chinese nurses to talk to. She wandered around the mountain, passing houses dotted here and there, but she did not venture far. Finally Miss Woodruffe was carried down the mountain, and Margaret was released to return to Kaifeng. The Jiujiang climate did not suit her; she had felt stolid and dull the whole time.

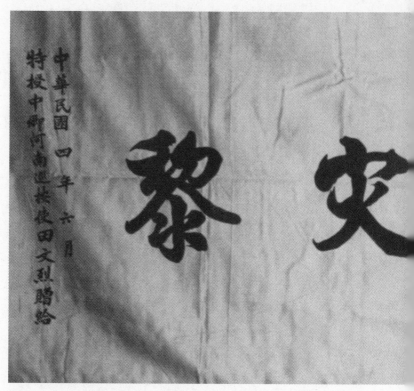

These four characters are embroidered on a sheet of blue silk, just under three metres long and one metre wide (approx. eight feet by three feet). The characters, read from right to left, may be translated as "Loving Kindness Shielded the Stricken."

The anticipated letter from Canada arrived, informing her that she was expected to fulfill her contract and that Canon Sydney Gould, the secretary of the mission board in Canada, was coming to look into the affairs of the mission. The mission board was quite concerned over the amount of illness incurred among its staff: appendicitis, smallpox, typhus, tuberculosis. One evening the bishop asked Margaret to attend a conference with Canon Gould, and they discussed Bishop White's plans for a ceremonial opening of the hospital with him as its president. The canon stated that none of this was essential for the smooth running of the hospital, so the scheme was revoked and Margaret was persuaded to withdraw her resignation. Early the next morning, she wrote a memo out-

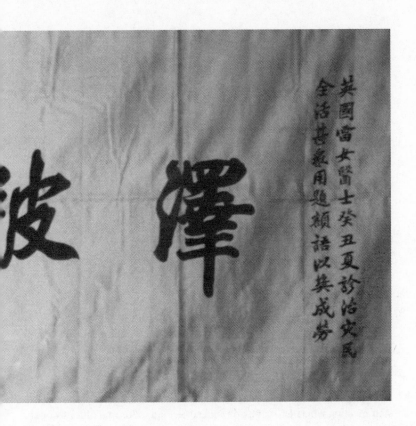

laying those decisions and sent it to Canon Gould for confirmation. He returned the document, saying that as far as he recalled, it was correct.

One day, as Canon Gould went round the hospital with her, Margaret amplified her views against opening the hospital with a formal ceremony, pointing out that it could foment bad feelings with the CIM. When the CIM helped her mission by buying the land for them, they had been unaware of any intention to build a hospital. The canon replied that could not be helped and Margaret must try to run the hospital on foreign lines so that, in effect, there was no competition. Margaret was unaware that the CIM was planning to build their own women's department, which was shortly brought into being. As her hospital was a foreign building, she went ahead with running it, not on Chinese lines, but like an English hospital. There would certainly still be room for both establishments.

Directly after Canon Gould left, the bishop began making further plans for the hospital, to establish a committee for hospital management with himself as chairman. This would have been reasonable enough but for the inclusion of certain administrative restrictions requiring Margaret to request his permission for everything she did, such as dismissing or engaging amahs and coolies—even her training agenda for the nursing staff. Since she would not think of interfering with the bishop's ecclesiastical administration of his diocese, she saw no reason why she should tolerate his usurping her medical authority in the running of her hospital. She did not trust him to act strictly as a chairman and nothing more. She told him that she would again tender her resignation as this was contrary to their agreement, whereupon he denied any written agreement. When Margaret showed him her memo, he then said he would leave it entirely up to her. And so he did. Plainly, Bishop White could no longer take advantage of her willing nature.

There was no public opening ceremony in November 1914—just a staff meeting where Margaret announced St. Paul's Hospital officially open.

♪*

MEANWHILE, the Chinese authorities were well aware of the benefits derived from Margaret's ministrations on behalf of the populace around, and in due course she received a handwritten letter from C. F. Hsiu of the Bureau for Foreign Affairs in Kaifeng, Henan, dated June 11, 1915:

I beg to inform you that the Civil Governor of this Province has conferred you 4 Chinese characters "ZE BEI ZAI LI" to be put on a board in appreciation of the famine work done by you. I feel sure that you are well deserving of this honour.

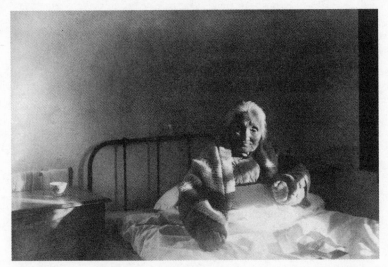

An elderly woman patient, in the newly constructed St. Paul's Hospital in Kaifeng, c. 1914.

Margaret received a handsome heavy board of black lacquer, 90 by 250 centimetres (3 x 8 feet) in size, with the characters in embossed classic Chinese calligraphy, as well as a facsimile in blue silk of the same dimensions with the characters hand-embroidered in black. This ensured that she had something less cumbersome which she could take with her wherever she went.[1]

♪✻

THE NEW HOSPITAL'S FIRST PATIENT was an old woman who must have thought she had died and gone to heaven. She took very kindly to her new surroundings, and after her broken leg had healed nicely, every time the subject of leaving the hospital arose, she found a new complaint. Finally, she had to be discharged before she produced something really serious.

Dr. Agnes Tso, the Chinese assistant, was most helpful, and she and Margaret got on well together. To have suitable training material to hand,

Margaret was translating Joseph De Lee's *Obstetrics for Nurses* into Chinese with help from Dr. Tso. From no trained Chinese nurse at first, soon there were fifteen in training, and they swept and dusted the wards. Six amahs did other cleaning and washed the green linoleum floor twice daily. The nurses had to be made to feel useful as soon as possible, therefore practical work was the main focus during the first year. Every morning Margaret took all the nurses round for inspection—including their own rooms. This hospital was as clean as any foreign one.

Every morning Margaret opened the outpatients department with a short service for outpatients and staff, including the men. She held morning prayers for the hospital nursing staff in the small prayer room, and whenever a difficulty arose, they met for prayer and conference.

Margaret preferred to examine her patients in quiet and privacy, but that was seldom possible, owing to the number of relations, friends and neighbours on the scene. A little polite firmness would reduce the numbers to about half a dozen. Sometimes she was called to attend a patient who had had a hysterical fit after an attack of temper and was lying seemingly unconscious—often a ruse to keep the parents-in-law under control, as the Chinese were terrified by anything abnormal such as unconsciousness. As the examination proceeded, a flickering eyelid would betray the insuppressible curiosity—the first step towards recovery as the patient's mind was diverted from its former upset. A soothing prescription and a loud suggestion that the patient might be better in an hour or so was generally effective.

Attempts at suicides were frequent. The favourite method was by taking poison—opium, lead (from face powders), arsenic, alkalis—or by swallowing the heads of several boxes of phosphorus matches and then drinking kerosene. Gold was considered very poisonous, and swallowing a gold ring was an aristocratic way of committing suicide. Hanging was fairly common. A dispensary patient who had been cut down in time was deathly pale, her neck ringed with an ugly bruise mark from the rope. Cutting one's throat was uncommon, but in a fit of rage a knife might be snatched up and the deed done with the intention of bringing some sort of retribution to the offending party. Margaret was once called to attend a woman who had cut her throat; her friends refused to take her to the hospital "for fear her head might drop off."

Margaret also attended any foreigners who required her services, mainly from the American Southern Baptist mission. Mrs. Harris, with her large family, being one who needed her most, usually sent for the doctor in good time, but when her youngest baby became ill, she waited too long. Margaret found the baby dying from pneumonia and could not save him.

♪❊

ON CHRISTMAS DAY, Bishop White invited the missionaries to dinner. During the meal Margaret began to have sharp pains in her appendix, which had grumbled for years, particularly during the past summer. She made some pretense at eating and sat quietly during the games that followed. Her fever was not high, nor were there any violent symptoms. She reported the situation to the bishop the next morning and said she would be all right after a few days in bed. He insisted that she go to Hankow to have the operation during the upcoming Chinese New Year season, when the hospital would be closed. He preferred not to risk an emergency operation in Kaifeng. In due course Margaret went to the Roman Catholic hospital, where a successful operation was performed and she was well cared for by the sisters. She recovered rapidly, and thoroughly enjoyed the good French food.

For her recuperation, Margaret moved on from Hankow down the Yangzi River to Jiujiang and spent a weekend with the missionaries there before proceeding farther. The river cruise down to Shanghai she found uninteresting. In Shanghai, she attended the China Medical Missionary Association conference, a large gathering from all over China. She had been invited to read a paper she had prepared, entitled "Treatment of Tuberculosis in China." Her audience was a significant, experienced group, and her description of pneumothorax treatment—the method based on her experience under Dr. Carling at the Berkshire and Buckinghamshire Joint Sanatorium—was most effective. Dr. H. Jocelyn Smiley of the Peking Union Medical College (PUMC) Hospital instituted its use in that hospital, where it was continued for many years. This lecture marked a crowning moment in Margaret's medical career, and fifteen years later she submitted a thesis under the same title.

Margaret returned to Kaifeng much refreshed, and she set to work with renewed vigour. In view of what had occurred over the year, she did not feel entitled to a long holiday. Instead she went into the country by mule cart to see her good friends, Rev. and Mrs. Simmons, who were stationed there. After that, hospital work continued apace till the end of the year.

♪✳

BISHOP WHITE HAD GONE TO CANADA, his third absence from his diocese within three years. The mission was in an unhappy state. One man had left for health reasons; another had resigned. One day, when Margaret was visiting the CIM, Dr. Guinness mentioned he had heard that her hospital was to be closed. She replied that he must be mistaken, but just before the year ended, the blow fell.

A letter came from the mission headquarters in Canada saying that on account of the proximity of the hospital to the CIM premises, it would be closed until after the war, then relocated to the nearby town of Guide (pronounced *Gway-der;* then known as Kweiteh). Margaret was instructed to close down St. Paul's Hospital immediately, and pack up all the equipment. The news was unexpected, despite the hint from Dr. Guinness. Margaret felt it was a wicked decision and altogether unfair without any sort of consultation, much less an opportunity to prepare. Similarly, she was stunned at the terms she was given: passage money to return to England, provided she went in six months, and three months' salary. After all that she had achieved for the good of the mission field over the past ten years, this poor recompense was little short of insulting.

Margaret found it hard not to suspect Bishop White's hand in this turn of events. It seemed unlikely that he had not been consulted. The hospital, which had been his idea in the first place, would no longer be a thorn in the flesh of the CIM, which as a result made this a sound political move.

The plunge from the pleasant glow of her award from the Chinese authorities to the chill of her virtual dismissal, all within a few months, was galling in the extreme for Margaret. Everyone thought the war must end soon, so she no longer considered offering her services in England. What would she do there? Her father had moved to New Zealand, for health reasons, and she did not want to become a burden to her family. Nor did she wish to be taken ill again, and as China suited her health, she thought it wiser to stay. But she baulked at the idea of letting the mission off so lightly. She had paid her fare to work for five years, and she had worked unstintingly, so she demanded the return of her passage money. She could not help feeling how much better fiscal sense it would have made to let the hospital justify its cost until her furlough was due, which would have been in another two years' time. She wondered whether, had they studied her first annual report (see Appendix D), the decision might have been reversed.

Margaret needed the demanded money, for she had spent all her salary in furnishing her home. Her salary was small, as for all single women workers, whereas unmarried male doctors received a considerably larger sum, to the extent that one could even afford to keep a pony. Margaret had previously maintained that all doctors should get equal pay, but the bishop scoffed at the idea, remarking flippantly that men needed more money because they did not know how to be economical.

Feeling disillusioned, Margaret did not wish to join another mission. For the next three months, she was busy dismantling the hospital and balancing the accounts so as to hand everything over to Mrs. Simmons. She also set about finishing the translation of Dr. Lee's *Obstetrics for Nurses.*

✻

HAPPILY, she did not have long to wait to find out what to do next, for the news of her imminent departure from Kaifeng had spread rapidly. Obviously no opprobrium had been attached to the humiliating treatment; in next to no time, no fewer than nine openings were offered to her. First came a telegram from the Canadian Presbyterian mission, north of the Huang He; then an invitation from Dr. Ida Kahn, who had a large hospital at Changsha in the province of Hunan—but Margaret feared for her health in that climate. Of all her options, Margaret felt the greatest draw to Peking, where she had been invited to teach half-time at the newly organized Union Medical College for Women. She knew the climate would suit her, and she could remain in touch with her own church.

She wrote to Miss Bowden-Smith regarding the prospect of private practice there, which they had discussed earlier in England. This, Miss Bowden-Smith still considered could present expectations as good as any. Meanwhile, she offered Margaret living quarters in return for a little science teaching, as she was short of teachers due to the war. This was to be a great help to Margaret while starting her practice, especially financially. She lost no time in accepting, thus giving up her life as a mission doctor, and starting a new life as a "citizen of China."

She sold most of her furniture, hiring a rail boxcar and a servant to accompany the rest. With no intention of allowing the closure of St. Paul's to adversely affect her staff, she brought along one of her nurses to enter the Methodist mission's training school for nurses; the others were placed in different hospitals. By the time she reached Peking, little remained of the passage money she had managed to extract for her severance, though that had to keep her going for some time. The pound sterling, which had once been as high as $12.00 Chinese, had deteriorated so much during World War I that for a long time she could only get $3.00 for one pound, and for a few days it was down to $2.50. Fortunately, food was cheap, and the housekeeping bills extremely moderate.

As always, she was confident that, if she was doing the right thing, God would see her through. While she felt sad and confused over the outcome of her hard work in the face of considerable hardship and jeopardy to her health, she recalled the words of William Cowper: "God moves in a mysterious way / His wonders to perform."

Indomitably, Margaret obeyed as best she knew how what she believed to be His will.

INFLUENCE

Where is the work that I did last year
In many hours of toil?
Is it forgotten and lost by all but me?
Was it nothing but waste
The work that I tried to do?

Work that is done with all the heart
Can never be lost or wasted.
It is moving on in unknown ways;
It spreads and enlarges as time goes on,
As the stone that sinks to the river's bed
Leaves an ever-widening circle.

Where are the words that I said last month?
Does anyone remember them now?
The words that I said to cheer my friend,
The words that my temper let fly;
Have they given him courage to face life's ills?
Have they left a wound that will never heal?
Is anyone better for those words of mine?

Words that are spoken are no longer mine,
Though mine be the praise or blame.
They are passing on from mind to mind;
I shall never know the harm they have done
Or the good, if that be possible.

Where are the opportunities I missed last week
Of kindness, service and happiness?
The little attentions that soften the way,
The words of love I forgot to say,
The kindness I meant to pass on?

They are lost forever, they have passed away;
The gaps they have left I never can fill.
I shall always regret those chances I missed.
Though the gaps be there I will not despair;
The lesson is mine, I must learn it well.

Where are the thoughts that I had last night?
Ah! There lies mystery too deep.
They are buried within the tracks of my brain,
For good or ill they are with me still.
They are only asleep, they will wake again,
Those thoughts that I had last night.

(E. M. P.)

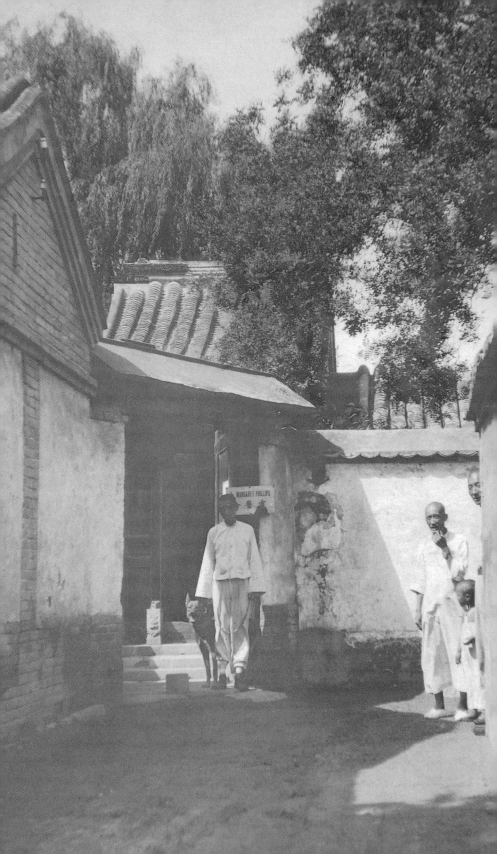

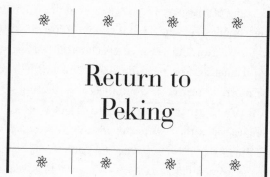

CHAPTER 13

Return to Peking

Ꮎ＊ Margaret's departure from Kaifeng was slightly delayed, as she had promised to assist Mrs. Harris of the Baptist mission with the birth of her child. The baby was safely delivered on April 2 and four days later Margaret left, accompanied by Wang Suqin, the nurse. Miss Bowden-Smith met them on arrival in Peking the following day.

Margaret and Miss Bowden-Smith, daughter of Lady Bowden-Smith, had first met in England while on furlough. Miss Bowden-Smith, then a teacher with the Society for the Propagation of the Gospel (SPG), had told Margaret that if she should ever consider a medical practice in Peking, she would gladly give her introductions to her Chinese friends. In desire for modern education, Miss Bowden-Smith had now rented part of a large Chinese house to establish her own day school, which taught both Chinese and Western subjects, and here Margaret would live and work. The rooms surrounded a big courtyard with two fine cypress trees. Leading from this courtyard were several side courtyards containing smaller classrooms, the staff living and dining rooms, and bedrooms. The great hall on the north side formed the main schoolroom. The pupils, all day scholars, were mostly from the official upper class of Chinese society.

Children of this class were usually taught at home by private tutors. Miss Bowden-Smith had spent many years in China teaching women and children in their homes.

On the evening of Margaret's arrival, Miss Bowden-Smith explained that two of her pupils were applying for Qinghua (Tsinghua) University scholarships to America and required coaching in chemistry, physics, physiology and English. The next day being Sunday, the two women attended the morning service at the cathedral. At teatime, Dr. Bryan-Brown and Bishop Scott with his niece, Miss Mary Scott, called to see Margaret. She walked with them to the mission for the English service at six o'clock, then stayed for supper at St. Faith's, which was still the residence of the women missionaries, as when she first went to China. The next two months brought many social calls and dinner invitations from various missions.

Classes began the next morning, easily filling Margaret's days. Looking back, she wondered how she managed to achieve all that she did, which included a good deal of church attendance. That evening Dr. Leonard of the Presbyterian mission came across the city to discuss Margaret's half-time work for the coming autumn at the Women's Union Medical College.

Soon afterwards, Miss Shebbeare, head of the Anglican mission girls' school, asked Margaret to attend to any pupil who became sick, as she had no mission doctor. Towards the end of the year, Bishop F. L. Norris, who had just replaced Bishop Scott on his retirement, wrote to ask if she would consider either joining the mission or becoming their visiting physician, which entailed attending the dispensary three times a week and looking after any sick women missionaries and their families. For this Margaret was offered half-time pay—hardly a generous offer, since missionaries lived rent-free and were entitled to furloughs and other allowances. But as it turned out, this was a better offer than either Bishop Norris or Margaret realized, largely because the families would pay her individually as private patients. Initially, the contract was for two years, which she gladly accepted. She pointed out, however, that although her relationship with the mission was happy, she preferred never to officially

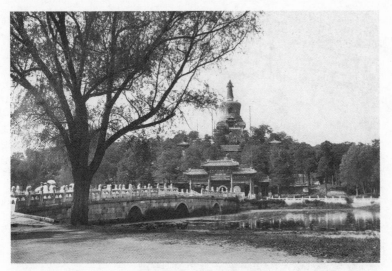

The Winter Palace in Peking. These lakes were artificially excavated and froze solid during the winter. During the summer months, the water was overgrown with lotus.

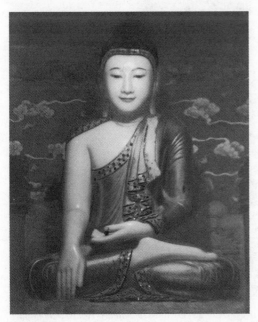

Just outside the entrance to the Winter Palace was a small temple housing the Jade Buddha, c. 1930s. The sash on the left shoulder was ablaze with jewels. The Buddha has since been robbed of this splendour.

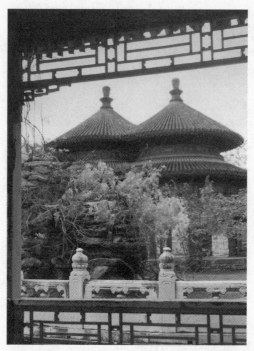

Unique to Peking are these two circular buildings with blue tiles which are by the lake of Zhong Hai south of the Winter Palace.

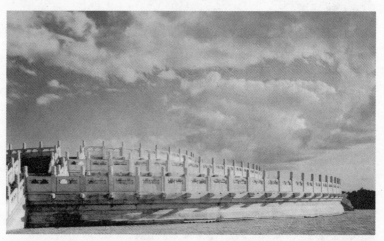

The Altar of Heaven. This three-tiered marble edifice resembles a vast wedding cake, 26 metres (approx. 85 feet) in diameter at the top. Here successive emperors plowed a ceremonial furrow after praying for a good harvest.

join a mission again. This arrangement proved entirely satisfactory and lasted more than twenty-five years.

Three times a week Miss Bowden-Smith went to the palace of the president, Yuan Shikai, to give English lessons to his son and daughter. Miss Waller, a mission friend, and Margaret persuaded her to request permission for them to see the famous South Lake (*Nan Hai*) of the Winter Palace, which subsequently became a public park. This was granted, and a pleasant afternoon was spent looking round a favourite palace of the empress dowager. It was so peaceful there.

∫*

MEANWHILE, the political situation remained the all too familiar seething mass of rumour, questioning and apprehension that Margaret had encountered on her arrival in Peking. Having thrown in his lot with the rebels led by Li Yuanhong, Yuan Shikai was largely instrumental in arranging for the abdication of the boy emperor, Xuan Tong (also named Henry Puyi). However, he overrated his own popularity when in 1916 he attempted to begin a new dynasty of his own. He felt that China was not yet ready for a republic, and he planned to install himself as emperor with the name of Hong Xian. Elaborate preparations were in place for the inauguration, with embroidered robes for himself and the chief courtiers, despite growing discontent and disapproval spreading throughout the provinces.

Matters came to a head when he went to the Altar of Heaven at the winter solstice, prior to Christmas 1915, to perform the ancient rites to the Supreme God of the Universe, a ceremony which was the sole prerogative of an emperor. A riot broke out in Yunnan Province, and the two earlier rebel leaders, Li Yuanhung and Zhang Xun, the Old Tiger, expressed total disapproval of Yuan's scheme; this spread throughout the nation. When Yuan realized the strength of the opposition, he hastily abandoned his ambitious program. He stated that since it was not the will of the people to revert to a monarchy, he would support the Republic with all his heart. It was too late, for the response to his repentance was the demand for his resignation since he had not been faithful to the Republic. His scheme had lasted only eighty-one days. In effect, this was the start of a drawn-out period of internecine war among the Chinese warlords.

This disturbing situation continued throughout May. It was rumoured that Yuan was ill, and that the French doctor, Dr. Bussière, had been called in to treat his disease. Margaret never found out whether or not he really saw his patient. Then came the news that Yuan had agreed to resign, repeating his regrets for having misunderstood the wishes of the people. He announced that he would leave the president's palace in the *Zhong Hai*, the Central Lake of the Winter Palace, no later than the fifth of the fifth moon, the occasion of the Dragon Boat Festival, one of the three most important festivals of the year. In 1916 this date, barely two months after Margaret's return to Peking, coincided with Monday, June 5, a general holiday, when all pupils were away. There were no newspapers, but there was an atmosphere of mystification and apprehension.

On June 6, the pupils returned to school. At 2:00 P.M., the death of Yuan Shikai was announced and excitement prevailed. The possible portent of his passing coinciding with the timing as announced was not lost on the public. Riots were expected, and many girls went home. The vice-consul called to tell the women to be ready for a summons to go into the British legation, so they packed their suitcases but had an uneventful night. As later events proved, Peking was a charmed city, passing calmly through every crisis.

June 9 was proclaimed a school holiday as a memorial to Yuan Shikai, after which the schools returned to normal. The vice-president, Li Yuanhong—the general who had led the revolt at Hankow in 1911 which precipitated the fall of the Manchu Qing dynasty and the establishment of the Republic—replaced Yuan. After five years of uncertainty, the crisis was finally over.

Yuan Shikai's funeral took place on June 28. Mat tents were erected at intervals along the route from the entrance to the *Nan Hai* to Watergate Station outside the Fore Gate (*Qian Men*), the route towards the Gateway to Heavenly Peace (*Tian An Men*) and again due south to the Fore Gate. These were resting places for the heavy coffin, which was borne inside a large palanquin, the two-tiered framework covered with beautifully embroidered curtains. This required no fewer than sixty bearers as part of a procession of three hundred, which included mourners, clad in white, who burned incense to Yuan and his ancestors along the route. Huge crowds lined the roadway for some two hours.

Margaret had waited near the Gateway to Heavenly Peace to no avail, as she was obliged to return to see patients at the Anglican dispensary. Understandably, there were fewer than usual, so when she had finished, she and Dorothy Bearder—who Margaret was happy to be reunited with in Peking—walked through the *Shun Zhi Men* city gate and along the embankment of the moat outside the city wall. It was a struggle to squeeze their way through the spectators waiting to see the train pass on its way to Yuan's family home in Henan Province. The two women finally reached the entrance to the station, which was guarded by troops. With not so much as a by-your-leave, they walked boldly up the steps. No one stopped them. They went right onto the platform. There they saw the coach containing the coffin, draped in blue (also a colour of mourning), and there they stood until the train steamed away.

♪⁂

MARGARET SOON SETTLED DOWN to a mixed routine of teaching, medical practice and social engagements. Her first call to outside patients unconnected with the mission was to see a girl who had recently had scarlet fever, which left her with a chronic throat infection. She had been given up on by Chinese doctors, but under Margaret's care she began to show signs of improvement almost at once. Margaret was allowed to visit her daily until she had quite recovered. Hers was a wealthy family with a large household. Nearly every time Margaret went, a new patient was produced till she must have attended most of the women and children in the house— sometimes as many as six in one visit.

About mid-June, Miss Alice Powell, nursing superintendent of the American Methodist Hospital for Women and Children, consulted Margaret about translating nursing training material into Chinese. Margaret told

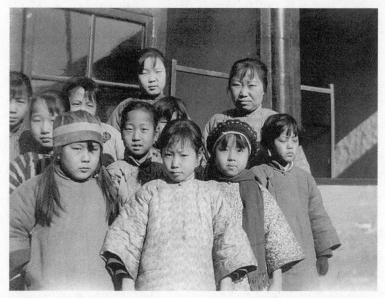

Upon returning to Peking, after World War I the care of children remained central to Dr. Margaret's medical practice.

her about her translation of De Lee's *Obstetrics for Nurses,* which she felt needed a good deal of revision. Miss Powell kindly provided Margaret with a good writer, so she went to the Methodist hospital nearly every day, sometimes twice, to create what over the next two months became almost a new translation. Final revisions saw it ready for publication after nearly six months. The nurses association purchased the textbook, and the proceeds from the sale allowed Margaret to lease a parcel of land in the Western Hills outside the city.

As promised, Miss Bowden-Smith took Margaret to call on some of her influential Chinese friends, while the mission, from then on, accepted her as one of their own. Nonetheless, she still preferred to remain independent. Miss Bowden-Smith was independent too, supporting herself and her school, though she was affiliated to the mission and consulted Bishop Norris about any planned new move. Her school, *Peihua*—the name meaning "cultivating the Chinese"—was between the boys' school and the mission, so callers frequently looked in. Visitors to the capital often stayed at one or the other of the mission houses. Though the East City was far removed from the west section, communication by rickshaw was easy and took less than half an hour, especially since the main cross-thoroughfare, *Chang An Jie* (Avenue of Eternal Tranquility), was now freely accessible to all traffic, an improvement since the Forbidden City was no longer the imperial residence. Bicycles were in general use by both women and men, including missionaries. Peking had become a city of schools, with boys and girls of all ages to be seen in the streets on their way to and from school.

When the summer vacation began at the end of June, the missionaries migrated to the St. Hilary's mission rest-house in the Western Hills or to the coast to avoid the humid heat of the July summer rains. There they recuperated, enjoyed family life and prepared programs for next year's work. Newly arrived missionaries continued their language studies. Margaret remained in Peking till the end of July, busy with her work at the Anglican dispensary and translating at the Methodist hospital. She did manage to have a long weekend at St. Hilary's, where she had last stayed more than ten years ago. The rather complicated journey there consisted of a long rickshaw ride to a railway station outside the north-west city gate, followed by a short but slow train ride to the village of Huang Cun, ending with an hour's walk across fields and up a hill. In contrast to Margaret's earliest visit, this trip was a considerable improvement.

During that summer break at the Hills, Margaret was asked to visit Mr. Gu, a sick man in the mission compound, who was a teacher at the Anglican mission boys' school in the city. He had been sent into the country to get sun treatment for the many enlarged glands in his neck. He was under other medical care but was getting worse, so after much persuasion she went to see him. She soon realized that the glands were not tuberculous; he was suffering from Hodgkin's disease, the first case she had encountered in China. Mr. Gu was getting worse rapidly, and as his wife demanded the truth, Margaret delivered the sad news. His wife then insisted upon a prognosis. Unwillingly, Margaret told her that if he continued to worsen at the current rate, he would probably live only about a month.

Mr. and Mrs. Gu returned at once to the city, where he "put his house in order" and made all arrangements for his funeral, a Christian one. One month to the day from Margaret's prognosis, he died. Margaret signed the death certificate. Mrs. Gu was able to claim a few thousand Chinese dollars, useful for educating her rather large family, though not so good for the insurance society as he had been insured for only a year. When Margaret enquired why he had taken out insurance, Mrs. Gu answered simply that he had not been feeling well—the disease was difficult to detect in the early stages—and thought it was a good thing to do. She told Margaret how glad they had been to know the truth in time to prepare for the future. A few months later, Margaret arrived home to find a small package on her desk containing a gold ring—a gift to convey the gratitude of Mr. and Mrs. Gu. The ring was heavy, for Chinese gold is nearly pure, and later she had it made into two rings. Whenever Margaret was asked if Chinese made grateful patients, she would answer in the affirmative, adding that one of her most grateful patients was one who had died.

At the end of the summer, all the missionaries returned home. Several patients awaited Margaret at St. Faith's. The following Sunday, the bishop held an ordination service at which no fewer than nineteen clergymen were present.

♪⁂

SOON AFTERWARDS Margaret made arrangements to rent a small separate court for twelve dollars a month from the landlord of Miss Bowden-Smith's Peihua School. The court had a separate entrance just inside the outer gate, making it convenient for Margaret's patients to reach her. She moved into her new compound in mid-September, though she continued to have her meals with Miss Bowden-Smith. The middle room was her study and to the right was her bedroom, while the left-hand room served as her consulting room. There were certain drawbacks. Margaret was asked to give houseroom to a double bed which Miss Bowden-Smith could not squeeze into any of her own small bedrooms and which was, in fact, rather a white elephant. So was the piano that Margaret also consented to accommodate. While it was nice to have a chance to practise on the piano herself, it was not so convenient when pupils came to practise or have lessons. Margaret purchased a nice couch for consulting purposes, only to find the room was too small. It was not long before she started to look around for a house of her own, which, as it transpired, was easier said than done. Eleven months elapsed before she succeeded.

In September, she began teaching medicine in Chinese, initially hygiene and embryology, at the Union Medical College for Women, for two hours three times a week. The dean, Dr. Eliza Leonard of the Presbyterian mission, was capable and down-to-earth. The senior class consisted of only four students. One of them, Marion Yang, became a leading physician in China, her career culminating in a position in the Ministry of Health. She too had a matter-of-fact, straightforward manner. Whenever they met, she always hailed Margaret as her teacher. Dr. Yang went on to establish a school of midwifery in Peking. Dr. Leonard died of cancer a few years later, and all her other teachers eventually left China.

Margaret's courses expanded to include pathology, public health and bandaging, and at times her classes had fifty students. In return for the use of obstetrics facilities, the Peking Union Medical College (PUMC) allowed her students to attend some of their courses, which allowed them the benefit of seeing live specimens. Since her students' English was inadequate for comprehending the PUMC's lectures, she attended classes with them and explained things afterwards.

♪✲

AFTER MARGARET MENTIONED to some Chinese friends that she wanted to set up practice in a home of her own, they asked their gate-keeper to find her a house. This seemed a strange person to ask, but in China nearly everything was done through a middleman of some sort (and, to some extent, it still is). Houses could only be rented through the middleman of the district, who formed the connecting link between one's servants and the servants of the future landlord. It was not necessary to even see one's landlord before moving.

Margaret's middleman, the gatekeeper, was quite optimistic and did his best to earn his share of the prospective "squeeze," or commission. Every day he arrived with a glowing description of a house that would be exactly right for her. She would accompany him to inspect some dilapidated-looking, worm-eaten, paint-lacking outbuildings in rows round a courtyard, more resembling barns and stables rather than any house. Finally, with some misgiving, after inspecting three discouraging displays of ruins covered with the dirt of ages, Margaret gave instructions to go ahead with negotiations. Her middleman then approached the other middleman to discuss the rent—always at first far beyond the value of the house, with the counteroffer far less than was intended to be paid; both gradually proceeded towards an agreement in middle ground. Then, just when everything seemed to be going satisfactorily, it was discovered that nothing would induce the landlord to allow a foreigner to occupy his house.

Margaret began to despair of getting a house, and to weary of those fruitless inspections. She implored her middleman to state plainly at the outset that the house was for a European, but this was not at all politic. However, everything in China comes right in the end. Mr. Ke, the husband of a Chinese patient, eventually found out that there was a house next door to his which the landlord would agree to let to her. He kindly acted as middleman and put through all the negotiations. The three-year lease, in Chinese, included a detailed description of the house: the number of rooms, doors, windows and even panes of glass, as well as the regulations with which Margaret was to comply.

After Margaret and the landlord had signed the lease, it was necessary to find a shop that would be willing to be her guarantor. This was not easy, for though the smaller shops were willing to oblige, they did not come up to the required standard. The larger shops did not anticipate her custom would suffice to compensate for the inconvenience of having the police nosing round their premises on the pretext of pursuing their enquiries. However, after many trials and disappointments, an obliging shop was found. This was achieved through Bishop Norris, who got his number-one boy to persuade the bicycle shop that the mission patronized to be the guarantor, and the lease was duly stamped with their business seal. Four copies of the lease—one each for the landlord and Margaret, and two for the police—were then sent to the police courts and to the Foreign Office for investigation and approval.

Three weeks later the lease came back and Margaret was allowed to take possession of the house. The rent book was produced, a concertina-shaped little book in a calico-covered case. She was required to pay three months' rent in advance, one of which was divided amongst the middlemen and the servants on both sides, and one credited to the last month of her tenancy. Although Mr. Ke was the real intermediary, the others having failed Margaret, the month's rent was shared between St. Faith's number-one boy, Miss Bowden-Smith's cook and a paperhanger. The latter was soon busy at work on the renovations, beginning with repapering the paper windows—essential maintenance twice a year. In the spring, the paper was affixed only at the top so that it could be rolled up, and netting was put on to keep out the flies and mosquitoes. In the autumn, the paper was pasted down to conserve warmth.

The next business was to make the place habitable. External repairs were the duty of the landlord, when he could be coaxed or coerced into doing them, but the internal repairs and decoration were the privilege of the tenant. A Chinese house may be altered to suit the convenience of the occupant, providing no alterations were made to the exterior structure. The landlord may require the house to be restored to its original condition when given back, and the rent would most certainly be raised in proportion to any improvements when the lease was to be renewed. So partitions were taken down in some rooms and put up elsewhere. All the walls were replastered, and the paper ceilings and windows renewed.

Moving in was a simple affair. No packing was needed, as all her furniture and belongings were carried on the backs of the coolies or in baskets slung from a pole supported on the shoulders of two men. They were dumped in glorious confusion, and then began the interesting task of settling in. The servants got to work with a will, and Margaret moved

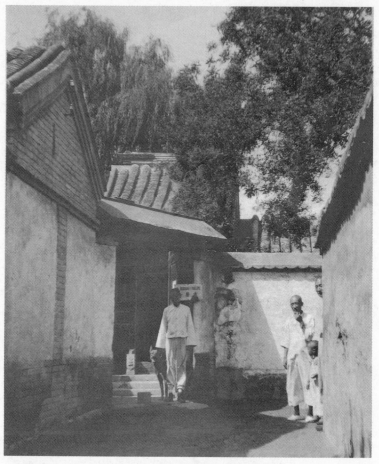

#13 Nanwantzu in Peking was to become Margaret's home as well as a comfortable resting place for many foreign visitors during the 1920s.

in on February 10, 1917. Bishop Norris loaned her some mission furniture for the dining room and bedroom, while she had furniture of her own for her study and consulting room. The rest she bought in stages when she could afford to expand.

An English house has the garden around it, but my Chinese house has the garden in the middle. For many months of the year the paved courtyard is my living room, and here in privacy I write or

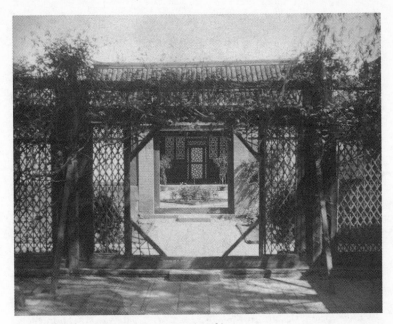

The middle courtyard at #13 Nanwantzu in Peking.

study and entertain my friends when they call…[S]everal trees… shade the stone flags from the blazing sun. The lilac bushes are the first to bloom, then the long white sprays of acacia unfold, the wild vine creeps over an old bamboo fence and is soon full of busy feasting bees. As summer advances the pink tassels of the "Glory tree" (mimosa) form a vivid patch of colour amongst the feathery green, but my favourite of all is the big weeping willow tree with its long streamers swaying with the breeze. Here the woodpecker finds many a savoury meal, and the courtyard echoes with his tapping. My flower beds are small, but gay with pansies, nasturtiums, snapdragon and many familiar English flowers. Here and there a few pots of pink and white oleanders give colour and fragrance…

Around the courtyard are the rooms, all with their windows facing the courtyard and their doors opening onto it. On the north side are the principal rooms…a large drawing room and dining room combined...the latter is partially separated by a screen of lattice work...[A] high-roofed verandah...keeps them cool in summer, but does not shut out the sun in winter...[Smaller] buildings... around the courtyard...are used as bedrooms. In some houses the side rooms are connected with the main building, so that one can pass from room to room without going outside, but in my house this is not possible, since indeed this facility is often obtained at the expense of light and air. Even in winter time it is good for the lungs to get some really fresh air and, if the courtyard is crossed at a run, one gets exercise too.

[A] dividing wall across the middle [of my large courtyard] ...[makes] the inner courtyard even more private. In a Chinese family the women all live in this inner courtyard where they are secure from the observation of callers or strangers. The wall is ornamented along the top with a border of tiles arranged in a conventional design. In the centre is a wide gateway surmounted by the same design in tiles on a higher level than the rest, thus breaking up the monotony of line. In a Chinese house a door fills this gateway, but I have taken away my four-leafed door so that I can see through into the courtyard beyond. For the same reason I have removed the wooden spirit-screen which usually stands inside to prevent the evil spirits (which are supposed to be unable to turn corners) from rushing straight through into the inner courtyard.

The roofs are much in evidence in the Chinese arrangement of a house, and are often very beautiful. Along the top of the roof of my main building is a high ridge which turns up at the two ends in a slender horn, and underneath the latter is a large carved tile of floral design. On either side of the ridge the tiles are arranged in careful lines alternatively convex and concave, forming deep channels for the rain. The edges of the roof are extended beyond the walls to form wide eaves which carry the water well away from the walls. On the projecting ends of each of the rafters an anti-clockwise gammadion swastika design is painted in white and green on the red of the wood, and on the supporting beams little pictures of flowers are painted which become very elaborate in some houses. The woodwork is painted a rich warm red which seems to suit the style of a Chinese house as no other colour would. The white paper of the windows, the green window framework, red doors, beams and pillars, grey walls and roof make a pleasing colour scheme.

The side of the house which faces the courtyard is entirely window from the roof down to the 3-foot wall which defines the space between window and ground. The lower half of the window consists of large panes of glass and the upper half is formed of a wooden lattice on which the paper is pasted. This lattice is made in many very artistic designs. In my house there are at least seven different designs, the most attractive being a "crazy" or "cracked ice" pattern. At night time the effect of the lit rooms showing up the lattice designs is charming . . .

Paper is pasted on the inner side of the latticework windows, some of it being left loose so that it can be rolled up like a Chinese scroll, around a little bamboo stick when it is desired to "open the window." This loose paper windowpane is kept in place by tightly stretched cords. A special kind of paper is used made from vegetable fibre, which is durable and yet allows a soft light to filter through...[P]aper windows are healthy as the ultraviolet rays can come through freely. There is the mistaken idea that paper lets in the cold. It is really warmer than glass and is more easily renewed. In the summer I take out the glass panes, tear off the paper, paste on netting and live in a birdcage.[1]

In the course of the next twenty years, Margaret moved house several times. Of all the houses she occupied during her residence in Peking, this was her favourite.

♪✳

MARGARET WAS HAVING A STRENUOUS TIME. She was working nine to ten hours every day, the varied nature of her work offering little opportunity for relaxation. Patients cropped up at any hour, including several with difficult confinements. Several letters arrived from her brother Frank; he had been fighting in France but was now back in England with rheumatic fever. A sharp attack of influenza pulled Margaret's spirits down. Miss Bowden-Smith was full of advice and criticism about teaching; this tended to discourage Margaret until she realized it was just "her way." It seemed to her that she had almost three full-time jobs.

In 1917, some medical colleagues signed up to join the Siberian Expeditionary Force for 1918–19. Margaret was rather keen to go, but she was asked to stay behind to help fill the gap created by the volunteers and to carry on with her teaching. She pondered whether she should go home and do more useful war work in England. However, in a letter, Frances, her sister-in-law in Sutton Coldfield, strongly advised her not to return because of the war conditions there. In the end, the fear of a breakdown in her health was the consideration that kept her in China. A restful long weekend at the beginning of the year at St. Hilary's in the Western Hills did the world of good to her morale.

That Sunday, four children of the compound caretaker, Liu, were to be baptized. Although he was not a Christian, the grandparents and the mother were, so the baptism was allowed. Just before the service Sister Edith asked if some of those present would sponsor the children; thus Margaret became a godmother to the eldest daughter, Meizhen, aged five. She undertook her baptismal responsibilities seriously, to the extent that she treated Meizhen as her ward, guiding and subsidizing her studies through to adulthood. As the girl grew up, Margaret was impressed with her intelligence and diligence, recognizing a kindred spirit and a similarity to her own progress some fifteen years earlier. She paid close attention to Meizhen's development and respected the girl's striving for a good education. Not surprisingly, her goddaughter subsequently took up the study of medicine.

Margaret's house was bigger than she needed, so with the extra accommodation available, she began to take in paying guests, or PGs, as she generally referred to them. This practice was sufficiently lucrative that she kept it up for two decades, the income subsidizing her charitable medical work as it developed over the years. Margaret's first boarder, Miss Fulton, arrived in March. Her parents were missionaries in Shenyang (then known as Mukden), and she had come to Peking to teach in Miss Leitch's School for English Children. It was partly because she needed somewhere to live that it occurred to Margaret to start such a venture.

That winter, Margaret experienced "one of the saddest events in my medical career." Mrs. Hughes had just given birth to her third child. Confinement was easy and her condition entirely satisfactory during the first two days, but on the third day she suddenly became acutely ill. Two doctors, called in for consultation, suspected haemorrhagic smallpox. Mrs. Hughes died, and only then, two hours afterwards, did the rash begin to appear. Five days later, the baby died of smallpox, the rash coming out abundantly after death. Margaret took two weeks' quarantine from teaching, though she seemed to have an unusual number of patients at the mission and in her private practice. Mr. Hughes's surviving children, Gilbert and Evelyn, and their nurse stayed with Margaret for a month until arrangements were made for them to go home to England.

One day in March, Margaret joined a group of friends on the city wall to watch a Miss Stinson "looping the loop" over the city. Then she was invited to a Chinese banquet where, for the first time, she tasted such delicacies as bird's nest soup and buried eggs (sometimes referred to as devilled eggs or thousand-year eggs). The eggs are buried in a mixture of lime and straw, and become almost gelatinous in appearance, with a flavour suggestive of almonds. They are cut up into slices, and with practice it is not hard to pick them up with chopsticks. Margaret found them "very palatable." Bird's nest soup is made from the nests of a type of swallow found on offshore rocky islands which feeds largely on seaweed. The nest consists of fibres held together and adhered to the rock by a jellylike mucilage the bird produces through its beak. This jelly, teased from the nest, forms the base of the soup, the flavour of which Margaret pronounced as "faint and not particularly interesting." This delicacy is often improved by the addition of pigeon eggs.

One day in the spring, Margaret was initiated into some of the niceties of diplomatic protocol. Miss Scott took her to pay calls in the British legation, one of the principal establishments in the Legation Quarter. She had not realized that it was customary (not just in Peking) for the new-comer to call upon the established residents first—this being to indicate to the latter that one had settled in and was ready to participate in the social scene. They had tea with Mrs. Turner, the consul's wife, and left cards on Lady Alston, the minister's wife, and Mrs. Lampson and Mrs. Brennan, the wives of other diplomatic representatives.

In May, a carnival was held at the American legation in aid of Red Cross relief. The highlight for Margaret was her first and only ride on a camel. Following common practice, she mounted the camel while it was kneeling on the ground. It was a curious feeling as the creature raised itself in two stages: first the front legs, which threw her backward, and then the hind legs, which threw her forward. She clung hard to the pommel and was relieved to be able to stay in the saddle, and even more so to get off.

Later that month, Mrs. P. M. Scott developed acute appendicitis. Telephones were out of order, so Margaret had to go first to the Methodist hospital to arrange for her admission and then collect her for the opera-tion, which proved rather troublesome; the appendix, which was adherent, had ruptured. After a struggle to convince the doctors to operate, Margaret administered the anaesthetic. For a few days Mrs. Scott appeared to be doing well, then she suddenly developed a high fever, and for many days she was critically ill. Margaret visited her constantly and once remained with her all night, as the nurses were unable to cope with such a critical illness. From time to time it seemed that she had stopped breathing, and Margaret had to bend over her to check. She had a peaceful night, but it had been touch and go. Mrs. Scott always declared Margaret had saved her life. She should have been operated on the first night, but in those days Peking hospitals were ill-prepared for working at night.

A while after Margaret had established her practice, she made a drawing of a nameplate, with her name in Chinese as well as in English. She then went off with her cook to a shop on Brass Street, in the Chinese City, to order a plate made to her specifications. By summertime it was ready and had been affixed to the wall outside the main entrance. That nameplate soon attracted attention. A policeman called to see her. After many polite remarks and questions about her birthplace, her age and family—all in keeping with Chinese courtesy—and how long she had been in China, he finally asked if the brass plate outside the gate was hers. Margaret acknowledged ownership, expressing admiration for its workmanship. Then he asked if she had a license to practise. No, she answered, adding that she was unaware of the necessity for one, or that she could get one. He replied most politely that she must have one if she wanted to hang up her brass plate, then went on to explain how this was done.

Until then Margaret had not realized that the Chinese regarded the practice of medicine on a par with shopkeeping or any other line of business: as a profit-making concern, far below the dignified profession of teacher. Mission hospitals and their doctors needed no licence, but for a brass plate which invited clients, a licence was required by law.

The brass plate was taken down, and Margaret went to the Peking law courts (*yamen*) to get an application form. After it had been filled out, she took it to be signed, only to be told that a photograph was needed. She had one taken, but when she went to collect it a few days later she did not recognize herself. Then she realized what had happened. Her hair, being a pale yellow, had come out white in the photograph. As this looked all wrong, her hair had been carefully blacked in. The photo certainly did not look suitable for identification purposes; nonetheless, it was accepted, and up went the plate once more. Peking was not a treaty port and foreign "business" was not legal, except in the Legation Quarter. But the *yamen* were tolerant—several foreign-run shops existed on Morrison Street (*Wangfujing Dajie*) and on Hatamen Street (*Chaoyangmen Nanxiao*). Margaret was delighted to get her licence. To the best of her belief, she was the first foreign doctor to do so. (Some years later, when a Ministry of Health was appointed, every doctor had to be registered.)

After that episode Margaret always had a nameplate outside her door. That summer she acquired her first Pekinese puppy. Her amah promptly named it Biqi, meaning "water chestnut," because it was round and black. Cute though he was, he was useless as a watchdog. One evening, her cook went outside the gate to take down her brass plate for the night, only to find it gone. It had been padlocked, but apparently not well enough to keep somebody from walking off with it. Obviously it was an attractive item to steal, if only for the metal, for being unique it was a useless item to sell. At least two others were stolen in the course of time, even though they were securely padlocked. Finally she had to be satisfied with an enamel plate, which served the dual purpose of marking her house as the residence of a foreigner as well as a doctor.

A friend loaned Margaret the use of a cottage for a month, located outside the city near the racecourse generally known as *Paomachang* (the name itself meaning "racecourse"). She took a young cook with her, leaving the amah in charge at home. The holiday was not very successful as it was unusually rainy, and she found it rather lonely with only the occasional visitor, such as Bishop Norris, who "donkeyed" out twice for tea. When the weather obliged her to remain indoors, she made use of her time knitting and writing letters. She also prepared a paper on a suitable hygiene syllabus for teachers for a forthcoming YMCA conference to be held at the Temple of the Sleeping Buddha (*Wo Fo Si*).

On the last day there, her cook was invited by neighbouring servants to a farewell breakfast. He was gone so long that Margaret wondered if he had returned to Peking on his own. When she went to check his room, he staggered out, saying that his friends had given him too much to drink, so would she get dinner for herself. He lurched violently, and after she managed to save him from falling into a flowerbed, she told him to go and lie down, then prepared her meal.

♪✳

IN THE SUMMER OF 1917, Bishop Norris wrote to Margaret asking her to take charge temporarily of the women's side of the little mission hospital; she recognized the similarity to twelve years previous when Dr. Aspland had given her the same responsibility. Miss Lambert was still the nurse in attendance, assisted by Dorothy Bearder. For three weeks Margaret attended the hospital daily, seeing outpatients as well as the inpatients, thinking that it was as well she had no teaching during the summer months, for schools closed for the hot months of July and August.

During July, two friends visited from the China Inland Mission (CIM) in Kaifeng, Miss Sollan, the sister of the CIM's Dr. Sollan, and Dr. MacDonald. During their few days together, Margaret found time to take them to the Temple of Heaven and the Central Park. At the end of the month she took a long train journey to Qinghuangdao (Chinhuangdao) on the coast, the port for British coal mines in Kailan. After leaving at 8:30 A.M., she arrived at 6:30 P.M., feeling delighted to be on holiday with the Reverend P. M. Scott, her host; Miss Waller, her school colleague; and Mrs. McDouall, with her three children. The Scotts' rented house was close to the sea.

In England, Margaret had seen little of the sea, and she had only paddled a few times. She had been given to understand that swimming was quite easy so long as one did not panic, so she took the first chance she got to go swimming with Miss Waller and a friend, who were unaware that it was her first time. At Qinhuangdao the beach is very flat, necessitating a long walk out before it gets deep enough to swim. Off they walked into the sea, Miss Waller and her friend leading, Margaret trailing behind, enjoying the sensual delight of wading through the warm water. Suddenly, to her utter alarm, she sank over her head. As much as she struggled, she could not right herself. Unable to shout, she feared she might not be missed until it was too late. She was feeling a bit drowsy when suddenly she was seized and pulled upright. Miss Waller asked, "Why are you standing on your head?"

She explained somewhat sheepishly how it had come about, then retired to bathe with the children in much shallower water. Later she was shown how to swim and float. At first she was none too successful, but finally one day she realized with pleasant surprise that she could float without assistance.

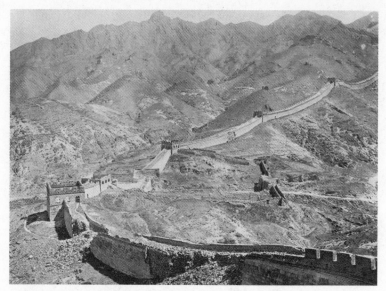

The Great Wall was an important destination for Margaret on her visit to Shanhaiguan in 1917.

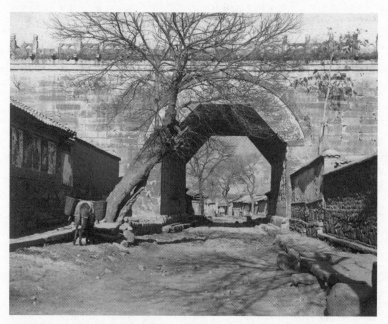

While the Great Wall was intended to be a barrier, it nevertheless had gates allowing two-way traffic at strategic points.

The highlight of the holiday was a trip to the Great Wall at Shanhaiguan, where it rises from the sea and makes its way inland over the mountain ranges. Margaret and Miss Pouley, a missionary from Korea, took donkeys to the station. In order to have a full day for the mountain trip, they arranged to stay for two nights at a Chinese hotel and spent the first day strolling through the narrow streets. Shanhaiguan was a typical high-walled Chinese city on the boundary line between the province of Hebei (then known as Chihli) and Manchuria, where customs tariffs were levied on merchandise crossing the border. The streets were uneven and muddy, with banks and steps up the sides leading to open-fronted shops, each with its high counter and the goods arranged in cloth-covered bundles on shelves behind. The Chinese had little need to display their wares since the long hanging shop signs outside portrayed, by picture or actual article, the nature of the goods for sale.

That evening they went early to bed but not early to sleep, for the hotel was noisy. The next morning Margaret felt rather ill and not up to the trip. Nevertheless, she decided to make the best of it, as her companions refused to go without her. After breakfast at the Railway Hotel, which served Western-style meals, they set off on donkeys with a hotel guide.

Leaving the city behind, they travelled a good distance across the plain before tackling a long winding climb up a mountain. The sturdy little donkeys were well accustomed to climbing those rocky paths. Margaret's indisposition turned out to be a mild attack of dysentery, so she prescribed for herself an aspirin washed down with brandy and distracted herself with thoughts on the events that had occurred here, leading to the downfall of the Ming dynasty. Near the top of their climb the party got soaked by a heavy shower, so they sheltered in the side room of a wayside temple, where they had lunch. On gaining the summit, they looked down at what resembled a perfect Chinese landscape painting. Far below lay a valley laced by a winding river emerging between range upon range of distant mountains that seemed to rise higher and higher into the sky, their tops disappearing into the mist. Afterwards, any time Margaret saw a Chinese landscape painting, she recalled that scene. She then fully understood the meaning of the old saying "First look for the picture in the mountains, then look for the mountains in the picture."

The next morning she walked along the top of the wall surrounding Shanhaiguan as far as a six-sided tower. She regretted that there was not time enough for her to reach the point where the Great Wall rose from the sea, as she had to be back in Qinhuangdao that afternoon.

Shortly after her return from the coast, Mrs. McDouall's youngest child, Hugh, barely six months old, died suddenly one morning after one day's symptoms of dysentery. It was a great shock to Dr. Bryan-Brown, who had seen him only the day before. He asked Margaret to attend to John, aged four, and Kenneth, aged two, who were also ill with dysentery. They were both sturdy little fellows, and John soon recovered. However, Kenneth's was a bad case and although his progress seemed satisfactory, Margaret visited him three or four times a day. Eventually she consulted with her friend Dr. Smiley at the PUMC, and only after that did she feel it was safe to go home to sleep. Even so, she maintained daily visits for nearly a month. In those days, she used emetine very carefully, especially for young children. Several missionaries also had dysentery.

Many of the schoolgirls had trachoma, so she instituted regular treatment with copper sulphate. She spent one night taking care of Mrs. Newland's youngest baby, Murray, who had some obscure abdominal trouble. She was very anxious for him, and was quite surprised when the whole family left her and went peacefully to bed. The next morning she called Dr. Smiley in consultation, who thought the child was doing well. By late afternoon, through her care and medication, Murray was recovering fast. "That was one reason why I liked attending young children," Margaret said. "They respond so quickly."

Rev. Brown died of uraemia, a kidney disease, and Mrs. Brown collapsed after all the strain and anxiety. She came to live with Margaret and was given the largest room, as she had brought her own furniture. She was a pleasant house guest, and Margaret missed her when she and Mrs. Scott eventually went home to England.

Margaret, having bought her dinner service and some pieces of furniture, including a piano, returned the items that had been loaned to her from the mission. She welcomed an invitation to join the newly formed Peking Choral Society; for many years thereafter this was her chief relaxation. She attended practices fairly regularly throughout 1917, and in January the choral society gave its first concert at the YMCA hall, a favourite place for entertainment. The main program consisted of songs of the Allies. Another pleasure was a weekly knitting group at Mrs. Lampson's house in the British legation, their activity consisting largely of making socks and comforters for the troops in Europe. An October meeting at Mrs. Aglen's house (Customs) led to the formation of the British Women's League of Friendship, an effort to link all British women, especially the lonely and friendless. A small lending library was started in that house, where books could be exchanged on certain days. In December, the league held a charity bazaar, an activity that became an annual social event.

In late autumn Margaret took her three PGs for a long weekend at St. Hilary's. The mission compound was well equipped, so all they needed to bring were provisions and a cook—the selfsame who got drunk in Paomachang. While not a satisfactory servant, she had kept him on, since her roles of teacher, physician and guest-house keeper left her no time to take on a cook's duties. Soon after the party reached the Western Hills, his attitude became erratic and he refused to cook. When Margaret insisted, he picked up a large kitchen knife and cried, "You can kill me if you like!"

This was rather disquieting, and may have been due to drink, but she said nothing to the others, and fortunately he behaved quietly for the rest of the time. There could be no question about keeping such a disturbed servant, so he was dismissed directly when they returned home. In China, a servant loses face if he is dismissed, so she gave him a present in lieu of notice in order to get rid of him at once.

In Shanhaiguan, Margaret gleaned her first inkling of the prospects of an ending to the Great War. A British garrison stationed there was commanded by a genial elderly colonel, who was glad of female company for a change. For some time he had been rather pessimistic over when the war would end. Towards the latter part of July, Margaret noted a distinct change of manner, to the point of his being almost jubilant, which she took to be a good sign even though security prevented the old soldier from divulging any information.

♪※

MARGARET MAINTAINED an eyewitness account of the political climate existing around her during the period leading up to and after the armistice. After Yuan Shikai's death, there had been a lull in political affairs. The Chinese parliament was meeting regularly in the parliament buildings near the Anglican mission in an effort to get China to join the Allies against Germany. Those in favour managed to get a majority vote in the face of great opposition. One day a rabble surrounded the parliament buildings to force the issue, but whether for or against Margaret did not know. In any case, most of the mob were paid agitators who caused much discontent with the government, leading to its ultimate dissolution. The president, Li Yuanhong, had little or no voice in the matter. He refused to resign and, as Margaret recalled, he had invited Zhang Xun, after time-honoured custom, to come to Peking to give advice and support.

October 10, the Double Tenth as the Chinese call it, was the anniversary of the establishment of the Republic in 1911. Since the restoration of the monarchy had been safely averted, it was celebrated with special fervour on this occasion. Large, decorated temporary archways (*pailou*) were erected across the main streets in front of government buildings, and a very large one with five arches was put up before the *Tian An Men* entrance to the Forbidden City. These were constructed of large poles wrapped in red cloth, the cross-sections thickly covered with paper flowers. All buildings displayed the Republic's new flag, with its five horizontal stripes—from the top: red, yellow, blue, white and black—representing the five principal groups of people comprising the Chinese nation.

On March 18, 1917, Margaret heard rumours of a great revolution in Russia, and it was confirmed the next day that the Social Democratic party had seized power. Fearing that ultimately there might be "trouble," some of the Peihua boarders left school at Easter-time. It was anticipated that the foreigners might be called into the Legation Quarter for protection. Miss Bowden-Smith obtained a note from Bishop Norris permitting her and Margaret to stay in the school because of their responsibilities to the parents of any remaining children.

On her way to church on Sunday, July 1, Margaret was surprised to see the old Chinese imperial dragon flags (a black dragon on a yellow background) flying over shop doorways. She was told that Zhang Xun had reinstated the boy emperor, Xuan Tong, on the throne to restore the monarchy. His troops, known as the Pigtail Braves because they had retained their queues (emulating their general), had occupied all government buildings.

A republican force was preparing to attack Peking, and aircraft had flown over the city dropping bombs on the Imperial City, most of which fell into the lakes of the Winter Palace. Zhang Xun resigned his post of chief advisor and remained in his house, just inside the south-east corner of the Imperial City. Late in the day of the eleventh, Rev. Scott called to say that the republican army was planning an attack during the night. He invited Margaret to take refuge in his house near the mission, but she preferred to stay put a little longer.

Because of the hot summer nights, Margaret had been sleeping in the courtyard. That night she woke up at three o'clock but heard no sounds of battle. At four o'clock the amah woke her, as she was alarmed by the gunfire coming from the Chinese City, in the south. The republican army was taking possession of the Temple of Heaven, but as Margaret was not alarmed, the amah went back to bed, apparently reassured. By five o'clock the noise was loud and obviously the action was very close, so Margaret got up and dressed. At six o'clock she opened the front gate to see if she could go out, as she was expected at the mission for breakfast.

The street was empty except for a line of soldiers across the road, creeping along or running from gate to gate for protection from the bullets whizzing down the street. They gesticulated to her to return inside and shut the gate. For some reason her telephone was not functioning, so she went through her neighbour's deserted courtyard to use their telephone to say she could not go for breakfast after all. On her return her coolie brought her a bullet which had fallen into the courtyard. Bullets were buzzing overhead and striking the roofs. Margaret went upstairs to get a view outside, but she quickly changed her mind when she saw soldiers hiding round the corners of houses, realizing that bullets could easily ricochet round the room. She found the amah laying out breakfast in the middle of the courtyard, but she hastily changed that idea, and keeping close to the walls they moved indoors.

Margaret's house was opposite the Ministry of Finance and several other government departments that were the first to be attacked within the Tartar City. The gunfire soon moved away from her neighbourhood, though it went on furiously in the distance till about one o'clock in the afternoon. Then Rev. Scott phoned to report that Zhang Xun had taken refuge in the Dutch legation and his men had surrendered. For a long time smoke was seen rising from his burning house (where, in later years, the Union church was built). Curiosity got the better of Margaret and she opened the gate again. She saw no sign of soldiers or traffic, but there were a few people in the street busy picking up spare cartridges, no doubt for the brass. Seeing the door open, a soldier rushed in but checked his pace when he saw Margaret and asked for water for his horse, which was gladly provided. The man was panting with excitement, and Margaret asked if this was the end of the battle. "Oh no, it isn't," the man exclaimed. "We are just beginning." Then he mounted his horse and galloped away.

At two-thirty Rev. Scott came to escort Margaret to the mission, where she was needed to attend to wounded civilian women, one of whom was seriously hurt with a bullet in the abdomen and had to be sent to hospital. The other woman had two wounds in her arm; a round had passed through her upper arm and killed her husband, sitting by her side in the house. Shooting had been erratic, causing more than one hundred civilian casualties, but there was no mention of whether any troops suffered injury. Bishop Norris thought Margaret should take refuge for the night in the mission for fear of looting or other disturbances. She accepted his offer of sending a soldier to protect her house. However, when she went home the next morning and asked her coolie if the soldier had arrived, he replied, "Oh yes, but I sent him away. I wasn't afraid." Evidently he thought the soldier was meant for his protection.

Walking home from the mission early the next morning, she saw policemen knocking on the doors of the shops, which were closed, saying "Hang up your republican flags." This was duly done as obediently as twelve days earlier with the imperial dragon flags. In this manner, law and order had always been maintained in Peking's times of crisis. As Margaret neared home, she saw a large republican flag being hoisted up a tall flagpole in the grounds of the Winter Palace, at the South Lake, where the presidents resided. Later she returned to the dispensary, but only four slightly wounded patients turned up. Bishop Norris told Margaret that he had been holding a service during the battle when a spent bullet came through a window in the church and fell at his feet.

Peking was at peace again. The imperial household had gladly relinquished the temporary glory, which they claimed to have not wanted in the first place. The president was automatically reinstated, and China joined the Allies in word, if nothing else.

♪✳

IN JULY 1918, Bishop Norris allowed Margaret to rent the parsonage at Shanhaiguan. She was badly in need of a break and glad to have two months' rest at the coast in lieu of the furlough enjoyed by her mission friends. She was very tired and often had the feelings in her throat that had preceded her previous haemorrhages, so it was essential for her to rest as much as possible. This time she accomplished her ambition to walk along the Great Wall from where it rose out of the sea. She met Mr. and Mrs. Varè, the minister of the Italian legation and his wife, through an introduction from a friend in England. Both were typically English. He had inherited some Italian property and was required to adopt an Italian name. Some years later, after leaving Peking, he wrote several books on his life in China, with unusual titles such as *The Maker of Heavenly Trousers* and *Tzu-Hzi: The Dowager Empress of China*.

The following April, Margaret had a short rest in the Hills, where she rented rooms in a temple for the summer to come. It was hard to do any effective work during the humid heat of July, the slackest time of the year. The Temple of Eternal Peace was the lowest temple in a fertile valley in the Western Hills. This area was well used by the legation residents before they built cottages for themselves at Paomachang, on the outskirts of the city. Most of these temples depended on the summer visitors for their upkeep. Margaret's rooms were in the main court, made attractive with oleanders and pomegranates, and two handsome ancient white pines, peculiar to North China. She painted a watercolour of one of these growing by the steps up to her rooms. (It remains as a treasured keepsake with her family in Canada.)

Throughout the rest of the year Margaret was kept busy, as her reputation grew, with a constant turnover of paying guests, but she rarely accepted anybody without a personal reference she could trust. Her erstwhile colleague from Pingyin days, Dr. Cunningham, kept her supplied with a constant flow of missionaries from inland China. Mr. and Mrs. Pourdell, missionaries from Shanxi Province, lived with her for several months while attending language school. There were also American guests from the Philippines sent by Mrs. Christman, who started Margaret's Manila connection. She made many American friends in this way.

Shortly after her summer break, Margaret fell while crossing the courtyard, which was slippery from the rain, and cut her hand badly from the teapot she was carrying. As there was a lot of dirt in the wound, she went immediately to the Peking Union Medical College Hospital to have it cleaned and stitched. No local anaesthetic was used, and it was extremely painful and ached all day and night—the kind of ache which experience told Margaret signified a broken bone. Neither the doctor nor she had thought of that at the time. Five days later she found that indeed she had broken the fifth metacarpal, but this did not deter her from her work.

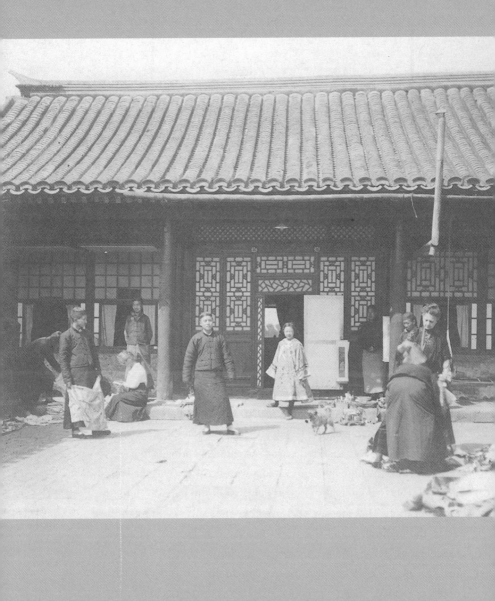

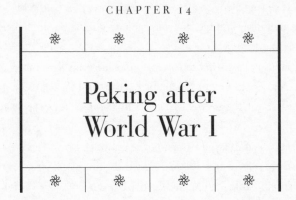

CHAPTER 14

Peking after World War I

ℐ❄ DESPITE THE TROUBLE brewing in the south, Peking remained at peace in 1918. The public event of the year was the enthusiastic reception of the victory over Germany in November. China was nominally an Ally, though contributing little to the war. The leaders pretended to believe the victory had largely been won by the consignments of the Chinese Labour Corps in Europe; in fact, the government had tried to prevent them from going, and those who went were practically smuggled away from the British-leased port of Weihaiwei. However, there was a great feeling of excitement and jubilation in the air. Margaret had certainly never seen the Chinese so keen about anything before.

Her first confirmation of the impending armistice was seeing the French soldiers busily stringing up electric lights over the gateway into the French legation. This she saw on November 11 as she passed by on her way to the medical school—before it had actually become an accomplished event, since Peking time was eight hours ahead of European time. During the next few days the excitement grew, rousing the whole populace. Victory *pailou* (ceremonial archways) were erected, and preparations for illuminations were made in all parts of the city. Legations held receptions for their nationals and hosted staff dinners. On the night of the twelfth, Margaret was called to a prolonged confinement case just as she was getting ready to attend the reception given by the British minister. Though disappointed not to be able to go, she put the needs of the patient first.

Margaret's bottled-up excitement broke loose on November 14, when she was crossing the city to the medical school and saw all the flags flying and heard about the events of the night before. The large stone lions outside the German legation lay toppled on their sides, and *"Der Tag"* had been chalked in large letters on the entrance gates. The French garrison, usually very restrained, had looted the premises. They also set fire to the German bank; fortunately, the blaze was extinguished before much damage had occurred. Finally, they attempted to demolish a stone *pailou* that had been erected as a memorial to Baron Klemens von Ketteler, the German ambassador who was killed on that spot during the Boxer Uprising. The Chinese authorities begged the French to remove the soldiers, promising to pull down the stone archway themselves. This was done immediately; it was later re-erected inside the entrance to the Central Park as a monument to "Allied Victory of Right Over Might."

Margaret was so stirred up that she could not think of lecturing. With the dean's consent, she invited her students to go out with her to see the sights. She had bought a small Union Jack at an Indian silk shop, which she carried leading a small procession of a dozen young people along Legation Street, then northwards toward the Forbidden City and eastwards along the Avenue of Eternal Tranquility (*Chang-An Jie*). They wound up heading south down Hatamen Street back to the Methodist compound. She thought it was brave of the girls to accompany her, but they attracted little attention since everyone else was equally excited.

That evening Margaret attended a mass meeting of the United War Work campaign at the Gateway to Heavenly Peace (*Tian An Men*), followed by a tour around the city to see the illuminations. By the end of the day she was weary, having walked a considerable number of kilometres.

This atmosphere of jubilation continued until the official victory celebration in the Forbidden City on November 28. The venue was the vast quadrangle in front of the Great Throne Room, where many great imperial functions had been held. In addition to the model Chinese army of ten thousand troops were the Allied garrisons in full strength, honoured as guests of China by having their national flags down the centre of the parade. Even then, there was space aplenty for the troops to drill and manœuvre during the ceremonials.

All foreign nationals received, through their respective consuls, invitations to attend, with a request to be in place by 9:00 A.M. The men occupied the side verandahs surrounding the vast court, while the women (requested to wear skirts) watched from three terraces on the south side of the Throne Hall. Margaret had a superb view from the middle terrace near a flight of marble steps. The day was sunny and windless, enlivened by aircraft circling overhead and dropping red congratulatory leaflets over the crowds—a new kind of excitement for Peking. At last the president, Xu Shichang, and various officials arrived. The bands struck up as he walked slowly across the court, up the steps past her and into the main throne room. About fifteen minutes later, the visitors followed and Margaret saw the Dragon Throne for the first time.

The vast bare hall was carpeted throughout. In the centre of the north side on a three-tiered carpeted platform, approached by three flights of balustraded steps, stood the throne like a great armchair, beautifully carved in red lacquer with no fewer than ninety-nine dragons. (It was claimed that when the emperor took his seat, he completed the mystical set of one hundred dragons.) Behind the throne stood a massive four-leafed red lacquer screen. Carved bronze lacquer dragons covered the lofty pillars supporting the roof beams. Afterwards, on the way home, Margaret watched magnificent illuminations and pyrotechnic displays in Central Park. The commemoration ended on November 30 with lantern processions.

Not long afterwards, all three throne halls were turned into museums and thrown open to the public. In years to come, Margaret saw that main hall many times, overfilled with art treasures. On the last occasion, in 1948, she found it quite bare, as the Nationalist administration had emptied it prior to evacuating to Taiwan. However, to her the Great Hall

never seemed so grand as on that first visit when it was furnished only
with the great carpets and the throne.

PEKING

Peking, thou Pole Star of a great Empire;
Home of a thousand Rulers;
Product of an ancient culture;
An age-long city set in a fertile plain,
Protected by chains of timeless hills
Adorned with twistings of the Great Dragon Wall.
Most cities grow but thou wast planned,
Lofty conception of a noble mind.
Thy walls and towers proclaim the greatness of past days;
What tales these walls could tell of wondrous sights
And glorious pageants of Imperial days.

Can you not see them as you pass
Along the thoroughfares and through the courts
Where once they trod?
And still within these massive walls the people come and go
And live their little lives and speak their ancient tongue.

The spacious courts, the lofty halls and gracious parks
Are free for all to wander in,
And even mount the Sacred Altar
Where once the Son of Heaven adored.
Long may thy spirit, Yung Lo, be undisturbed
In the fastness of thy sealed tomb;
Yet may thy spirit so inflame thy people of today
That China, like the Phoenix, shall rise glorious again.

(E. M. P.)

*

FOR THE STUDENT MOVEMENT, 1919 was a memorable year. Much indignation had been caused by Japan's presentation of the Twenty-one Demands in 1915, which China agreed to under compulsion but made no effort to fulfill. The death of Yuan Shikai, the "Strong Man of China," had precipitated a power struggle amongst the various warlords whom he had placed in charge of the provinces. In the ensuing state of confusion, Japan began to undermine Chinese resistance by a system of financial intrigues with the Anfu clique, then in power in Peking. The Anfu (meaning "appeasement") clique offered China's industries and mineral resources in return for lavish Japanese loans.

At this time, the peace conference was underway in Versailles. The Allies wished to transfer German properties and rights in Shandong to Japan, since Japan had defeated the Germans there without help from China, but Chinese delegates in Versailles refused to sign. This provoked tremendous resentment in China, especially in the higher schools and colleges. On May 7, students forced their way into the residence of one of the pro-Japanese Anfuites and attacked him, laying havoc to his premises. Many were arrested and sentenced to be executed. The students then organized a giant demonstration against both Japan and the Anfu collaborators on May 17, a day named National Humiliation Day in memory of China's capitulation to the Twenty-one Demands. Margaret read these demands in the press, the gist of which gave Japan special privileges and preference, and almost full control of China's resources.

An uproar swept the country. Students everywhere went on strike, holding constant demonstrations, speaking in marketplaces and temple squares, calling on merchants to boycott the Japanese and trying in every way to arouse opposition to the traitorous Anfu government. They succeeded. The chambers of commerce and merchant guilds declared a nationwide shop strike, not to be lifted until the imprisoned Peking students were released, and the pro-Japanese cabal dissolved. On June 4, Margaret saw a procession of women students en route to beg the president for the release of the one thousand students arrested the day before for holding meetings. For ten days banks remained closed, business halted and government revenues stopped. Peking then capitulated, dismissed some Anfu traitors, released the arrested students and instructed the Paris delegation not to sign away Shandong Province.

The students, however, were not satisfied. They persisted in their anti-Japanese campaign by organizing boycotts of Japanese merchandise. They entered shops and hunted for Japanese goods, which were taken away and publicly burned. Many Japanese shipping and export firms went bankrupt. Japan not only lost the promised loans, but at the Washington Conference in 1922 was forced to withdraw the Twenty-one Demands.

Thus China's youth set democracy and national self-consciousness to work in China to a greater degree than any other force had done, even the Revolution of 1911. However, the student movement, like many revolutionary movements, carried on too long. In succeeding years it became almost an annual event to strike at examination time, on some pretext or other. As Jean Escarra, author of *China, Then and Now*, put it, "It has been described as a pretext—more than anything else—to escape from discipline." He also said, "The Student Class formed part of an elite circle which believed that it alone, like the Scholar Class under the old regime, was entrusted with the mission of national reconstruction and of directing the national destiny."[1]

Although China had been a republic since 1912, the parliament that existed in Peking when Margaret returned there in 1916 had not been elected by the people, thus a democracy it was not. If Yuan Shikai had been less pro-Japanese, she believed he might have been able to fulfill his ambition to create a new dynasty. Certainly the country became more divided after his death and the parliament faded out over the question of joining the Allies. Under mob pressure the vote was taken, and China achieved Allied status. District and village governments maintained order in local areas, although after 1918 the schism between North China and South China became more marked.

As before, China was actually controlled by the governors of the provinces, then referred to as the *Jun Fa* (literally, "military caste"), but later known as the Warlords because they kept their own armies and struggled against each other for possession of Peking. There the leading officials were chosen to suit their own interests, and presidents and their cliques fled at the approach of the army. This state of affairs was entirely distinct from the anti-Japanese demonstrations, though the students were exploited to rouse popular feeling against a president who refused to budge. A state of general unease pervaded, until it became apparent which hands held control of the nation. For some while the possibility of evacuating foreign residents existed, to avoid any repeat of the uprising at the start of the century. Margaret took the precaution of consigning a caseful of her more treasured possessions to England into the safekeeping of her brother Frank.

∮✻

THROUGHOUT THIS TIME, Margaret maintained her busy schedule with her teaching and medical practice. As well, three evenings a week she gave English lessons to two Chinese women doctors who wished to improve their conversational abilities. She also served as treasurer on the committee of the Peking branch of the China Medical Association and arranged the regular monthly meetings, held at one of the clinical hospitals or at a doctor's house. At one meeting, the topic for discussion was the recent epidemic of influenza—a mild type, although it later spread to America and Europe in 1919 and became more and more devastating. Margaret was also making preparations for the next annual meeting of the China Medical Missionary Association (CMMA), to be held in Peking.

She was actively engaged with examinations of both medical and nursing students. With the help of her nurse colleague, Miss Brown, it took six hours non-stop to prepare the nursing exam according to her requirements. Most of the nurses showed a high standard of practical nursing. By the end of May, sixteen senior nurses had passed their written and practical examinations, but the junior students, who had been preoccupied with the anti-Japanese demonstrations, were allowed to postpone their examinations until the autumn. This was a bad precedent, and in the following years it was tried on several occasions by the students of high schools and colleges. Two students failed in medicine, and Margaret thought they should not be allowed to graduate without further study. However, at the June faculty meeting, after much discussion, she was overruled on the grounds that they should have been turned down before the final stages of the course. Eventually, all eighteen graduated as M.D.'s.

With so much regular medical work, Margaret had to fit in her private practice as best she could. Many patients were outside her mission commitments, so she gradually dropped a number of obstetric cases, as the Presbyterian and Methodist hospitals were meeting the need. At that time Chinese patients seldom sent for a doctor for their confinements unless something appeared to be going wrong.

On December 31, at 3:15 A.M., Margaret was called to attend a confinement. Mrs. Yun had engaged her services in November, when she was eight months pregnant. She already had eight sons and was anxious for a daughter. She had not had a doctor for childbirth before, and her confinements had all been normal. Margaret arrived within a half-hour and found confinement well on the way, but complicated by a partial placenta praevia; she was greatly relieved when the baby was born at 8:00 A.M. Everything was going well when Margaret visited Mrs. Yun again in the afternoon. How delighted the mother was with her little daughter, but how worried Margaret was in later weeks when she refused to have the baby vaccinated. The Chinese method of live-virus vaccination made them fear it for children under a year old, hence many died of smallpox in infancy. Sadly, this was the case when this baby was only eight months old.

As the British legation doctor was still away due to the war, Mrs. Lampson, wife of the Chargé d'Affaires, consulted Margaret about her little girl and also about a small cyst on her own eyelid, which Margaret removed. Several English personnel in the Chinese customs service consulted her regarding their children, and from time to time she examined applicants for insurance.

Her most distressing case was a young Chinese woman who had become insane. During the Boxer Uprising, when she was a baby, a Boxer had wantonly struck her head with his sword, deeply cutting her forehead. Surprisingly, she recovered and appeared normal until about seventeen, when she became gradually insane, thought due to scar tissue in the brain beneath the cut causing pressure. In those days, an operation was considered too risky, and she became more and more violent, to the extent of having to be tied down. Her exhausted father begged Margaret to take her under care, but as the girl shouted and raved all night she was returned home. She was never brought back for treatment.

Margaret was once called out to pay a house call. The symptoms described suggested a breast abscess, so she prepared her bag accordingly and arrived at the appointed time. Not only was she unexpected, she was told no one was ill and that she was the fourth doctor to have called that day, whereupon the door was slammed in her face. Later she learned that the hoax was a common means of giving annoyance, or wishing bad luck upon someone. Sometimes a coffin would be delivered on New Year's Eve to bring bad luck. Margaret's friend said he had never heard of a foreign doctor made use of in that way. It occurred to her that the incident was meant to portray particularly bad luck, since it was only too often that a Western doctor was called in too late to help the patient.

Another patient, her landlord's muleteer, had been kicked by his mule. The injured leg was septic and becoming gangrenous from frostbite. He refused to go to hospital for fear of amputation. Margaret thought he had good reason for his fear, so she tried to do what she could for him. Over four months she visited him no fewer than ninety times and saved his leg. There were no sulpha drugs in those days, but potassium permanganate won the fight. The only cost for this treatment was for the dressings. The victory was sufficient reward.

In 1919, Margaret made a special study of the causes and treatment of tuberculosis, in preparation for a thesis for her M.D., which she had not had time to do before leaving for China in 1905. Her reading time for this was generally in the evening, when the house was quiet. At that time Peking had several women doctors who had trained at the Canton Women's Medical School. One especially, Dr. Zhang, had a large practice among official people. In those days, Chinese women definitely preferred a female doctor, so she asked Margaret to do a minor operation on the president's wife. She was taken to see Mrs. Feng Guochang to arrange for the operation. The president had left for his native home that morning, leaving five of his seven wives at home and taking with him his latest concubine, a girl of sixteen.

The Chinese had as many concubines as they could afford to keep, but only one official wife. His first official wife had died. Margaret's patient, his senior concubine, took her place. The wives all lived in one compound and had their meals together. They were quite excited by this visit from a foreigner and had dressed in their best, and all talked together animatedly. They invited Margaret to make a tour of the whole complex of court-yards, known as compounds, which some of them had not seen before. They thoroughly enjoyed the tour and babbled happily about which rooms they would choose for themselves.

April 18 was the date fixed for the operation, but Dr. Zhang sent word that Mrs. Feng wished to postpone it for a day. That day was not a "happy" or propitious one. The next day Dr. Zhang gave the anaesthetic while Margaret worked quickly and hoped for the best, for the circumstances were not at all suitable or convenient. Dr. Zhang visited Mrs. Feng daily, and Margaret went again before the week was out, then once more to remove the stitches on April 27. The operation was successful.

♪✳

FOR MARGARET, 1920 was one of the busiest years of her life both professionally and socially. She completed the translation of the two-volume book *Materia Medica for Nurses,* and in the evenings continued working on her thesis. For several years she had made careful notes of every case of tuberculosis coming under her observation, and this pro-vided the basis of her paper.

The great medical event of 1920 was the medical missionary confer-ence held in the newly built, but yet to be completed, Peking Union Medical College (PUMC) Hospital, owned by the Rockefeller Foundation. This took place over the Chinese New Year season, February 23 to 27. Margaret was on the hospitality committee looking after the delegates, and she spent much time meeting trains and shepherding delegates to

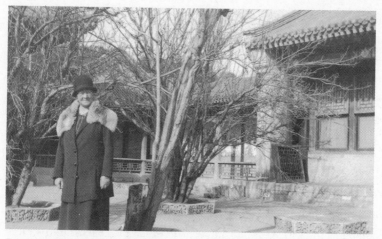

Dr. Margaret dressed for winter weather, c. 1920.

their various accommodations. Saturday, February 21, was the day of the Spring Festival and, appropriately enough, the occasion for a grand reception. Six hundred invitations in Chinese had been sent out to Chinese officials, prominent community members and diplomatic representatives. A record number of members attended due to the growth of medical organizations in China.

The CMMA was China's first medical association; most foreign doctors were connected with missions, exclusive of the legation doctors, while a few operated in the large business centres, such as Shanghai and Tianjin. Since China was opening up, a wider organization was needed, so on March 24 the Peking International Medical Society came into being. Margaret attended meetings of both groups. Initially the CMMA had accepted only Chinese doctors with full Western training. Margaret had joined when she first arrived in China, and much appreciated the monthly *China Medical Journal.* Years later, China-trained doctors of long standing were permitted to join, including graduates from the PUMC and other medical colleges in China who received their M.D. degree at the conclusion of their course, in accordance with American custom and in contrast to the current English practice. Since Margaret had not had time to prepare her thesis before leaving for China, she remained an M.B., although she was preparing to rectify the situation with her thesis on tuberculosis.

Eventually all groups merged into the China Medical Society. Some useful clinical meetings were held, and some papers were given in French. Dr. Howard presented an interesting study of the condition of hospitals in Japan, which he and a colleague had made during a holiday tour that summer. Japanese doctors were in the forefront as far as diagnosis and scientific medical research was concerned, but hospital conditions were deplorable and the nursing inefficient.

Xu Shichang hosted the conference's closing reception in the president's palace in the Central Lake (*Zhong Hai*) of the Winter Palace. He shook hands with each individual, after which they passed into a room with a long table down the centre, well loaded with rich confectionery. After a closing meeting at the PUMC and another tea, followed a farewell reception to Sir John Jordan, the erstwhile British minister to China, at the British legation. Dinner was at the Army Medical College, and the long day ended with "moving pictures."

♪✲

THE THIRD DECADE of the century began quietly enough, but Margaret's pace hardly slackened, although she sensibly started with a short holiday in the Western Hills with a few friends. The weather, though cold, was kindly, so they made an expedition to the Mummy Temple of *Tian Tai Shan*, where they saw what was purported to be the mummy of Shun Zhi, the first Manchu emperor of the Qing dynasty, who abdicated the throne in favour of his son Kang Xi and retired to this temple, as a brokenhearted man, to become a monk.

By now Margaret was firmly established as a Peking resident, both socially and professionally, with an enviable reputation in the Chinese and foreign communities alike. One evening, at nearly bedtime, her servant announced a Chinese lady. Supposing her to be a patient, Margaret received her in her study, only to find that she was not ill but asking for accommodation for the night. She was a secondary wife who had run away because she was afraid, and she wanted some place where the first wife could not make trouble. She thought she would be safest with Margaret, and seemed so distraught that Margaret did not ply her with questions, putting her to bed without even asking her name. The next day she was gone before Margaret was up. She was never heard of again.

Margaret's landlord, General Jiang Chaozong, had rented to her part of his own ample establishment, so he lived nearby. Still, they had yet to meet, since all the arrangements for her lease had been made through intermediaries. Although unsure of the correct procedure, Margaret felt it was her duty to call on him in due course. She recognized that his social status was higher than hers, for he had held a high position in imperial days, and as mayor of Peking he had kept peace in the city during the difficult days of 1917.

She sent her visiting card by hand of her servant, with instructions to ask when seeing her would be convenient. The reply was that he would be glad to receive her at once. Margaret walked round to the front gate, where a sentry was on guard, and she was immediately ushered into the living room, where she was received in a most cordial fashion. After a pleasant conversation over a few cups of tea, Margaret was taking her leave, when the general said he would now call on her. She well knew the correct etiquette was to return a call in good time, but she had not expected anything quite so prompt. He and his wife came on foot since it was only a short distance, although ordinarily he always drove out in his light four-wheeled carriage accompanied by mounted outriders.

The Chinese couple were pleased to see how Margaret had arranged and furnished the house, and they left with many expressions of good-will. The general told her that foreigners had lived in the house before, including Dr. George Ernest Morrison, the London *Times* correspondent. The lovely carved screen-work in her study came from the general's home. Margaret felt he had fulfilled every requirement of courtesy. The draw-back to sociability and courtesy in China was that it took up so much time. Being so busy, Margaret was unable to form any real friendships, though she was on friendly terms with many Chinese.

Later that year, General Jiang invited her to a banquet, a grand affair with many important foreign guests, held in a vast dining room adorned with numerous ornate gilt clocks, most of which were gifts from the empress dowager, who had a weakness for collecting. Margaret remembered little of the elaborate menu with its traditional dishes, as she was too busy making conversation with strangers. The old general was a genial host, and after dinner he showed his guests his magnificent collection of porcelains. He gave Margaret the name of a reliable curio dealer, which later she found useful.

Eventually Margaret got to know the head of the Peking gendarmerie, General Wang Huaiqing. He occasionally invited her to dinner parties, particularly when he was fulfilling his social obligations to foreigners. Margaret's knowledge of Chinese was frequently put to work for interpreting since his English was limited. He resolutely excused himself from conventional wine-drinking with the decorous platitude *"Zai li,"* which meant that he was being "sensible" in the interests of sobriety. This was not to say, however, that he never imbibed. After dinner, Chinese jugglers provided entertainment. Margaret admired their skill at sleight of hand and juggling, but was less appreciative of fire-eating. This consisted of eating a roll of smoking paper, pretending to swallow it, then belching forth clouds of smoke and flame. The climax of the performance was usually a somersault, landing with a large heavy bowl containing live goldfish, which had been concealed under the juggler's long gown. On one occasion something went wrong; water ran from the bowl and streamed across the floor. The somersault did not take place, but no notice was taken of the mishap in accordance with the Chinese habit of maintaining a stoic calm in the face of an awkward situation.

Margaret gradually learned to put aside more time to enjoy life. A particular pleasure was attending a performance of *The Marriage of Kitty* by Marie Tempest at the Peking Pavilion. Her favourite relaxation, choral practice, continued on Monday evenings; she managed to attend quite regularly and to participate in a number of concerts. Still, the messages from her throat indicated that she needed to regulate her enthusiasm. More than once she sensed the early warnings of haemoptysis. She dared not cough, but by careful heeding of those dreaded "feelings," she was able to avoid any catastrophe.

The British Women's League was expanding its membership and usefulness, so it seemed advisable to have a definite constitution. Hitherto the committee had asked for funds as needed and was not required to give a public account of spending. Parliamentary law was studied, and after two hours of animated discussion, a constitution was formed. The annual bazaar for various charities was held at the Wagon-Lits hotel. All British children looked forward to the annual children's sports, hosted by the League on Empire Day (May 24) on the British legation grounds, with prizes and tea. With little time for social hospitality, Margaret got to know most of the British community by attending league meetings, and she developed a good friend in Mrs. Richardson, wife of the deputy commissioner of Chinese Maritime Customs. She was glad to find time to attend the garden party at the British legation, held annually in celebration of the king's official birthday. The minister to China, Sir Beilby Alston, and his wife Lady Alston received guests under the great open-sided Chinese pavilion in front of the residence. "It was a really, truly, British at-home," Margaret noted. She never lost her pride in England, despite that she had spent less than half her life there.

Early one June morning, Margaret saw a huge fire: the well-known Morrison Street Bazaar blazing away. The Chinese fire service was in an elementary stage and could do little more than create a firebreak by knocking down neighbouring stalls. Buckets of water were trundled hastily along the street on trolleys. Soon the Italian legation's fire engine arrived to lend a willing hand. Only after the whole of the interior was gutted was the fire extinguished, but the shops opening onto Morrison Street were saved. The bazaar had been one of the sights of Peking, and it was sorely missed. It was revived bit by bit, though not until several years later was it completely restored.

Margaret spent a refreshing escape from Peking's summer heat at Beidaihe (Peitaiho) Beach, where she improved her swimming skills and enjoyed beautiful strolls over the nearby Lotus Hills. This was a favourite gathering spot for many missionaries from the Interior, providing an

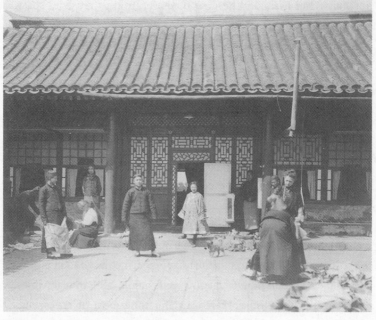

The weekly merchant market inside Margaret's courtyard became known as "little Lung Fu Si."

interlude with a taste of home life, and supplying an opportunity to rendezvous and mingle with colleagues from other missions.

Her private enterprise of running a guest-house was thriving. Her household was becoming thoroughly international, including Russian, Danish, French, American, Canadian, English and Australian visitors for varying periods of time, with all getting on happily. The guests had to amuse themselves, but Margaret would oblige with sightseeing advice and engage selected rickshaw-pullers by the week or the month to be at their disposal. With a good cook and number-one boy, and judicious supervision of the staff overall, Margaret managed the housekeeping well. Meals were served fairly punctually, and there was usually a social time after lunch and dinner. Her one attempt at establishing this as a full-time venture did not work out, likely due, she thought, to her having engaged the wrong person as manager.

That winter Margaret's servants had a narrow escape from coal-gas poisoning when her staff of five almost succumbed to carbon monoxide emanating all night from the Chinese stove heating their room. Seemingly, one man had got up to go to the latrine, and on his return collapsed unconscious, which is often the effect of fresh air after carbon monoxide poisoning. His prostrate body had prevented the door from closing, and eventually Margaret heard loud moaning. With some difficulty, she managed to wake the other servants. It was lucky she was there in time, as all could have died before morning. She insisted that a foreign stove be installed, though the staff did not like it as well as their own.

There were occasional burglaries, including the theft of some carpets and her electric power meter. As demand for power exceeded the supply, meters were hard to come by. The ingenuity of her servants enabled her to identify the culprit, and the police soon returned her equipment.

On Saturday afternoons Margaret permitted dealers to come into the main courtyard to display their wares for the benefit of her guests. At two o'clock, they would rush in with their bundles and, in groups around the courtyard, arrange their treasures of silks, embroideries, porcelains, mixed curios, cases of bead chains and jewellery. This became known as little *Lung Fu Si*, after the old temple courtyard where a famous bazaar was held every nine days, with one section devoted to curio stalls where treasures were often found.

As Mrs. Richardson was planning to leave China, Margaret was asked to replace her as chairman of the management committee of the old men's home, a large committee composed of Chinese, American and British women, and difficult to preside over, as several of the Chinese did not understand English and others knew little Chinese. The bilingual committee was apt to become disorderly. While Margaret was interpreting to the Chinese members, the others naturally began talking to each other and vice versa, so business moved slowly. An important Chinese official, Cao Rulin, offered new rent-free quarters for the old men's home: two compounds on either side of an imposing entrance to extensive grounds surrounding a handsome foreign-style house that he had built for himself. In a sense this was a political move, as he was not in favour with the students because of his pro-Japanese tendencies; he was one of those who had virtually agreed to the notorious Twenty-one Demands of the Japanese. He doubtless thought that serving as an official residence for old people might be a protection for his house, which had been broken into during previous student riots.

Five committee members inspected the compounds and found them full of tenants, who were urged to move out before the Chinese New Year, when their rents would be increased. This ploy proved effective, for when Margaret went to visit, the old folk were already in their new homes, one for married couples and the other for old men. A formal opening took place, with the compounds looking very spruce. A middle-aged man was appointed as a paid warden. One of the old men became the cook; others had various jobs assigned to them according to capability.

Two committee members were appointed to visit the homes once a month. The old people seemed to appreciate the attention and took pride in keeping their rooms and courtyards spick and span. They could go out for walks as they pleased, but had to be back punctually for meals and at home by six o'clock, when the doors were bolted for the night. Sometimes the old men were found begging from the shops. When this was discovered, all were given a badge to wear on their blue cotton outdoor coats, and all shops were requested not to give them anything. They were allowed a little pocket money for the main festivals, and visitors kept most of them supplied with small change. Only men older than sixty who were destitute and without a son to support them were admitted. Still, it was remarkable when an old man lay dying if no son turned up to be near him at the last. As Margaret was the physician to the homes, she visited them frequently, considering this her contribution to the social service of Peking.

She continued to teach at the Union Medical College for Women. As pathology and medicine were her chief subjects, she attended several autopsies on subjects of Western nationality. In China, it was considered essential to be buried whole and complete; autopsies were a new procedure being introduced gradually, as a necessity for medical education.

During this year the YWCA unofficially adopted Margaret as their doctor, and she made frequent calls at a house where several American secretaries lived while studying the language. They started coming to her for their annual medical exams, a practice they continued for a number of years. Spring was a favourite time for vaccinations, and to her surprise eleven clerks from the Asia Banking Corporation arrived for treatment as well.

Early in May, Margaret paid the first of a number of visits to the wealthy Li family in Tianjin, consisting of five brothers and sons or grandsons of Li Hongchang. Her connection with them was due to her attendance on their married sister in Peking, Mrs. Yun—the patient with eight sons. Although the distance was 130 kilometres (80 miles), the train journey took four hours due to the long stops en route. One of the brothers met the train, and Margaret felt important when he brought the car right onto the platform alongside the train.

The patient was an eighteen-year-old slave girl in an advanced stage of pulmonary tuberculosis. It was impossible to do anything for her, and Margaret was horrified to find her living in a room in the middle of the family. Slave girls in China were usually bought from impoverished country families. They took the family name and lived with the women of the family, who required a great deal of personal service. Later they might be married or become concubines. In a Chinese house the rooms communicate, and this girl was living in a central room through which the family had to pass to go from one room to another. The family acted on Margaret's advice and isolated her immediately. She died a month later.

After a pleasant Chinese meal with the ladies, who were delighted that Margaret could use chopsticks, she was escorted to the station by the same Mr. Li, arriving in Peking before dark. Over the years, Margaret made several train trips to Tianjin at their request to attend to various female relatives of the Li family.

∫※

ON THE SPRING HOLIDAY in China known as *Qing Ming*, meaning "clear [and] bright," which corresponds generally with Easter, people clear their family grave sites to celebrate the renewal of life. Margaret had arranged for a stone wall to be built surrounding the plot of land she had acquired below St. Hilary's. She spent this short holiday in the Hills while construction took place, experience having taught her that it was as well to keep an eye on progress to ensure the best results. She hoped to build her sanatorium here, and she had offered it to Bishop Norris for that purpose.

In the middle of the year, Margaret had to have all twelve of her remaining upper teeth extracted—an unforgettable experience. She engaged a nurse for the day, and together an English anaesthetist, Dr. Cormack, and an American dentist, Mr. Smith, got to work. An hour later, just after the doctors had left, Margaret came round from the chloroform to find her mouth full of blood. The profuse bleeding would not stop. She asked the nurse to telephone the doctor, but his response was to send for the dentist. Ultimately a reply came from the doctor that the dentist said it would do the gums good to bleed, but to call again if the bleeding had not stopped by four o'clock.

It was after five before Dr. Cormack arrived, by which time Margaret was feeling weak and desperate, since her mouth was constantly filling up with blood. As soon as she spat it out, her mouth started to fill up again. The doctor was alarmed when he saw her mouth full of clots and a big basin of blood at her side. When he asked how long this had been going on, Margaret held up seven fingers. After she emptied her mouth again, she explained that the basin's contents were only from the past hour. He found that the bleeding was due to a small torn artery, and he had to ask Dr. Chapman to assist him to plug it. Remarkably, Dr. Chapman had been in the building the whole time, but had not wished to interfere. Margaret then had a fairly good night, but when she opened her mouth the next morning she was startled at how colourless a tongue could look in a living person. It took her two weeks to recuperate, after which she paid several visits to the dentist to be fitted with a plate.

Two months later, a faith healer, Mr. Hickson, visited Peking. He was invited one day to hold a service of healing in the legation chapel. The little church was full, and many people went up for him to lay his hands on their heads while he uttered brief, beautifully expressed prayers over each one. Margaret had previously had a short interview, telling him about her work, and at his invitation she went up for a blessing.

As he put his hands upon my head a curious thrill passed through my whole body. I did not hear of any startling results of his mission, but I am sure there were, for I believe in faith healing when the faith is there.

Margaret's belief in faith healing was based on several instances during the course of her wide practice.

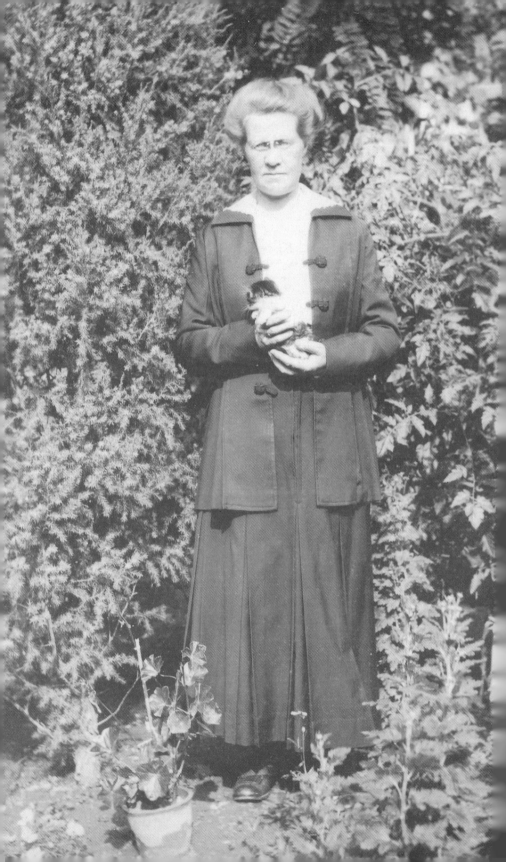

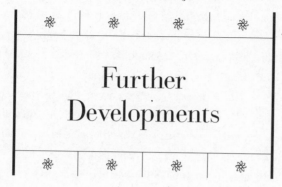

CHAPTER 15

Further Developments

♪* MARGARET KNEW that she could never bear a child, after her hysterectomy while at university, but she hoped that someday she might adopt one. When the Great War broke out, she wanted to return to England to help, and at the same time look around for a child who needed love and care. However, the Canadian Church Society would not release her just then, so she had to content herself with the thought that she might adopt a war orphan when her next furlough became due. Though circumstances changed and she did not go to England, Margaret still harboured her heart's desire.

"Why wait till you go home? Why not send for a baby?" a friend one day asked. "A child under the age of two can come out passage-free." This idea delighted Margaret, and shortly afterwards she read in the *Church Times* about the work of the National Adoption Society, started in England during the war to find homes for orphaned babies. Margaret sent the cutting to Mrs. Mosse in London, who promptly offered to visit the home where the babies were and choose one for her. Since there was little hope of getting back to England and she was now forty-five, Margaret felt that it was a case of now or never. Peking was a good place to raise a child, with two good schools, one American and one French, as well as an English boarding school in Yantai. A friend who had just gone home on furlough was willing to bring the child back with her.

Margaret allowed Mrs. Mosse to decide on a boy or a girl, and soon a letter arrived telling Margaret that she had adopted a lovely boy on January 31, his first birthday. Margaret declared it "the greatest event of my life." Mrs. Mosse had chosen a boy, as it was easier to find homes for girls because a boy's education was more expensive. "He was such a beautiful child that I fell for him immediately and, though he already showed signs of a strong will, I knew that you would be able to cope," Mrs. Mosse wrote. "His name is Clifford, after his grandfather."

There turned out to be some difficulties over an escort after all, so Mrs. Mosse advertised in the *Daily Telegraph* and engaged a lady who was returning to Shanghai. "On August 18th I received a cablegram saying that Clifford was sailing on a French boat which would be in Shanghai on September 17th," Margaret wrote in her journal. "What a thrilling telegram! I went round the house telling all my guests." She decided to take her summer holiday by going to Shanghai to meet him, arranging for Dr. Yang to hold the fort.

The unusually heavy rain of that summer's wet season continued into mid-August, and the bridges on the railway line between Tianjin and Shanghai were washed away. Repairs would take several weeks. Coastal shipping was fully booked, and Thomas Cook's informed her that it might take three weeks to secure her a passage—too late for Margaret to meet the ship. Finally, friends in Tianjin, Mr. and Mrs. Nichols, booked her a passage on a Japanese steamer en route to Shanghai via Dalian (Dairen) on September 7.

That ship was delayed, so Margaret had two restful days with her friends. She was the only foreign passenger and had a four-berth cabin all to herself, with courteous Chinese stewards to wait on her. At Dalian she ventured ashore to avoid the dockside racket of the loading and unloading. She hired a horse-drawn carriage for a drive to Star Beach, a popular summer resort nearby, and she enjoyed being able to converse with the driver, who could speak Mandarin as well as the local dialect.

Margaret joined the captain for meals, intrigued to see him enjoying the foreign menu, especially how he liberally applied marmalade at every meal. Near Shanghai, they encountered rough weather and she spent a whole day in bed. Two doses of chloretone kept off the sickness, but she had nothing to eat for thirty-six hours. When the ship anchored in mid-river at Shanghai Margaret waited, thinking that they would presently draw up to a quay, only to be informed she would have to get herself ashore on one of the *sampans* hovering about. She did not feel like entrusting herself and her luggage to one of those, so she said, "My ticket is for Shanghai, not for mid-river. What is that launch doing?"

"That is the Customs launch. You can't go in that."

"Oh, can't I? Boy, take my trunk to the launch." And down the gangway she went with the steward following. No questions were asked, and Margaret got to the customs jetty, where she hailed a wheelbarrow to take her luggage, then got into a rickshaw. Fortunately, the rickshaw-puller understood Mandarin—the Shanghai dialect is quite different—and in due course she arrived safely at the missionary home. She had expected someone to meet her, as she had booked a room and given the name of the ship. The excuse was that the ship was late and they did not know when to expect her. Her accommodation had been given away, but if she did not mind waiting till evening there should be a vacancy available. "Not very cheering," Margaret thought, "but one learns to make the best of things in China."

After lunch, she went out to seek news of the ship, which was due to arrive the next day—the date of the Mid-Autumn Festival (the fifteenth day of the eighth lunar month), one of the major festivals of the Chinese calendar and on which all shipping offices were closed. Happily, Thomas Cook's office, being English, was open, and there she was informed that the ship was delayed for another six days.

Margaret settled down to enjoy her holiday. After tea, two former guests of hers, Mr. and Mrs. Runyan, came for her in their car and took her out to dinner at the Baptist mission. She filled her time as best she could, sightseeing, window-shopping and looking up other friends. On Sunday she enjoyed the morning service in the cathedral and an evening sermon at the Union church. The Runyans again took her in hand, and they visited the spot where the willow china pattern originated. Margaret was disappointed that there were no longer willow trees or a pagoda, and that the site was so enclosed by buildings that only the zigzag bridge suggested the original scene.[1]

By September 23, she was restless. The menu at the home was arranged to cover three days—the average duration of a guest's stay. Margaret had had three rounds of that fare and she did not wish to eat a fourth. Finally, the next day the shipping office notified her that the ship was due at the Huang Po wharf at 3:00 P.M. After waiting for over two hours, Margaret was cold so she headed home for a coat, hurrying back by taxi just in time to see the great ship drawing up to the dockside.

As soon as the vessel was made fast, she rushed up the gangway into the crowd on deck, asking for Clifford. He was nowhere to be seen. She appealed to the purser, who obviously knew about baby Clifford, and he suggested another deck where she might find him. Breathlessly she rushed to the nearest companionway, and on the next deck—at last!—she spotted Clifford in somebody's arms, but certainly not the woman she expected. Margaret took him without any fuss and went into the saloon, found his official escort and panted, "Can I take Clifford now?" Margaret was so afraid that she would not want to part with him, but the woman said, "Please do. I will come round tomorrow with his things." Margaret never saw her again, though his little parcel of clothing was delivered the next afternoon. Margaret wrote later from Peking to thank her for bringing him, but received no reply.

After tipping a steward to carry Clifford, who was too heavy for her to handle down the gangway, she got him into a taxi, and they were on their way. "He was such a lovely, cuddly, happy baby and did not mind a stranger at all."

When they arrived at the home, Margaret gave him supper and put him to bed on pillows laid on two opposing chairs. They had a fairly good night albeit his being a little restless, while she was almost too excited to sleep, "for he really was a beautiful child." Although then twenty months old, he had only just learned to walk, and, though vocal enough to definitely make his wants known, he could not yet talk properly.

The next day, Sunday, Margaret hired an amah for the day and they took turns looking after him. That afternoon they visited the Qinsan Gardens, where he was intrigued by the other children. One child had a scooter which Clifford was determined to try for himself, so Margaret persuaded the owner to let him have a ride. She then firmly took him off to the station to buy tickets for the train—the railway having been repaired—back to Peking and to reserve a sleeper. After tea, leaving Clifford with the amah, Margaret went to the cathedral evensong with a heart full of joy and thankfulness.

The journey from Shanghai to Peking involved a ferry crossing over the Yangzi River at Nanjing. A change of trains went without a hitch, but Margaret literally had her hands full—carrying a heavy baby and hand luggage—at the same time trying to produce tickets from her handbag while holding onto Clifford at the barrier. They had just settled down when some French sisters passed the compartment and recognized the baby from the ship. They asked to come in and began at once to make a fuss of Clifford, which he enjoyed, for he evidently knew them. They told Margaret that he had been very popular onboard ship and his escort had had an easy time looking after him. All went well until about six o'clock, when the nuns relinquished him to Margaret in order to say their prayers. Clifford had strong objections to maintaining silence during that time.

At Jinan, the mother superior joined the train, and she helped to amuse Clifford, as it was apparent that Margaret—as yet unused to his demands—was getting tired. The Nichols met the train at Tianjin, where the nuns departed. When the train reached Peking, it was eleven o'clock. As Margaret gathered her things together, she spied a bag under the opposite seat which she knew had been left behind by the sisters, so for safety's sake she took it with her. Clifford was carried off in triumph by three of Margaret's house guests, who had come to meet them.

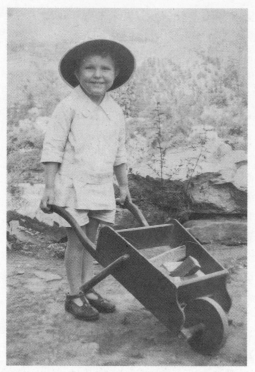

Clifford with his pushcart at the family's cottage in the Western Hills, c. 1925.

The next day Margaret returned to the station to collect the luggage and deliver the salvaged bag to the station-master. He was greatly relieved and said that mother superior would be a happy woman to recover it, for the bag contained some valuable documents.

♪＊

Before Mrs. Richardson left for England, she called to see Margaret and Clifford, and left several things for him, including a cot with a good mattress and mosquito net, a pushcart and some clothes. That afternoon she took Margaret to view an empty compound which she thought would serve well as an annex for PGs, helping to build up a nest egg for Margaret to take a furlough one day. She insisted on Margaret accepting a loan of one thousand dollars to launch the new project.

Margaret lost no time in getting back to her busy routine. She spent her scarce spare time trying to establish the annex, which did not work out as well as hoped. Ultimately she leased a house at the north end of Morrison Street, opposite the Salvation Army headquarters. The landlord, the Chinese Independent Church, had named it *Ping-An Fang* (House of Peace), which Margaret translated into "Rest House." By the end of the year, all formalities had been taken care of, Margaret engaged the services of a prospective hostess, Miss Saxild, a previous house guest who would be satisfied with a home in lieu of salary. This time Margaret already knew the person, and things worked out well for the next few years.

Within a couple of months, there was a constant stream of guests in both houses. Margaret frequently took meals at the Rest House, and she planted trees and flowers in the courtyards. Permanent guests included a dressmaker from the English Outfitters who stayed for three years, a young Russian studying Chinese and English, numerous missionaries learning the language and a succession of secretary-typists from the British legation.

Roads in the Far East often led to Peking, much as roads in Europe were said to lead to Rome. Hoards of American officers and their wives came from the Philippines to escape the damp heat of the rainy season, finding Peking refreshingly cool while the locals were gasping in the July heat. Margaret made them welcome and helped them to enjoy Peking as much as she could. They made few demands, as they understood that she had little time to spare.

Clifford did not take to amahs, and Margaret could not find anyone satisfactory to mind him while she got on with her professional duties. He was getting fretful. When she left him to go to dinner, he would grizzle till she ran back from the dining room to speak to him. Margaret thought this was being naughty, and to convey her disapproval she gave his hand a little slap. Soon she would find him standing in his cot with his hand held out in readiness. Better to be slapped than to get no attention, seemed to be his attitude.

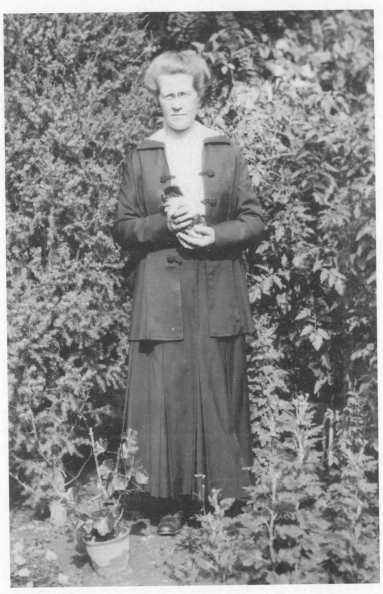

Dr. Margaret with a kitten in the 1920s.

Life was developing into such a rush for Margaret that she felt unable to give Clifford proper attention, so she looked around for a nanny. A young Russian girl, Miss Alexandra Bashkiroff, was highly recommended. Shura—as she liked to be called—spoke poor English, but this improved rapidly. The two got on well together which was a great relief to Margaret, knowing that she could leave Clifford in good hands should she ever need to be away for any length of time.

♪*

PEKING HAD SUCH A PROLIFERATION of women's clubs that they were becoming cliquish, so to combat this tendency a Federated Council of Women's Clubs (later known as the International Women's Clubs) was inaugurated. Margaret's social desires were adequately met with her interests in these clubs and her committee work. Her paying guests, another source of social intercourse, enabled her to live in a larger house than she could have otherwise afforded, and to keep a good table. She took pride in her accomplishments, feeling privileged to have an adopted child, educate her Chinese goddaughter and run a charitable institution for TB sufferers—all on the income pulled in from her many activities. She was immensely grateful for the timely assistance and support of loyal friends.

On the political front, changes were occurring, although with little impact on the city's way of life. At one stage when railway traffic became disrupted, an Allied military train plied between Peking, Tianjin and Shenyang for the purpose of preserving communications as laid down in the Treaty of 1901 after the Boxer Uprising. To prevent Chinese officials from taking refuge in the Legation Quarter, a special guard of armed police was maintained at the various entrances to this walled international settlement. Plainclothes detectives conspicuously loitered nearby. However, there was no apprehension in Peking, since every "takeover" occurred peacefully. The side that manoevered its armies into the better position paid the other side compensation money to move away.

One night a nearby arsenal exploded. Two days later Zhang Zuolin, the ex-bandit governor of Manchuria, arrived to take possession of Peking. In dense silence the crowds watched him gallop by on horseback, closely flanked on all sides by mounted guards. Cao Kun, the next candidate for the presidency, arrived on a later train and drove by in a limousine.

A year later one of the most popular warlords, Wu Peifu, came north to drive out Zhang Zuolin. In April the railway line between Tianjin and Shanghai was cut. Soon people became used to the sound of distant artillery gunfire, continuing with their daily round of business, for there seemed to be a mutual desire to keep the fighting well outside the city. The firing gradually came nearer and became more continuous at night, but it ceased during the day. By May the firing was so incessant that Margaret could not sleep, but then word came that Zhang was in full flight, and peace and quiet were restored.

The missionary association met monthly during the winter. On one occasion the speaker was the so-called Christian General, Feng Yuxiang, a colourful warlord and recent Christian whose nickname arose from his zeal. He virtually commandeered Mr. Gailes of the YMCA to teach his troops, and rumour had it that he arranged for his soldiers to be baptized by the thousand with the help of a long water hose. The general criticized the missionaries for spending too much time attending meetings and conferences, instead of focusing on evangelistic work. With a Bible tucked under his arm, he paced hastily back and forth. Margaret sensed a touch of fanaticism or religious mania in his behaviour. Years later he spent some time in Russia and was said to have become a communist. After the Japanese surrender, the Nationalist government sent him on a diplomatic mission to America and Europe. He died returning home in 1947 as the result of a shipboard fire in the Mediterranean.

♪﹡

FOREIGNERS WERE OFTEN DISTRESSED by the cruelty to animals at the hands of the Chinese, who seemed to think that animals had little sense of pain. Deaconess Edith Ransome of the Anglican mission started a small SPCA, and Margaret was roped in one day with other speakers to give a talk on the subject of animal care to the Anglican and London mission combined girls' schools. As the years went by, the Chinese treatment of animals certainly became more humane.

North China experienced a severe famine that winter, and in February the Chinese held a fête for famine relief in the Central Park. Each entrance ticket bore a lottery number for scrolls of four characters written by the president, Xu Shichang. Margaret's ticket was one of the lucky ones, and she long treasured the "writing" she had won. The Chinese value calligraphy above all the arts, as for them it was the first and the writing of scrolls was a profession. Samples of the best writings of bygone days are engraved on stone and displayed in the oblong pavilion at the *Bei Hai* of the Winter Palace. Facsimiles of these are used in schools as models for students to copy by tracing. By this method, they learn the feeling of a well-written character.

♪✳

MARGARET BEGAN TO TEACH an English class twice a week at the law school, tempted by the good pay and the fact that her guests were fewer during the winter; tourist season was over, so she only had her long-term PGs. She taught a class of fifty young men, but it turned out to be a futile effort which she later regretted. Certain students gave all the answers; others seemed to have done no preparation. Near the time for the annual exams (the school year ended in February at the Chinese New Year), the students began their political strikes. One day Margaret arrived at her class to find no one there. The students had all gone to a demonstration at the Foreign Office. On December 21, the school was actually on strike. A few of her keener students showed up, but as the principal was locked up in a nearby room and furiously kicking the door all the while, it was a case of teaching under difficulties. It was obvious by the timing that the students were making trouble in an attempt to evade the end of year examinations, so Margaret never returned.

By 1923, political events had begun to liven up again, again with little effect on Peking's inhabitants, who were getting somewhat case-hardened. Troops frequently moved about, and trains were irregular. One Sunday morning in September, Margaret saw several thousand of Feng Yuxiang's troops marching northwards. This may have been a manœuvre to oust the young emperor and to force his retinue to leave the Forbidden City. There was a tendency to panic, however, when Feng continued to pour troops into the city. On November 22, three of China's key men were all in Peking on the same day: Zhang Zuolin, the warlord governor of Manchuria; Feng Yuxiang, the army strategist in power in Peking; and Duan Jirui, the president.

♪✳

A NEW MISSIONARY, Mr. Braund, on his way to China, was taken ill with bronchopneumonia and hospitalized in Hong Kong. When he was somewhat better, he went on to Peking, but he was still so seriously ill that he was admitted at once to the Peking Union Medical College (PUMC) Hospital. It was found that his pneumonia was due to extensive pulmonary tuberculosis. Recovery was out of the question, and under pressure for hospital beds, the medical superintendent requested that the mission make other arrangements. Rev. and Mrs. Scott kindly agreed to receive him, and the bishop asked Margaret to care for him. She fetched Mr. Braund by ambulance. Though obviously he had not long to live, she visited him frequently, if only to make him as comfortable as possible. No nurse could be found for him until two days before he died. After the funeral service in the cathedral, the coffin was carried on men's shoulders through the Chinese City to the British cemetery outside Peking's West Gate (*Xibian Men*), the mourners walking in procession behind.

En route, Margaret overheard a Chinese passerby say, "What little boxes the foreigners use to bury their dead." The Chinese use large, thick coffins which hold many of the deceased's belongings for use in the hereafter. The coffin provided by the PUMC looked insignificant by contrast.

During the summer months, whenever the opportunity arose, Margaret played tennis with guests before breakfast. Clifford was then the main interest in her life, and she had a quick peep at him every time she entered or left the house. He played in the courtyard all day, and slept in a room adjoining hers. She put him to bed at night, dressed him in the morning and usually took care of the afternoon nap as well.

♪✳

MARGARET STILL HOPED to open a sanatorium for TB patients in the Western Hills. Dr. Hopkins of the American Methodist mission had established a small one for men, but, as so often seemed the case, there was no place for women and children. TB occurred so frequently amongst teenage schoolgirls that Margaret found it advisable to examine every boarder very thoroughly at the start of each year. She took her idea to Mr. Robert Greene of the PUMC, who seemed quite interested. He promised at least one thousand dollars towards her project but wanted a more definite scheme. But then at the end of the year he said the PUMC would not collaborate, as they now had their own plans for anti-TB treatment.

A month later Margaret received a letter from Miss Ida Pruitt, the PUMC's director of social services, inviting her to call. She had heard of Margaret's desire to open a sanatorium. When Margaret told her that she had been unable to get any support, Miss Pruitt encouraged her to make a start in Peking and promised to send her patients. The upshot was a small home that Margaret set up near the Anglican cathedral, which was convenient for her to look in on every time she attended St. Faith's, at least three times a week. It held six patients and a woman to cook and look after them while Dorothy Bearder, from the mission dispensary just across the street, came over to take their temperatures. Little equipment was required, as the patients supplied their own bedding and eating utensils. They paid only for their food, and where there was no money, Miss Pruitt's social service department paid for them. Margaret's lifelong campaign against the scourge of tuberculosis had begun.

That year she was elected to sit on the medical board of the Anglican mission. She was interested in hearing details on the progress of the mission hospitals in Hejian, Qingzhou and Datong. With her tuberculosis home just getting under way, she was encouraged when the board donated $150 towards its upkeep.

It had been long agreed that the Union Medical College for Women should not remain in competition with the PUMC, and the Rockefeller Foundation, through its China Medical Board, had promised substantial help for the college to join the Cheeloo University medical department in Jinan. The move meant that Margaret gave her last lecture in medicine after seven and a half years of consecutive teaching. Soon afterwards she stopped her translating work. To fill the resulting gap in her income, she taught English at the Peihua School. Her private practice was still active.

Margaret's friend, Mrs. Heal, whose imminent miscarriage had been averted the previous November, gave birth to a healthy daughter at the end of May. Margaret discovered that Clifford had not been baptized, so she and the Heals agreed to have their children baptized together. On Sunday afternoon, November 26, Helen Heal and Clifford Harold Phillips were baptized by Rev. Gilfillan of the Anglican mission in the British legation chapel. Mr. Heal became Clifford's godfather, and Margaret godmother to Helen. Margaret asked her old friend from Kaifeng, Canon George E. Simmons, to be Clifford's godfather *in absentia*. After the service, the Heals held a tea party in their home.

∫※

ONE MORNING, just before Christmas, a policeman came to take Margaret's cook, Yang Huating, away for questioning. It turned out to be a trumped-up charge of misconduct by a disgruntled amah. With the help of a good Chinese lawyer and Margaret's testimony, Huating was released several days later. The case was dismissed, on the grounds that the woman was a bad character whose accusation was unsubstantiated. An official regretfully told Margaret that, since the start of the Republic, Chinese women could bring such charges against men. Had it not been for Margaret's support, Huating would have likely had a long stay in prison. She found it an interesting experience of Chinese justice; the case had been well handled. Margaret respected Huating, who was honest, literate in both English and Chinese, and invaluable as a cook.

Before Clifford's third birthday, Margaret decided to take him to Dr. Cormack's private nursing home for a "necessary operation," a circumcision. The day was cold, and the room was heated only by a small oil stove. She gave the anaesthetic, becoming anxious when the doctor seemed slow and kept him exposed too long. That night Clifford developed a fever, and he remained quite ill for several days.

About that time, Shura had an attack of haemoptysis and was taken to the French hospital. Margaret was sorry to learn that this was not her first attack. Neither Shura, nor those recommending her, had dared to tell Margaret this before. Dr. Sudakoff begged Margaret to take Shura back, as she had nowhere else to go; White Russians were the displaced refugees of the new Bolshevik regime, and North China was flooded with them. Margaret knew well that haemoptysis was not infectious, and she believed Shura had a better chance of keeping well in the open-air life of the Chinese courtyard of her home. As she was more reliable than any amah had ever been, Margaret grudgingly allowed her back—so long as she did not cough. Just the same, Margaret rarely felt at ease with her, especially whenever she heard a tiny cough. She was relieved when Shura got married four months later to a minor official in the Russian mission.

ſ*

MARGARET WAS BUSY SUPERVISING the building of a five-room cottage on her land in the Western Hills. Though small, it was strongly constructed of stone blocks from a nearby quarry. By the middle of the year, the place was fully furnished and equipped for occupation as a handy retreat from the city. The mission caretaker, Liu, did the cooking, while one of his sons brought up water from a spring in a nearby gully. This was the family of Margaret's goddaughter, Meizhen, which made it

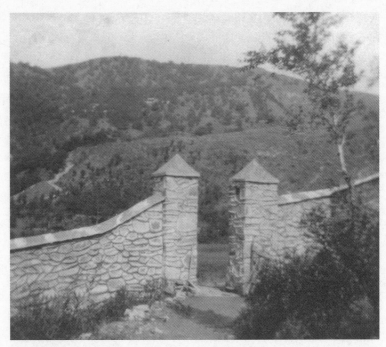

The entrance to the Phillipses cottage in the Western Hills.

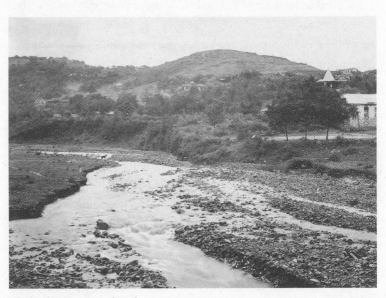

The landscape surrounding the cottage.

easier for Margaret to observe the young girl's progress with her schooling. Margaret enjoyed being able to ease her packed program with a series of short breaks in the Hills. The view from the terrace by the cottage was extensive and very pleasing, and Margaret painted a watercolour of that scene.

A recently arrived missionary, Mrs. Cox, a young war widow, consulted Margaret about her throat. Her tonsils were much enlarged so she was referred to the PUMC for a tonsillectomy, but it was decided to be unnecessary. One morning a little later, Margaret found her in bed with a sore throat. Two days previously she had been on an expedition to the Great Wall, and she must have picked up a germ in the crowded train. At first she did not seem very ill, but the next day she had signs of pericarditis and the sinister spots of septicaemia. Margaret asked for a consultation and a PUMC doctor came to see her, and the following day a second doctor came, but the patient was doomed from the first. Margaret remained with her in the mission for the next three nights until she died. Margaret remembered in time to have her sign an impromptu will, which she and the nurse witnessed. However, they had omitted the important words "in the presence of each other." Margaret was called by the consul to render an affidavit that they were both together and had signed at the same time. Her diagnosis had been septic pericarditis, and subsequently the postmortem proved her to be correct.

♪✽

CLIFFORD ENJOYED PLAYING with the caretaker's youngest children and their friends, and he quickly learned to speak Chinese. While adults seldom learn to speak the language well, children learn easily to emulate their playmates and speak Chinese perfectly. Clifford found it much easier to speak than English, so that he was inclined to be lazy over his mother tongue. It was not uncommon for English parents to speak to their children in Chinese, but Clifford soon discovered that he had to learn English if he wanted to speak to his mother.

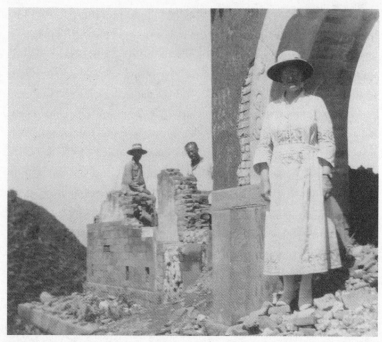

Margaret standing in the ruins of the old Summer Palace (Yuan Ming Yuan) in the summer of 1929.

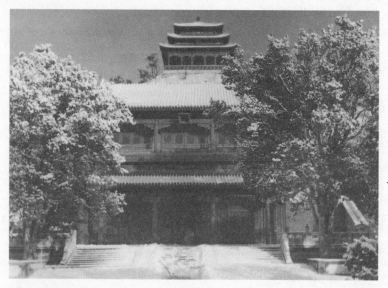

The new Summer Palace, located west of Peking, in wintertime.

Life in Peking was gradually developing a style appealing to tourists. In those days, cruises on oceanliners brought sightseers in droves to China, where Peking was the main attraction. With her growing network of connections and sponsors, Margaret was able to offer her guests a type of accommodation in her Chinese-style homes which contrasted immensely with the great hotels. Her personal touch was much appreciated. Margaret once took a guest, turned patient, by car to the hot springs at Tangshan for a week's complete rest, returning the following Saturday with two friends. They spent the night at the hotel, enjoyed the baths, and all returned to Peking the next evening. She often took guests to the Temple of Heaven park, which encloses the Altar of Heaven, treating the group to a picnic on a clear night beside the moonlit altar—a beautiful sight. Occasionally, if any guests were at loose ends and she had a free afternoon, she would guide them round some of the better temples, or the Moslem mosque in the Chinese City. No hotel could match that sort of care, and these brief interludes benefited Margaret too.

Late that summer Margaret had an unfortunate mishap. The Betteridges were house guests for a couple of weeks before returning home on furlough. Margaret and Frances Betteridge (*née* Cunningham), her former colleague in Pingyin, planned to visit the ruins of the old Summer Palace (*Yuan Ming Yuan*), which had been wrecked by the Allied forces after the Taiping Rebellion in 1860 as retribution for the cruel treatment of British envoys to the court. At breakfast Margaret kicked over a kettle of boiling water which was on the floor by her chair, badly scalding her right foot—her good one! Naturally she preferred to stay home, but the party would not go without her, so she agreed to go. Having never visited that place, she was unaware that it entailed a long walk over wasteland, and that little was left to see other than the remains of an Italianate villa. For all that, Margaret was glad she went, because quantities of carved marble were being carried off bit by bit by the warlords who in turn had occupied Peking.

From there they went on to the Jade Fountain, then to the Temple of the Sleeping Buddha, where Margaret remained in the car. When they returned home, it was time for Margaret's clinic at the mission girls' school. The Betteridges went out to the Hills for the next ten days and Margaret joined them with Clifford, thinking it would be a rest for her foot. However, it got worse, so she consulted Dr. Cormack, who was rather puzzled and advised bed-rest. She was getting the most severe cramps when she stood up, so that she had to rest her foot on the wash-stand while getting dressed. When she noticed little patches of black on her foot, she knew that gangrene was setting in. After five days in bed and dressings of potassium permanganate, good healing began. Because of the demands of her practice, she was soon again hard at work.

One day Margaret went to the *Lung Fu Si* fair to buy wallflowers for her garden, but as yet there were none in bud—the stage at which the Chinese market their plants. Disappointed, she turned into an alley where pets were sold and promptly fell in love with a beautiful black Pekinese dog, a year old, and probably stolen from some household. He took to Margaret at once and snuggled up on her lap. She felt he would make a good playmate for Clifford. The dog was named Fishy because of his goggle eyes, plume-like tail and fringed paws, which reminded her of the black goldfish in the Central Park—especially when he lay spread-eagled, his back legs stretched straight out behind him.

♪✳

ABOUT THIS TIME the Peking Club came into being, starting off as the local branch of the Overseas League. It was originally known as the League of Patriotic Britons Overseas, to which Margaret had belonged during and since the war. The members were mainly businessmen who found it useful as a meeting place. This became very much a men's club, with a separate women's section.

The arts were very much part of Peking's social life. The Choral Society was active for nine months of the year with impressive performances, thanks to some good soloists in the community. Plays such as *The Bat* by the Amateur Dramatic Society and *The Dover Road* by the American College Women's Club were well attended. Among the more distinguished visitors to Peking that year were interesting speakers such as Roy

Chapman Andrews, the world-famous archaeologist, lecturing about his discoveries in Mongolia. He showed slides of his excavations where he had unearthed dinosaur eggs and expounded his theory on the close relationship between Mongolians and North American Indians, claiming that a land bridge connecting Asia to the American continent had enabled the Mongolians to find their way eastwards.

Margaret belonged to yet another Peking society called the Things Chinese Society, started by her friend Mrs. Richardson, who felt it would be good for Westerners residing in Peking to learn more about Chinese history and customs. Several meetings took place in Margaret's house, once when seventy people came to hear Mr. Bertram Lenox Simpson, an authoritative correspondent otherwise known as B. L. Putnam Weale, talk about his experiences during the Boxer days. Many listeners spilled over onto the verandah. The last speaker of the year was Mr. J. E. Baker, an adviser to the Chinese government on the industrial development of China, which was just beginning. There was no lack of interest in China's history and progress.

Mr. and Mrs. Whymant, from Japan, came to stay at the Rest House. While there, Mrs. Whymant had a severe attack of malaria, but she recovered quickly, and they extended their stay so she could see something of Peking. On September 1, a terrible earthquake struck Japan. Had it not been for Mrs. Whymant's malaria, the couple would have been back in Tokyo and could have lost their lives, as did many others. The news of the damage was appalling: Yokohama had been nearly wiped out, and Tokyo was not much better. The Royal Navy and the US Navy poured all available stores into the stricken areas, while the US Marine Corps dispatched a contingent to help with rescue work. Margaret offered her services to the Red Cross to do relief work, but she was not needed.

On National Day, the Double Tenth (October 10), Cao Kun took up the office of president after having spent enormous sums to bribe his electors. (In the end, he was not in power for long.) The occasion was celebrated enthusiastically, and the Forbidden City was illuminated in the usual fashion. Two days later, for the first time, Coal Hill was opened to the public. A small entrance fee was levied as a contribution to the

Japanese Earthquake Relief. Swarms of Chinese clambered up the steep pathway past the five pavilions which gave an impressive all-round panoramic view of the city. Down the other side, they passed the tree from which the last Ming emperor, Zhuang Lie, had allegedly hanged himself when the Manchus were attacking his palace gates.

♪✲

THAT MONTH Margaret's mother died in Bridgwater, though Margaret did not receive the news from her two brothers till mid-November. In those days mail travelled via Siberia and took nearly two weeks to be delivered. Margaret grieved as much for Bert as for her mother, for she knew they were very close. The two women had almost given up corresponding. Margaret had been gone for more than ten years; she felt she had been neglectful about writing to her mother.

Soon after Clifford's fourth birthday, Margaret took him to school. She reluctantly decided to have his long, curly fair hair cut; the barber was unwilling to cut it until he was assured that Clifford was indeed a boy. The kindergarten at L'École Sacré Cœur was run by a French convent. At first he was shy and took shelter under the sister's desk, largely because he could not understand French. However, the mother superior's soothing manner soon persuaded him that he was among friends and thus started him on the road to speaking French with a good accent.

Before the year was out, Clifford had a mild bout of whooping cough. He only managed a little whoop or two, the sound of which rather intrigued him, but when he tried to practise it Margaret firmly discouraged him. She had a strong aversion to all types of coughing and was of the steadfast opinion that, whenever possible, people should restrain the urge to cough.

Since Shura had left to get married, Margaret had been on the lookout for a replacement. She came across an advertisement from a Miss Amy Bradbury, who was looking for a home with a missionary family where she could be useful by looking after a child. No salary was required, so Margaret answered the request and Miss Bradbury quickly replied that she would be pleased to come to Peking. Years earlier she had come to China as a missionary under the China Inland Mission, but she could not get on with the language. As her health was poor, she had returned to England, where she taught in school for fifteen years before retiring with an invalid's pension. Then she had returned to China as a nursery governess to a missionary family with four young children in west China. She had been with them for two years and wanted a change.

Miss Bradbury had written what seemed to be "a well-educated letter in good handwriting," so when Margaret met her, she was shocked to hear her speak with a pronounced Cockney accent. However, to Margaret's relief, Clifford was unaffected by her accent, and for the next two years Amy was a great comfort. Margaret relied on her to run domestic affairs smoothly regarding the guests, although her primary job was the care of Clifford. Occasionally, Margaret and Amy took turn and turn about in Peking or the Hills, thus freeing Margaret to visit more of the country-side and the temples thereabouts.

Near the end of the year, the lease for the Rest House expired, and Margaret felt it was time to give it up. Similar establishments were springing up, and she did not wish to compete with them, which would have demanded more time and energy. She was still hosting PGs at her home, and even with Amy's assistance the enterprise was taking up all her spare time, although she enjoyed cosseting guests with special tours, particularly to temples.

♪⁂

GENERAL FENG YUXIANG had decided that the situation of an abdicated emperor of China, still living in Peking in the imperial quarters of the Forbidden City and holding court there, was anomalous. In his usual impulsive fashion, Feng went one morning to the palace and ordered Xuan Tong (Puyi) to leave at once. There was no option for Xuan but to retire to Tianjin, where he lived in a very comfortable style as a modern playboy.

Dr. Sun Yat-sen was not getting on well with his party in the south, and he had come to Peking to look into the state of affairs in the north. When he arrived, he was already a sick man. It may have been the new PUMC Hospital that attracted him, for there was no other establishment as good nearer than America. Mrs. Wellington Gu, wife of the Chinese ambassador in England, had placed her house at Sun's disposal, but he had not occupied it for long before he went into hospital for observation. For a time the PUMC had to find outside nurses for special cases, as the supply of nurses was inadequate and the newly trained nurses were not yet ready. A few foreign nurses in Peking undertook private nursing, and they were in great demand. One of these was Miss Gardner, who lived with Margaret while doing night duty for Dr. Sun from November 29. She was still with Margaret on Christmas Day, when it was finally ascertained that Dr. Sun was suffering from cancer of the liver. He refused to believe this and left the hospital, returning to Mrs. Gu's home, where he sent for Chinese physicians.

Miss Gardner found him a difficult patient, and his wife, the revolutionary Song Qingling, even more so. She discharged Miss Gardner on January 29. One of his special day nurses, Miss Ho, was a friend of Margaret's. At dinner one evening, she mentioned that it had been arranged for her to live in the French hotel—which was conveniently near the hospital, making it easier for Sun's Russian friends to keep her under surveillance. All her movements were questioned, and she told Margaret that they knew where she was dining and when she would be returning. She had no doubt she was constantly being followed.

By February 12, another English nurse, Miss Tamkin, who was doing night duty for Dr. Sun, had come to stay with Margaret. Margaret supposed this was because living near the hotel made her movements more easily observed. Miss Tamkin left on March 11, and the next day Sun's death was announced. He was to be embalmed and reverenced like Lenin, and it was reported that a glass coffin would come from Russia.

On March 19, Sun Yat-sen's body was taken to the Central Park. Margaret went to see the procession. After a memorial service in the

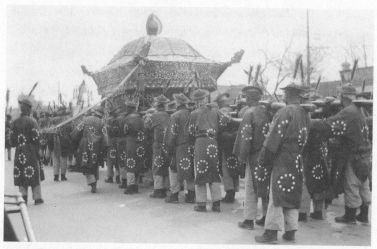

The catafalque and the rear of a funeral procession for Dr. Sun Yat-sen, March 19, 1929.

PUMC auditorium, a simple foreign-style coffin was carried on the shoulders of his followers with none of the trappings of a Chinese funeral. A long line of mourners followed, mainly students and Russians led by Lev Karakhan, the Soviet consul-general. The next afternoon Margaret went to the Central Park to see an exhibition of paintings by Miss Yang, an artist friend. People were crowding into the park to see where Dr. Sun's body was lying, and looking through the windows of the pavilion by the Altar of Grain and Harvests, Margaret saw his coffin on display.

She accompanied a friend to the Central Park on March 25 to see the actual lying-in-state. The park seethed with people. In the central enclosure, where the altar stood, the crowd was densest, but orderly and quiet. A line of people slowly advanced to the pavilion where the coffin lay. Guards directed them inside, where they passed slowly round the coffin and were kept on the move. A pane of glass in the coffin allowed a view of Dr. Sun's head and shoulders. Margaret thought he looked "quite small and rather grey." People then passed through another door to see the many memorial scrolls displayed in the long mat galleries that had been erected to accommodate them. Day after day, long lines of students headed to the park: first college students, then middle school groups, later even the primaries. All wore black armbands, according to foreign fashion, and white rosettes on the chest, a Chinese sign of mourning.

This continued for about three weeks. On April 2, the coffin, accompanied by a monstrous procession of students, was moved to the Azure Cloud Temple (*Bi Yun Si*) in the Western Hills, which became a place of pilgrimage for officials and other visitors while Sun's mausoleum was being constructed in Nanjing. After Dr. Sun's removal from the Central Park, a special memorial service was held every Monday morning in the pavilion where he had lain in state. Obeisance was made to a large oil painting of his head and shoulders. A similar painting hung over the central arch of the *Tian An Men*. Every school opened with a memorial chant and three bows towards his portrait, and the same procedure began any programs in the cinema and all public meetings. The graduation ceremony at the PUMC opened in the same way, with the addition of two minutes' silence.

The worship of Sun Yat-sen seemed to be making good progress and Margaret began to wonder whether she was seeing a new religion in the making, but within a few years the fervour had slackened. At a PUMC graduation ceremony Margaret attended then, Sun's portrait hung in the position of honour at the back of the platform. Everybody stood and bowed as instructed by the emcee, who then ordered, "There-will-be-two-minutes-silence-please-sit-down," all in one breath. "*Sic transit gloria mundi*," thought Margaret, knowing it was fading. For a few years the portrait in the Central Park pavilion remained in position and the chairs in place, but eventually the picture was turned round, and after a time the hall was in use again for exhibitions and other meetings without it. However, the park still retains the name *Zhong Shan Gongyuan*, which it had been given at the time. *Zhong Shan* (Central Mountain) is the name of Dr. Sun's ancestral home in South China, and accorded to him as an honorific title.

AT THE START OF THE YEAR, Margaret's small tubercular sanatorium was crowded with six adults and four children. After the recent death of a child, she seldom missed a day visiting, though, sadly, the patients were usually too far gone for hope, but at least they were not spreading the infection. When any improvement came about, the patient was naturally eager to return home, but often far too soon.

Margaret paid a short visit to Tianjin to read a paper to the Women's Social Service Club on social service in a Chinese home. She stayed with Mrs. Goodrich, who took her to visit the Bei Yang Hospital, provided a delicious Chinese dinner and took Margaret to see her orphanage. Mrs. Goodrich belonged to a well-known American pioneer missionary family of North China. The next day Margaret gave her lecture to twenty-two members at the club.

This club supported a little girl at Margaret's TB home for several years. The child was orphaned and homeless during the great famine of 1920–21. Under Margaret's care she had lessons, and learned to knit stockings and make her own clothing, including her cotton shoes. In time she recovered but was then found to have a rather unusual blood disease, which was cured by the removal of her spleen. When she was quite well again, she was sent to the Anglican mission school. Margaret learned that after she left school, her benefactresses at the Social Service Club had successfully arranged a marriage for her.

Later that year Margaret appreciated a course of lectures on paediatrics, given by a celebrated American specialist on diseases of children, who the PUMC had invited for a short term of office. For three months, two weekly lectures and a Saturday morning lecture-clinic were open to all Peking doctors. The clinic was held in the lecture room, and patients were wheeled in on their beds for examination. Many, like Margaret, were only too glad to have this refresher course. She felt she could not have stayed away from England so long but for the help provided by the PUMC in keeping her up to date. While she was about it, Margaret "rubbed up" her medical knowledge with a comprehensive review of diseases not frequently encountered in Peking, including leprosy—rarely seen in North China, though she had had patients with it in her Shandong days. The daily routine involved morning ward rounds, afternoon lectures and practical work. Apart from films, the syllabus included blood tests, stomach tests, sputum examination, transfusion, X-rays and postmortem.

This hospital was becoming increasingly appreciated by the local populace, which tended to diminish Margaret's private practice. As the disturbed conditions in China discouraged tourism, she decided to take up private teaching, initially giving English lessons to Yuan Shikai's relatives. The Chinese were keen to learn English, and many foreigners had a pupil or two, often in exchange for lessons in Chinese—a useful way of getting to know the Chinese and making friends. Mr. Britland from the mission made the introductions, and they were invited to lunch—an informal meal at a large round table with the whole family, elder and younger of both sexes, eating together. Margaret's four pupils were three of Yuan's teenage grandchildren, a boy and two girls, and their aunt, the youngest of the old man's children. After the meal, Margaret was taken to see the oldest Mrs. Yuan, his widow, who kept to her own apartments.

Margaret was to teach for two hours on Monday, Wednesday and Friday afternoons. Her pupils were responsive, so the lessons were enjoyable. They liked Margaret to play the piano for them, and eventually the young aunt asked her for music lessons. During tea, which is always served to teachers and visitors, they loved to produce some tasty Chinese dish. Despite this pleasant routine, Margaret was none too pleased with herself for taking up this kind of work, for it amounted to little more than "a potboiler."

She started to look round for more meaningful medical work, recalling that when she first came to Peking, Dr. Gray had invited her to assist with an operation at his hospital for indigent Chinese in the Chinese City. That, of course, was many years ago. After he left during World War I "to do his bit for England," the army surgeon for the British garrison had replaced him. Now that Dr. Gray had returned, Margaret wrote to ask if he could make use of her services at the British Charitable

Hospital, so-called because no fees were charged in the early days; support came mainly from contributions by friends in the British community.

Dr. Gray replied kindly that his hospital was small, primitive and short of funds. He did not consider it worth troubling Margaret to go so far, for the hospital was located deep in the southern part of the Chinese City. In reply, Margaret asked him to remember her if he should think of any way in which she might help. A month later he wrote saying that he had reconsidered her offer. As the women and children in the outpatients department were increasing and the women's ward was always full, he thought it would be helpful if she could be a visiting physician. He would give her complete charge of both departments, for a small monthly honorarium, if she attended three mornings a week, from ten to twelve-thirty, with breaks when the hospital closed for the Chinese New Year, and also the whole of July. Margaret was happy to accept, and this arrangement continued until December 8, 1941, when the Japanese declared war on the Allies.

Margaret was now pretty much on an even keel again, fully occupied mornings and afternoons three alternate days a week, the other four days attending to her mission responsibilities, TB sanatorium and private practice. This kept her evenings free for meetings, committee work and infrequent recreation or socializing, which invariably included the Choral Society and the British Women's League. The next four or five years passed rather quietly.

♪※

ABOUT THIS TIME Clifford acquired his Chinese name. During a summer holiday in the Western Hills (Xi Shan), Margaret took him for a walk across the valley to visit one of the temples for which the area is known. Most of those temples were nothing more than sightseeing spots, but this temple was an active place of worship, with an abbot and a small group of monks. Clifford was fascinated by the large red carp in a sizeable pool. Margaret was well known and respected in the neighbor-

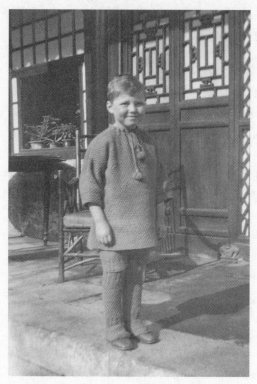

"Shao-Ye": the Little Master, c. 1926.

hood, and soon the abbot appeared to bid her welcome. Noticing Clifford at her side, he asked his name. Without hesitation Clifford replied, *"Shao-Ye,"* which means "little master."

Margaret hastily explained that her small idiot of a son did not yet have a proper Chinese name, so he knew no better than to give the name he was used to hearing. All his Chinese associations, from domestic servants to village children, addressed him by this honorific. The abbot was gracious over the gaffe, and offered to compensate for this lack by creating a name. Margaret was grateful for the venerable monk's understanding. A scholar, the abbot was aware of the weight of his responsibility in naming the young boy before him. He knew that Margaret's Chinese surname was Lei, which is indicated by a Chinese character consisting of the "rain" radical over the character for "field." Gazing across the fertile fields in the valley below, the old man said:

Rain falling on the fields below makes them fertile, even as Thunder quickens the seed in the ground. The answer is plain. With the surname Lei, he shall be named Hou-tian [which may be translated as "Abundant Fields"].[2] ·

By the age of seven, Clifford had progressed to a boys' elementary school, L'École St. Michel. Now the proud possessor of a green canvas satchel for his books, he was allowed to walk unescorted to school, a distance of about a kilometre and a half (1 mile). When the weather was bad, he had the luxury of a rickshaw ride.

For the next couple of years life continued along these lines at No. 13 Nan Wan Zi, Margaret's home for almost ten years. In September 1929, Clifford transferred to the Peking American School, which provided a full curriculum of primary and secondary education. It had begun as Miss Leitch's School for English Children soon after World War I. About three years later, it was taken over by an American educational organization based in California, and it became one of a chain of such schools around the world, catering primarily to children of professional or diplomatic families. This school was fee-paying and coeducational, attended by children of ten or more nationalities, including a few Chinese. All teaching was in English, except for foreign languages on the syllabus. The principal, Miss Alice F. Moore, maintained an enviable standard of excellence throughout a tenure of about thirty years. She was invariably fair, and constantly encouraged her pupils to do their best.

∫※

IN MAY 1929, Dr. Sun Yat-sen's coffin was moved from its temporary resting place at *Bi Yun Si*. His earthly remains were to be transported to the great mausoleum on the slopes of the Purple Mountain in Nanjing.

During a three-day memorial service at the temple, officials, diplomatic representatives and other foreigners paid their respects before the coffin. Finally, his widow, Madame Sun Yat-sen, his only son by an earlier marriage, Mr. Sun Fo, and other close relatives paid their homage. The body was then removed from its casket, re-embalmed and dressed anew before being transferred to a bronze coffin.

The entire operation from the temple took fifteen hours to cover a distance of 70 *li* (27 kilometres or 22 miles) for the cortège to reach the *Qian Men* station. A 101-gun salute heralded the start of the proceedings in the very early hours of the morning. A mounted guard of honour led the procession of one hundred soldiers, with a rearguard of another cavalry escort. Throughout the day the procession was joined by many students until finally the whole column extended over more than three kilometres (2 miles), lined by spectators all the way from the city limits to the station. Clifford was able to catch no more than a glimpse of this activity from the city wall overlooking the railway station. At 4:30 P.M. another 101-gun salute signified the imminent departure of the funeral train, and a half-hour later the train was on its way. At each major city en route to Nanjing, starting with Tianjin, a ceremony was held to show respect for Dr. Sun until the coffin reached its destination. On June 1, the final entombment took place at Purple Mountain. The magnificent mausoleum is visited by thousands of Chinese and a constant flow of tourists every year.

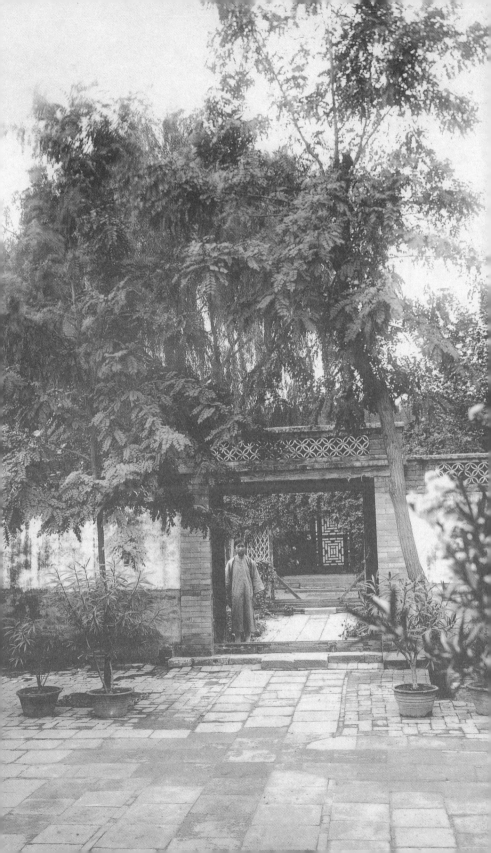

CHAPTER 16

Interregnum

♪﹡ PEKING WAS NO LONGER THE CAPITAL of China. Despite the power struggles and internecine warfare among warlords in North China, authorities were trying to clean up the city. In step with China's other major cities, Peking was finally realizing the benefits of the twentieth century, thanks largely to the foreign influences in its midst. All the big nations who traded with China still had legations there, and the British, American, Russian, Japanese, French, Dutch and Belgian legations had troops attached in barracks. When Chiang Kaishek had transferred the capital to Nanjing in 1927, their diplomatic protocol was extended to embassy status. The German legation lost those privileges due to World War I.

Since 1860, the world powers had been investing steadily increased amounts of money in China for several large enterprises that the Chinese could not undertake for themselves. The French built the railway from Peking to Hankow, and a great bridge over the Huang He. The British built the railway from Peking to Shenyang, which the Russians extended across Manchuria to the Siberian border. The Japanese built yet another railway for their own purposes, to the east coast through Korea. The

British worked coal mines near Peking and Tianjin. Foreign concessions were granted to Tianjin, which became a major port for North China. Similar enterprises existed in South China, where the great port of Shanghai was being raised from the mudflats on piles. Dredging enabled steamboats to navigate the Yangzi River beyond Hankow, while other shipping lines plied the entire length of the China coast.

The British had organized a postal service and a joint maritime customs service with the Chinese, and in many ways helped China to assume the role of a modern nation. The Americans helped largely with education, developing schools and universities, providing teachers and hospitals with training for Chinese doctors and nurses. Peking particularly saw great improvements in road construction with urban bus services and trams as well as an adequate supply of electric power for the city. River conservancy became organized, prison reform was started and scientific appliances were developed. Particularly dear to Margaret's heart was the significant reduction in infant mortality. Modern conveniences began to appear: telephones, modern plumbing, motorcars, aeroplanes.

Margaret believed that much of this development could be credited to missionaries of all denominations, who gave the Chinese Christianity and education, as well as to the traders, business people, engineers and diplomats who played their part in proving the benefits of international co-operation, proper administration and the use of taxation—all of which contributed eventually to a higher standard of living.

Peking became a desirable place to live. Two dozen years earlier, when Margaret first lived there, the city was marred by the dilapidation wrought during the declining years of the Qing dynasty. A few years later China became a republic, and Peking began to rise from the ashes, as it had done several times during its long history. People were better fed, and the streets were again a kaleidoscope of motion and colour. Smartly dressed Chinese women and more soberly dressed business people and students mingled with the poorer people wearing garments of indigo or grey. The country folk and minority peoples were easily recognizable by their colourful costumes and head gear. Cinemas had a growing appeal, as did the radio, generally at maximum volume.

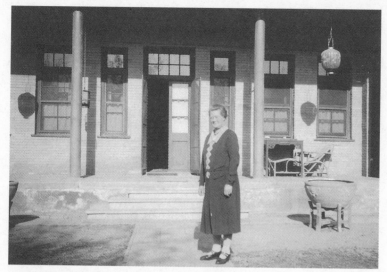

Dr. Margaret standing outside her new Peking home.

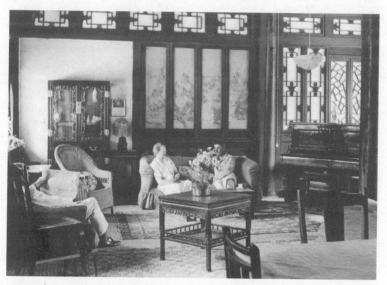

Margaret's new home in Peking was able to accommodate up to two dozen visitors at one time.

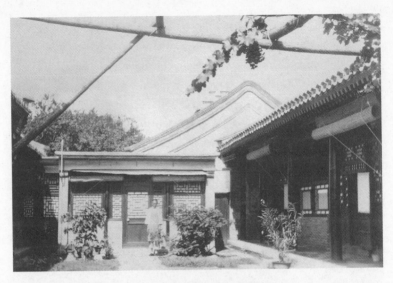

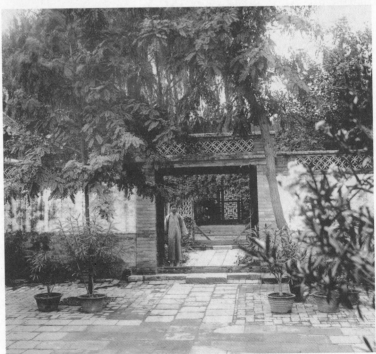

In the 1930s, Margaret and Clifford moved to a larger home in Peking which was noted for its modern plumbing and large inner courtyards.

Much of Peking's charm resided in its main streets, where lay evidence of an ancient civilization coupled with historical associations. Camel trains still presented a picturesque sight, but mule carts and sedan chairs became scarce. Rickshaws and bicycles remained the most useful means of getting around town. The Chinese rarely walked if they could afford to ride, and rickshaws were cheap and plentiful, competing with trams and buses, until later replaced by pedicabs. Rickshaw-pulling required no training or capital, and was the last resort of the unemployed and uneducated. The old, decrepit, lazy and very young swelled the ranks, contributing their strength and energy at the likely cost of their lives—particularly during the harsh winter months. Squads of rickshaws waited at the main street corners ready for hire, the pullers resting between the shafts. Fares were always negotiated by brisk bargaining before stepping into the vehicle.

Clanking streetcars, noisy motorcars, trucks and buses vied for attention with a cacophony of horns. One car was fitted with no fewer than five musical appliances. Serious accidents were remarkably rare. Bicycles were the pedestrians' greatest danger and the thoroughfares swarmed with both. Cyclists zigzagged along the streets, darting heedlessly in and out of traffic. With the increase in numbers, they realized that obeying traffic regulations was essential. Bent and broken bikes were often seen being taken home by rickshaw.

The Peking mule cart, formerly the most fashionable conveyance, was now used mainly by country folk. Its successors became numerous: small four-wheeled carriages resembling glass boxes on wheels, usually drawn by a weary horse that would trot but not run, often at a slower pace than the rickshaw-pullers. The driver sat in front, clanging a foot bell incessantly; on a step behind stood a runner who jumped down when approaching a corner. Running ahead to clear the way, he would seize one of the shafts to guide the mild-eyed Bucephalus round the bend. In previous times, family servants on horseback preceded and followed as escorts when the master ventured out.

Heavy carts conveying huge loads of grain, coal and all sorts of bulk materials were expected to keep to the soft shoulders at the edge of the macadamized roads. In muddy weather, which was fortunately infrequent, the sick-looking mules had great difficulty in dragging the carts through the deep ruts. Commandeering of carts with their beasts by the military was so common that much transportation was carried out by human labour: four or five men pulling and pushing heavily loaded carts.

In the midst of the city traffic, often in the early morning or afternoon before mealtimes, strings of camels ambled along with a majestic gait and a supercilious air, bringing burdens of lime, coal and other loads from the country districts, conjuring up visions of ancient caravans that for countless centuries were the only form of transportation over the desert wastes separating China from the West.

Wheelbarrows never carried passengers in the city, but trundled along with vast loads of farm produce or merchandise. They were much in use for hawking vegetables, ice and coal. A modified version still conveyed much of Peking's water supply, while the honey cart remained the means for removing the population's excrement. Happily, as modern plumbing became more established, such odious conveyances appeared at one's front door less frequently.

All this traffic increased the local dust, so street sprinkling went on nearly all day long, usually in the time-honoured manner of casting water over the street from a close-woven basket attached to a long pole. Clifford admired the men's great skill in distributing the water evenly and far. Modern motorized water tanks appeared from time to time, when the police had sufficient funds for the service.

The sedan chair of dynastic days had disappeared, except in wedding or funeral processions of the more affluent citizens. In weddings, a sedan chair conveyed the bride to her new home while more modern carriages followed with the guests. For funerals, the sedan "spirit chair" preceded the coffin to escort the body to its resting place. Funeral processions were striking, the grander ones an extravagant blaze of colour. An approaching funeral procession, stretching up the street as far as the eye could see, was an imposing sight, with the cortège of coloured banners, symbols, embroidered umbrellas, huge wreaths of paper flowers, and life-sized paper figures of servants, horses and carriages for use in the afterlife, followed by an enormous embroidered catafalque bearing the coffin. Sometimes bands of Buddhist priests in crimson or saffron robes played ancient musical instruments. When the seemingly grand procession drew closer, Clifford was often disappointed at the sight of irreverent ragamuffins—often beggars hired off the street for the occasion—carrying the symbols. Children, hired to carry the lighter articles or noisily beat drums, chattered and shouted, without concern for the solemnity of the occasion.

The chief mourner strolled along heedless of his surroundings, playing his part with dignified solemnity. Dressed in a robe of coarse white cotton, he preceded the coffin with downcast eyes yet stumbling feet, holding a tall staff in one hand and supported on either side by a friend. At specific intervals he knelt, facing the coffin, on a white mat in the middle of the street, and kowtowed three times. This break in the advance of the procession provided the coffin bearers with a brief respite. White circular paper money was thrown in the air, he rose, gongs were beaten, the bands played and the procession moved on.

The catafalque consisted of a framework of poles in the shape of a rectangular tent in which the coffin rested, covered with a vast, imposing curtain of red embroidered silk; five-year-old Clifford thought it resembled a moving Chinese temple. According to its weight, it was borne by thirty-two or more bearers—sometimes as many as eighty—all clad in dingy green livery. Behind followed the white-robed women mourners in carriages or mule carts draped in white. Funeral and weddings only took place on auspicious days, thus several processions might be seen following or passing one another. Occasionally, as many as three got mixed up together, and it seemed remarkable that they could ever get sorted out.

Wedding processions were far less imposing than funeral processions and, strangely, the music was melancholy by contrast. A distant wedding procession was instantly recognizable by the dismal drums and mournful pipes. The same ragged and decrepit symbol bearers wore similar dingy green livery, but this time with red Double Happiness (the wedding symbol) medallions stamped all over the garments. The leader, in a high cone-shaped hat of scarlet felt, beat a gong to direct the procession and clear the way. Then followed the lamp-bearers, though for ornamentation rather than practical purposes as most weddings took place by day. Behind came the symbol bearers and ceremonial umbrellas, followed by the bridal chair covered with scarlet embroidery. A second chair, often of richly embroidered green silk, carried the matron of honour. Behind her the guests—each decorated with a large red rosette—rode in red-draped carriages. In more fashionable modern weddings, the chair was replaced by a gaily decorated carriage or motorcar, perhaps preceded by a red-uniformed fife and drum band, providing more cheerful music.

Clifford discovered much of the colourful Chinese lifestyle while walking to and from school. Innumerable street hawkers identified themselves and their wares by their distinctive calls, intended to carry through to the inner courtyards of the distaff. To this end, the vendor raised his voice to a singsong pitch rather than a shout. The scissor-grinder employed metal clappers and the itinerant barber, a gong. Their services were well patronized by Chinese housewives or servants in their daily bargaining. Chinese cloth shoes did not need to be blacked, but they often needed to be mended, and the wayside cobbler was a great convenience. So was the travelling barber with his simple equipment, suspended from a pole across his shoulders. He could set up at any spot, and for a few coppers be ready to give a shave, haircut and a refreshing wash. The umbrella man, the tinsmith who soldered leaking pans and kettles, and the skilled artisan who repaired broken crockery by riveting the pieces together were much in demand. This last was an anathema to Margaret, who loathed the sight of cracked crockery on her table, however skillfully repaired. With no way of identifying the clumsy culprit, she stacked all offensive pieces in a cupboard. Once a year Clifford was told to carry the repulsive crockery into the backyard, where he had a wonderful time hurling each piece against the back wall, watched by an embarrassed servant who Margaret then instructed to clear up the debris.

Food stalls lined the outer edges of the sidewalks; the aroma alone was enough to guide one to a quick hot snack. A whole kitchen's equipment, including a stove, would be packed into a hand barrow, and the cook did a brisk business. Other vendors, like delicatessens, presented a variety of tasty cold cuts. During the winter the man with his large semi-circular cauldron roasting chestnuts in a mixture of sand and coarse brown sugar was not to be missed. Another popular stall sold baked sweet potatoes, which gave off a tempting redolence. Shandong Province was said to grow the best sweet potatoes. These two treats Clifford was allowed to buy off the street, but he also indulged in others which Margaret never suspected.

A particular favourite at New Year was *tanghulu*, sugar-glazed crabapples impaled on bamboo skewers like a kebab. A tasty alternative was Chinese dates or *zaor* (jujubes), the fruit of thorny trees prolific in North China, pitted and dried for winter consumption. Thousands of rickshaw-pullers fed on the streets, and many other Chinese also took their daily meals at these little stalls. Clifford often watched enviously as schoolchildren congregated round the toy and candy stalls with shrill cries of excitement to spend the coppers probably intended for more substantial meals. Young clientele often cut their teeth in the gentle art of bargaining with itinerant vendors of various small, inexpensive toys.

At the roadside, a fortune-teller might attract interested spectators as he cast the horoscope for a client and gave advice concerning future undertakings. Artisans created a variety of handicrafts on Peking's streets. Another street occupation was lumber sawing. A large log set up at an angle was sawn into planks by two men hauling on a large cross-cut saw—a slow and laborious process, but the resulting planks were remarkably even. The man on top skillfully guided the great blade as he hauled it up, while the job of pulling the blade down and getting covered in sawdust fell to the man below. Ropes were made, baskets and mats woven, pails and kettles and stove-pipes soldered, bicycles mended and even furniture built or repaired. A blacksmith worked in his open-fronted forge, with two sturdy posts and a cross-piece outside. The hapless horse would be securely roped to the posts before the smithy was willing to shoe it. Invariably a small crowd gathered round to watch.

Street fairs were frequent and popular. Goods of endless variety—old shoes, tins and bottles, spectacles, lamps of all sorts, toothpowder and soap—spread along the edge of the sidewalk, were much sought after by the country people. Piles of secondhand clothing were brought out for sale in front of pawn shops, which frequently attracted the most customers. Like the pawn shops, nearly all shops were identifiable by the signs and symbols suspended from the eaves over the entrance to the premises. A study of these alone could occupy a tourist with a camera for a long time. Better still, paintings of those symbols on rice-paper made a striking souvenir.

While the Chinese were not renowned as pet lovers, they delighted in breeding varieties of colourful goldfish in large earthenware jars. Many homes kept flocks of pigeons, which could be heard as well as seen, because the lead bird had fastened above its tail feathers a light bamboo whistle with a distinctive, clearly audible note. A popular practice was to try to lure someone's birds away from their home loft, then see how long it took to get them back. In many neighbourhoods this form of overt poaching provided a constant source of amusement. A dignified bird fancier might stroll along the streets, proudly displaying his birdcage containing a colourful and tuneful pet—often a rubythroat. A few people carried their birds openly on perches, off which they were launched to retrieve particles of food tossed into the air.

Beggars—blind and crippled, or with unsightly injuries—lay in full view on the sidewalk. Police vigilance gradually diminished their numbers, and certain temples were turned into refuges for these unfortunates. Nevertheless, the mendicants had an unerring eye for the tourist and gathered round to solicit alms in the most piteous fashion. Numerous charities dealt with the destitute in Peking, especially in the wintertime when porridge or soup kitchens were set up. Many beggars were not destitute but belonged to powerful guilds, and some professional beggars deliberately mutilated themselves to solicit sympathy. Horrified yet sympathetic tourists were more affected than the locals.

More deserving of largess were the strolling players and minstrels who eked out a meagre living with their street performances, varying from puppet shows to a lesser form of Chinese classical opera. A noisy orchestra of drums, cymbals and pipes helped draw an audience. The high-pitched falsetto voice assumed for Chinese opera is said to have derived from the need to be audible over the general noise and hubbub of the fairground. These and the itinerant storytellers, often blind, considered themselves fortunate when they were invited into a private courtyard to entertain an affluent household. On Clifford's birthday, as a treat for him and his friends, Margaret once hired a Chinese juggler to entertain the party. The children were riveted to watch at such close quarters.

Well aware that Clifford was often distracted by the activities on Peking sidewalks, Margaret worried he might be relating too closely with that influence. She preferred that he behave more like a proper young Englishman—not realizing how standards had changed over the twenty years that she had been away. Her ground rules were along the following lines:

- An Englishman is a gentleman at all times, noted for his good manners and always polite to all people.

- An Englishman's word is his bond. A promise is a firm commitment not to be undertaken lightly.

- An Englishman is a protector of the weak, including the opposite sex, and defers to females of all ages. It is not nice to be pushy.

- An Englishman is God-fearing, and loyal to the king and his country.

At times Clifford felt the rules were quite unfair, if not discriminatory—such injustices as having to sit on the floor because girls had occupied all the seats available, or missing out on the goodies on the party table because the girls had gone off with the best pickings.

Young Clifford was absorbing a considerable dose of Chinese culture by osmosis. He would amble as long as allowed through the Morrison Street Bazaar, *Dong An Shichang,* a large, popular marketplace, *inter alia* delighting in the jugglers, acrobats and wrestlers. Margaret did not give him pocket money, since she provided for all his necessities and knew the perils of unsanitary food. So he would scrounge a few coppers from his friend the cook, Yang Huating, although this was strictly forbidden. Huating, like Clifford, subscribed to the principle of the eleventh commandment: Thou shalt not be found out. He also understood the "little master" would lose face if he could not make a contribution when the hat went round after a street performance. With or without Margaret's approval, the Phillipses' honour was maintained.

For the past few years, since changing schools, Clifford had been feeling something of an oddity. He was growing up to be a loner. Margaret insisted that work come before play, and he had to return home to do homework before there was any question of games, much less sports. Most children were allowed to stay an hour or so after school to play before going home, and did their homework after supper. Clifford also dressed differently. Though none of his schoolmates wore shorts, Margaret believed a young English boy ought not to wear full-length trousers until he was twelve. What a great day that was! He endured much teasing and many scraps, which Margaret seemed to regard as part of growing up. Once Auntie Eve (Mrs. Heal) remarked, "It's a pity Dr. Margaret doesn't understand little boys."

Margaret upheld the creed that to spare the rod was to spoil the child, and she had no intention of allowing that to happen. Caning might occur two or three times a year, but it came to an abrupt stop when Clifford was fourteen. He had been disobedient, and disobedience and lying were two sins Margaret would not tolerate. Clifford had assumed the required position over the edge of the bed, biting his lip so as not to give the satisfaction of knowing that the punishment was having any effect. Suddenly a stroke landed across the back of his neck. He reared up and snatched the cane from his mother's hand. Breaking it over his knee, he cried, "Don't ever do that to me again!" She never did.

One day Margaret came in late for breakfast, having spent the small hours of the morning over a difficult delivery. The baby had died an hour after birth, but Margaret was gratified that at least she had been able to baptize him. What was the point, Clifford asked. The water used had not been blessed, and Margaret was not ordained and therefore had no

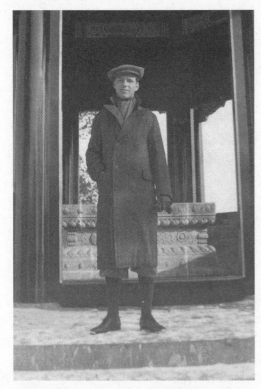

Clifford, in front of a gazebo on Coal Hill, winter 1935.

authority to perform a baptism. What about the millions of other babies that died at birth? Margaret, with the best will in the world, could not ensure that each and every one would enter the gates of heaven, which was her prayer for this infant. Refusing to dignify Clifford's outburst with a rebuttal, Margaret got on with her breakfast. Obviously she knew what she was doing, even if he didn't.

As Clifford's adolescence progressed, Margaret decided that his moral development would be improved by the influence of the Oxford Group movement. He attended a session of meetings in Beidaihe during the summer of 1934. Emotions ran high during evangelistic calls to come forward and be counted, but Clifford resisted. He did, however, respond to the need to unburden his soul. The mentor to whom he entrusted his confidences was attentive and consoling, and afterwards Clifford felt uplifted. What induced the man to repeat his whole confession to his mother some time later, Clifford never knew. He felt betrayed and bitter when she approached him with a view to "working things out." The result was a rift between mother and son which took a long time to repair.

Margaret never saw fit to teach Clifford anything about the facts of life. He, however—like his country playmates—had long acquired the basic facts of human reproduction, if only by watching the antics of dogs in the street. He took drawing lessons on Saturday mornings, and once showed his mother a poster he had designed, portraying Columbine pirouetting in a stage setting. She immediately objected to the dancer's bust, insisting that Clifford erase it at once, since "drawing that sort of thing was not polite."

It never occurred to Clifford to think of his mother as prudish, though she once embarrassed him terribly at the cinema. Margaret bought two balcony seats, and Clifford noticed a number of school friends sitting nearby. Preceding the main feature was a travelogue, in which the Paris tour included the grounds of Le Petit Versailles, noted for its fountains and statuary—mainly large, scantily clad female figures, some even with water spurting from the nipples of their ample breasts. The ensuing splutter of giggling—Clifford dared not join in—did not go down well with Margaret. Unnecessarily loudly for her son's liking, she said disapprovingly, "How very graceful!" A sudden silence resulted; the proverbial pin drop would have been thunderous throughout the cinema. Clifford was mortified, to say the least.

In villages in Xi Shan, full-breasted women commonly nursed their babies quite openly. Clifford had the grace to clear off when he once came across a woman, naked from the waist down, who had just given birth. She was cleaning up both herself and the infant at the edge of the field where she had been working. His presence could have been taken as an ill omen more than an embarrassment.

♪

CHINESE WOMEN were enjoying an incredible degree of emancipation. Over the two dozen years since Margaret came to China, they had become better housewives, mothers and helpmates to their husbands, and much of this was due to missionary influence. Margaret was eager to now promote a wider awareness of social service, which she defined as "helping others in special ways intended for their benefit and betterment."

The aim of the YWCA was to help the young women of China achieve higher standards of health, education, spiritual power and social relationships, so that they might become wiser citizens. Hampering that goal was the sheer magnitude of the task, the need for funds and the difficulty of changing existing conditions, or of influencing the ignorant and conservative. But Margaret firmly believed that the hope and possibility for a better China lay with women and their influence in the home. Why did young Chinese women crave higher education? Not necessarily due to a thirst for knowledge, she thought, but rather to escape restrictions and especially the dullness of home life.

In many wealthy homes, women suffered from a lack of occupation, being surrounded by swarms of servants who performed every service. Their babies were taken care of by amahs and fed by a wet nurse. Their only outlets for mental or physical activities were social duties and feasting. Such restricted mental life was often injurious to bodily health, leading to a high degree of stress. Margaret was called out one night to see a wealthy Chinese lady who was dying from heart failure brought on by anger. Another patient's fits of vehemence caused severe bouts of asthma. Happily, such conditions were changing as many Chinese women looked for a role with the YWCA, the Chinese Red Cross or another of the numerous philanthropic institutions. Margaret was convinced that those women were happier and healthier than if solely wrapped up in their own affairs and pleasures.

In the houses of the poor, Margaret was often appalled at the state of misery. Even a small degree of cleanliness was beyond their means, for water was expensive and difficult to obtain. Overcrowding was widespread, and landlords were not obliged to repair their properties. Tenants became used to discomfort and lacked the energy of good health to improve their conditions. Middle-class homes were also lacking in sanitation and cleanliness, often containing cheap foreign-style furniture, dirty matting and rugs covering the floors, and filthy curtains keeping out the light and collecting dust and germs.

Margaret believed the focus of social service work fell under four main headings:

1. Charity Organization Committee
2. Guild of Health
3. Mothers' Club
4. Home Training School

The Charity Organization Committee had the widest scope. Margaret insisted that the organizing committee be aware of all possible sources of assistance, for when it was not possible to raise adequate direct funding, even from other agencies, help could still be provided in the form of clothing, employment, medical relief or small loans on the recommendation of the nurse or other visitor. An intimate knowledge of Chinese homes was required, making home visits essential and necessitating a firm commitment by the membership. Chinese workers could do this with the utmost tact, knowing the most suitable time to call, how long to stay and when to leave, as well as how to interpret the conditions of the home and the responses of the people. One community social service agency alone reported two thousand visits in one year by their nurses and visitors.

Most hospitals in China charged more than the poorest could pay, thus the payment of those fees by charity would often mean a life saved. The primary problems were poor nutrition and tuberculosis. Tubercular patients needed to be taken from their surroundings, not only for their own better treatment but also to prevent infecting others. Margaret believed development of sound social services was the best way to combat the scourge of this disease, and she applied her energies wholeheartedly to this objective.

When hospital patients returned home, they were often too weak to return to work—if indeed they had any. Here the subcommittee on employment would find them a position. The child-placing committee had a list of people willing to adopt orphans, and the blind or crippled would be found suitable institutions. Visiting in middle-class homes was more difficult, but by dint of lectures, at homes, entertainments and health clinics, excuses would be found for follow-up work, especially concerning hospitals.

An easier task for the Charity Organization Committee was arranging sewing meetings to repair garments for the poor, or distributing such work as employment for poor women. Many workrooms were started in this way; for example, the Peking Exchange began with five women, developed into an industry of two hundred workers and carried on as a model industry. Women were also taught cleanliness, industry and a tranquil living style that must have affected their home life.

Margaret felt that fund-raising for a specific need was more effective than soliciting fixed annual subscriptions. She had often been struck by the remarkable hospitality shown by the Chinese, and felt sure this could be encouraged and directed for the betterment of the dissident. She did not consider handouts to be true philanthropy. Soup kitchens, poorhouses, orphanages and foundling homes were run largely by the police.

The Guild of Health also had a large task. No one visiting Chinese homes could fail to realize the need for improved hygiene. The courtyards of most Chinese homes were littered with all kinds of rubbish— decaying vegetables, ashes and dirty water. Peking's sanitation had improved, but only the main thoroughfares were kept clean; side-streets left much room for improvement. Many houses dumped their garbage outside their main gates, where it lay waiting to be collected. Under the Ministry of the Interior, responsibility for public health fell to the Department of Health; the police had the duties of controlling garbage collection and keeping the streets swept and watered. However, the city's public health was often at the mercy of the Guild of Scavengers over which the police had little control. In the rainy season the scavengers often failed to appear, sometimes due to sickness. Householders without septic tanks could be in great difficulty. Disease soon spread under such conditions, and only the glorious sunshine and dryness saved the Peking residents from epidemics of typhoid and cholera. Dysentery remained terribly prevalent.

The Council on Public Health of the China Medical Missionary Association held public health exhibitions, providing literature, and urging health instruction and better sanitation in schools, but extending the improvements into Chinese homes required additional help. The Chinese delighted in guilds and societies, and Margaret believed a guild of health would be a feasible means of bringing about better home sanitation. A similar society had been started in Kaifeng some years ago, though she did not know if it still continued.

Everyone, including children, would be eligible for membership in the Guild of Health, with the requirement that each member:

a. follow certain rules of personal hygiene, specially regarding spitting

b. keep the courtyards clean

c. remove excreta and keep latrines clean; if possible, these should be fly-screened

d. ensure kitchens are fly-screened

e. conduct regular monthly housecleaning

f. if a landlord, undertake to keep property in repair; if a tenant, promise to protect such property

g. agree that everyone in the home, including servants, be vaccinated

h. attempt disinfection after any occurrence of infectious diseases [After a death, a common practice was to move house, leaving germs for the new tenant.]

To achieve a higher public profile, each guild member would wear a distinguishing badge. Regular meetings would be held, with reports on homes inspections and overcrowding, in which case landlords would be notified. Prizes would be awarded for the cleanest homes. *Wei sheng,* meaning "sanitation," was a term in frequent use at the time, especially in advertising.

Mothers' clubs were a means, Margaret believed, of bringing greater happiness into the home, which would require some changes in home customs. The existing Peking Mothers' Club had evolved from an earlier Bible class, and it had about fifty members, mainly from the Western-educated, English-speaking upper class. The bimonthly meetings were always held in Chinese homes. Though the speakers were usually for-eigners—as requested by members—few foreigners attended, to permit the Chinese women greater freedom of expression.

Margaret was impressed with how openly they discussed their prob-lems. Subjects chosen for study included:

a. how to make the home attractive
b. how to keep the husbands at home
c. management of the home
d. care of the mother during pregnancy
e. care of the baby
f. nursing of the sick
g. moral training of children

Margaret felt that the formation of such clubs with their free discus-sions would lead to the desire for reform of social banes in the Chinese home. A subcommittee had already risen to work on certain problems—improvident marriages, forced marriages, concubinage, quarrels, suicide, gambling and extravagance (an issue which included the ostentatious weddings and funerals out of proportion to the family means, and the customary giving of presents)—which required the consideration of serious-minded women before they were to turn their attention to politics.

The Peking YWCA established a mothers' club for lower-income fami-lies, with a membership of about sixty. They met in the Chinese Independent Church every week for Bible study and talks about health and home matters. Margaret's dream was that the more affluent women involved might agree to lend their homes for such meetings; the practical example of a clean, refined, well-ordered home would be worth more than many lectures.

A Home Training School also required the principle of practical demonstration. During a score of years' service in China, Margaret had witnessed a marked improvement in general living conditions, especially in the towns. Contributing factors included improved communications, trade and the increasing Western influence due to more Westerners in China and more Chinese going abroad for education and other reasons. Margaret also credited the influence of years spent in mission schools, and the examples of foreign homes in China. Former schoolchildren were now married men and women. It was not so much the education that raised the standard of living as the domestic habits to which they became accustomed during their years in the mission schools. Theirs were the homes with which foreigners were most in touch, and from which the present-day student class came.

Margaret's concept of a home training school involved small classes in an ordinary Chinese house so that students could be, as much as possible, under conditions similar to their home life. She thought that the missions' current approach to education resulted in half-educated girls unsuited to become teachers, yet who considered themselves above manual work because of their education. In the Home Training School, students would focus primarily on practical work, with a secondary emphasis on subjects such as reading, writing, arithmetic, general knowledge and sanitation. Such schools would be arranged according to the general attainments and social standing of the students, but Margaret was most concerned about the requirements of the humbler homes.

Some nursing training was essential, for Margaret believed more lives were lost in China through mismanagement and lack of nursing rather than by actual disease. She cited a case of a young baby with pneumonia who refused milk, but for several hours no attempt was made to give him water. He needed to lie still, with his lungs as free for breathing as possible; instead he was carried around by the amahs with his chest compressed, and as he was a heavy child he was constantly shifted from one

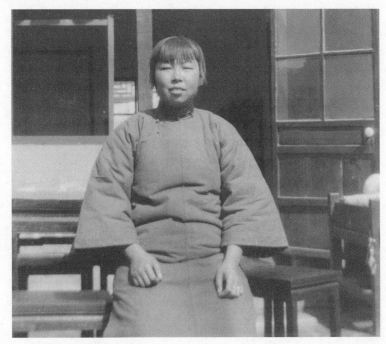

A nurse in front of one of the Peking sanatoriums. Dr. Margaret was an advocate for increased nurse training in China.

position to another, his breathing further impeded by heavy clothing. Thankfully, the parents were persuaded to take him to a hospital, and there, with proper nursing, he recovered.

The Home Training School taught commonsense care of the sick, emphasizing feeding and cleanliness as more essential than medication. The students learned how to wash up properly, to use clean water and not a stagnant ditch, and how to mend clothes. They were taught that even a small house could be clean and tidy. Nothing should be thrown on the floor. Separate washbasins and towels must be provided; the sight of the communal towel made Margaret shudder. Emphasis was placed on the value of open windows, changes of clothing and fresh bedding. Her program showed clearly that these things were not learned so much from teaching as by actually seeing and doing them. Environment affected formation of character, she believed, and methodic cleanliness provided

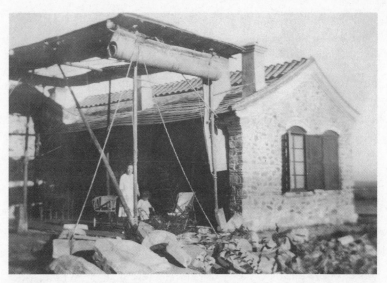

In the summer, mother and son would retreat to Xi Shan (the Western Hills).

happiness and enlarged the intelligence as much as book education, and thus was of more practical help to the women of China. She was certain that girls who received this training would be more sought after as wives than college graduates, for they would be the real homemakers.

Margaret firmly believed in working together for the good of others, and that doing this benefits the one who gives even more than the one who receives, since spiritual benefit is greater than material. The Peking Community Service Group arose from a band of about forty Chinese and foreign men and women of various qualifications. Many people were drawn together in a spirit of friendliness, gaining a wider knowledge of one another's customs, habits and needs, and inaugurating activities of many kinds. While Margaret was not alone in promoting social service, her influence and contribution were immense.

♪✳

MARGARET WAS WELL AWARE that working at her pace made relaxing occasionally essential. A cottage at Xi Shan (the Western Hills) had long been her retreat, where she and Clifford could spend uninterrupted hours of quiet and fun. One sultry late summer afternoon, a fast-moving dark cloud in an otherwise cloudless sky descended into the valley. Obviously this was nothing new for the villagers, who quickly prepared to deal with a marauding plague of locusts, and Clifford just as quickly joined in. The women produced large needles threaded with ninety-centimetre (3-foot) lengths of stout cotton with a matchstick knotted at the end. As the hoppers landed on everything green, everybody got to work threading the insects by skewering them with their needles. When the lines were loaded, the women handed out new lines to collect more locusts until the fields were more or less rid of them. Much of the crops were salvaged, but the bare trees presented a woeful sight.

That evening the exhausted villagers and Clifford gorged themselves. Large iron cauldrons of water were brought to the boil, and thousands of locusts were cooked alive. The result was quite edible, tasting rather like spinach. The wings, legs and heads were readily peeled off, not unlike shelling prawns. There was little rejoicing over the repast, as the country folk felt they had consumed their harvest prematurely, with no profit to show for it.

Across the hills were two or three quarries, where Clifford watched the stonemasons creating millstones. Eventually he was allowed to roll some stones down the zigzag tracks to the villages below, achieved with the help of a three-metre (10-foot) pole inserted into the central hole of the grinder.

One day mother and son were strolling down a path beside a field. Margaret's practised eye noticed a farm worker with black plaster round the calf of his leg. The man told her that several days ago he had a boil treated by the local medicine man in the traditional fashion. The plaster was never removed, the boil festered and the man admitted to a painful tenderness right up into his groin. Margaret warned him that his wound was on the verge of becoming dangerous. If he came to the cottage—all the locals knew where Dr. Lei lived—as soon as he was free, she would see what she could do for him. On returning home, Clifford was told to whittle a short stick, then cauterize his penknife in boiling water.

Margaret had only a kidney dish, cotton wool, iodine and her son's knife as equipment.

Later in the afternoon, the patient arrived. Margaret removed the plaster, revealing a nasty sight, for the boil had been pustulating badly. After cleaning it, she lanced the boil and released most of the pus into the kidney dish. She wrapped a wad of cotton wool round the end of the stick and proceeded to cauterize the wound under the skin with iodine. Small wonder that the poor man grunted and squirmed. Another wad of cotton wool was placed over the wound, then Margaret bandaged it with a strip of sheeting, advising the man to come and see her every evening. Within a week, the leg was healing well and the pain in his groin was gone. Clifford had watched the proceedings in horror, and when Margaret returned his knife, he hurled it as far as he could, declaring that he would never be a doctor.

Many winter and spring weekends Clifford spent at the Hill-Murray Blind Institute in Bali Zhuang (Eight-Mile Village), about halfway to the Western Hills and run by the Reverend Walter Canner and his wife. They had two children, John, who was the same age as Clifford, and Mary, who was about two years younger. The establishment consisted of two schools. Mr. Canner was the principal for the boys' school, while Mrs. Canner was responsible for the girls'. Apart their basic education, the boys learned carpentry and leatherwork, and the girls, how to weave and knit. Mr. Canner ensured that John and Clifford had a good grounding in woodwork and could use a variety of tools.

Like his mother, Clifford developed the attitude that any obstacle to his desire was nothing less than a challenge. When he was about twelve, he badly wanted a bicycle. Margaret was not keen on the idea, and thought to defeat his notion by ruling that he could have one when he could afford to buy it himself. The cost of eighty dollars would take about two years to save, based on a rough calculation of a dollar a week being enough to cover outlay expenses. Clifford decided to make jigsaw puzzles.

Thanks to Mr. Canner, he could handle a fretsaw to good effect, so he set to work. Using his meagre savings, he bought fine sandpaper and a sheet of good-quality plywood, then scrounged sizable coloured pictures from a variety of empathetic sources. As he could not provide a miniature of the pictures, he learned to type, then pasted a brief description on each container. To cover these boxes—specifically made by the Hill-Murray Blind Institute in varying sizes—he bought rolls of coloured paper, on a credit basis since he was well-known to management. The interlocking puzzles pieces had to be fairly even in size; the smallest puzzles averaged 150 pieces and the most ambitious, roughly 400. When completed, the puzzle could be lifted by the top corners without falling apart, so Clifford was confident of the quality of his product. The price per puzzle was one cent a piece, rounded up by roughly ten percent to cover overheads. Three months later, his money box started to show proof of his industry.

Surprised to learn how much was in the box, Margaret instructed Clifford to keep an account book of expenses and income. Later, after examining his accounts, she announced she would no longer provide him with money for offertory in church. A deal was struck when he agreed to donate a half-dozen of his better jigsaw productions for her stall in the upcoming British Women's League bazaar, while she would continue to subsidize his lesser offerings to the church.

Having achieved his objective, Clifford still needed his mother's approval of the bicycle model. She insisted on a carrier rack for packages, and an adequate light. As Clifford had depleted his earnings, Margaret relented and subsidized this last item, on the condition that he help out by taking specimens to the laboratory.

Summer holidays were a pleasure both Margaret and Clifford looked forward to. Long weekends or short breaks were spent in Xi Shan. The big treats came when Margaret took Clifford to the coast at Beidaihe or Weihaiwei, generally for the whole of July. In 1936, Clifford graduated with an American high school diploma. That summer's holiday—to be the last with his mother—was spent at Weihaiwei. Margaret had a five-year contract to serve every July as the resident doctor at the Queen's Hotel. The Royal Navy had a base nearby for their summer cruises and manœuvres, and Clifford enjoyed visiting the aircraft carrier HMS *Hermes*. Unhappy about his ensuing strong American accent, Margaret had

Clifford read aloud for an hour twice daily from Dickens's *Tale of Two Cities* while she worked on improving his diction, to the extent of rattling a pencil between his teeth to loosen up his "wooden jaw." This taught him to enunciate better and did succeed in overcoming his accent.

That September, Clifford left for England to further his education; he would stay with Uncle Bertie, who was appointed as his official guardian. As he set off on a ten-day train journey to London via Siberia, neither he nor Margaret could have guessed that they would not see each other again for almost a decade.

YOU WILL WIN THROUGH

Oh, it is good to be young, to have the best of life before you.
To face the unknown future with hope and confidence,
To let ambition plan the way to fame and power
and cross the stepping stones of difficulty towards the promised land.
To lend a hand to those beside you,
To struggle on through storm and darkness,
To go boldly forward when all goes wrong...

(E. M. P.)

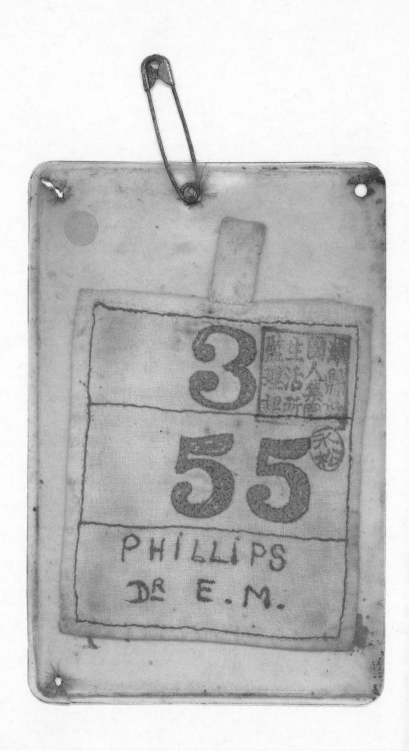

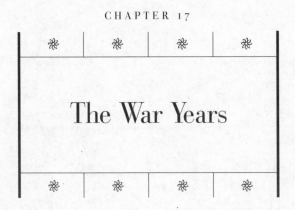

CHAPTER 17

The War Years

♪❋ JUST WHEN CHINA MOST NEEDED support from the Western powers, Europe was preoccupied with the invasion and occupation of Ethiopia by the Fascist forces under the leadership of the Italian dictator, Mussolini, and more apprehensive over the Nazi movement under Hitler than with what was taking place in China. While Europe was distracted, Japan launched military incursions in 1935—this time a two-pronged operation, from the north into Manchuria, and in the south into Shanghai.

In the summer of 1937, the Marco Polo Bridge incident in Peking signalled the start of World War II as far as China was concerned. Shanghai was occupied, followed by the Rape of Nanking. Still the Chinese forces alone were left to combat invading Japanese armies, whose objective was clearly to subjugate the nation. The Chinese wartime capital was set up in Chongqing (Chungking), and so it remained till the end of hostilities in 1945.

Incredibly, Peking appeared to be unconcerned over what was occurring in the south. Life in the north proceeded as usual, as in previous years during the Warlords' power struggle. Margaret now had a TB sanato-

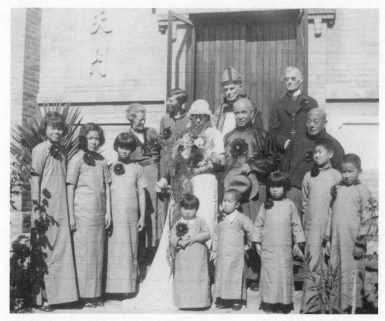

In 1938, Dr. Margaret attended the wedding of Miss Ho, one of the nurses at the Conquest Hill Sanatorium, Bishop Norris officiating.

rium in the Western Hills, in premises rented to her for the past four years at a nominal figure by Bishop Norris, which was fully occupied by twenty or more patients, who during the day lay outdoors on beds. When visitors asked about this, she replied, "The patients like it; it's the relations who do not." In the summertime the patients were moved to the north verandah, and many slept out all night with mosquito nets fastened overhead to bamboo poles. When it rained, all hands set to work to move the beds indoors.

At first, Margaret visited the sanatorium once a week, as cars were cheap to hire then. Later a bus service was inaugurated, conveniently stopping at the foot of the hill. As the climb to the sanatorium took her half an hour, Margaret decided to name the place Conquest Hill Sanatorium. It soon became necessary to acquire another compound to accommodate the rising numbers of patients.

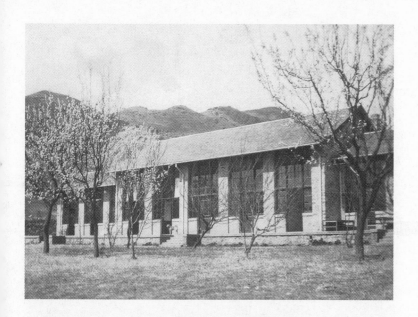

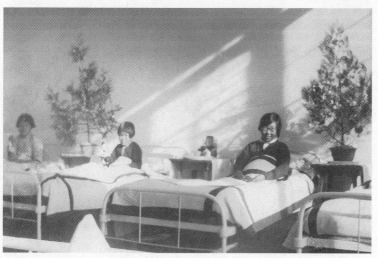

Outside and inside views of Margaret's brand new tuberculosis sanatorium, which she named Conquest Hill, c. 1935–39.

Margaret visited Weihaiwei for the summer of 1939, little knowing that it would be for the last time. She started her return to Peking at the end of July, just when the Japanese occupation of Peking took place. All shipping was held up, so it was the latter part of August before she returned— only to be told that her TB patients were marooned outside the city, waiting to be brought home. All the other sanatoriums had already been closed, so there was no chance of transferring any patients, and all had to be labouriously taken to their homes.

This heralded the end of Margaret's TB work, although applications continued to be made to her even in 1946. Again her work in China seemed to have reached a dead end, but Margaret had learned that the result of her work was not hers, nor did anything come to an end. It simply went on in a different way. Furthermore, she knew well that as one door closed, another would open.

Soon afterwards the Anglican mission girls' school was also closed— partly due to Japanese influence—so there was no more health inspection work for her. However, she still attended the mission workers, Chinese and foreign, but the Chinese dollar had depreciated so much her monthly salary was worth no more than one pound sterling. Then the Japanese purchased the whole Danish compound, and Margaret was asked to leave. This was painful since she had recently renewed her lease, and the house, a modern foreign-style building, had enabled her to charge her occasional guests higher terms; it was also convenient and economical to run. The Japanese were swarming into the city, taking up every available house. Margaret was offered an inducement of one hundred dollars if she would leave within a month. As this would be a great help with moving expenses, she did her best.

She got in touch with a Mr. Alabaster, who she heard was leaving Peking. His landlord, an absentee in western Free China, had left the property in the charge of a Chinese bank, where Margaret had an account. The bank manager agreed to her tenancy on the same terms as Mr. Alabaster's. He moved into a hotel two months before the expiration of his lease so Margaret could move in. In this way she avoided a lease which would have to go through the law courts. The place—obviously an old palace pavilion—was charming with a garden and nice green lawn, flowering shrubs, some old trees and a hill with a cave. Unfortunately, the bedrooms were tiny so accommodation for PGs was poor. Margaret felt her affairs were certainly on the downgrade.

Her last guests were seemingly nice people, a German and his American wife, but he was, in fact, a keen Nazi. At each meal Margaret was instructed in Nazism; she tactfully replied she felt sure that other nations might emulate anything worthwhile. No reference was made to ethnic cleansing nor were there any anti-Semitic remarks, or she would not have bothered with tact. After the guests left, Margaret was sorry to discover that her old cook, Yang Huating, had advanced TB. She sent him home with a pension.

That August, there was a bad flood in Tianjin, and many people sought refuge in Peking. A Danish couple found their way to Margaret's place, took a fancy to it and asked to sublet the whole house. Feeling obliged to agree, she moved into a separate building in the garden, sharing the kitchen and a servant who cleaned her room. This arrangement did not work well, so when the landlord's brother demanded double the rent, which the Danes were willing to pay, Margaret decided to move again.

With the current unsettled state of affairs, Margaret decided to deed her cottage in the Western Hills to a dear friend, Olga Lee, a Swiss national married to a Chinese. Under Chinese property laws, a foreigner was not allowed to own land, but with her cottage situated next to St. Hilary's, Margaret had been safe. She now felt that the property rights were best protected by being in the Lees' hands. Olga being her closest friend, Margaret was happy to donate the cottage to her, while her husband could rightfully own the land it stood on.

She felt fortunate to be allowed to rent a little mission house next to the East City branch church. For one person it was spacious, though the two courtyards were tiny. She had decided to give up taking in any more PGs, but she needed a consulting room, so there was no question of sharing her place with anyone. She was tired of struggling with Chinese servants, so she decided to do her own cooking and to retain just one. Old Bai was a treasure. He did all the housework, and tended to the fires and

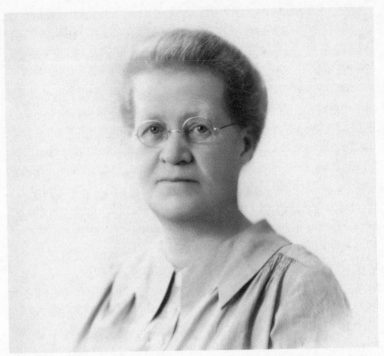

Dr. Margaret Phillips, just prior to the unsettling influence of World War II in China.

daily shopping. At first Margaret prepared all her meals, but soon Bai took over. He was always respectful, diligent and taciturn.

Presently he asked if his wife could come to live with him. As his quarters were intended for two servants, Margaret felt she could not deny him, but she did not appreciate it when his seventeen-year-old daughter turned up later and joined them. She had been living with relatives who were doubtless glad to get rid of her, as she was an unpleasant person with an exalted idea of herself. She wanted to work as a waitress in a restaurant, or at a hairdresser's, but her parents would not allow this. Instead she loafed around or went out with her girlfriends. The girl was an annoyance, but thankfully she kept out of Margaret's way.

Margaret was surprisingly comfortable living alone. Though gregarious, she enjoyed the respite from the perpetual need to supervise servants, or entertain and cater for guests. A friend had left her a radio set, something she had never felt a need for in the past, mainly because she knew someone would have it on all day long. Now she tuned every day at breakfast to hear the news from the United States and sometimes from England. She never felt lonely, and as she had to go out so much during the day, she was glad to be quiet in the evening, occasionally inviting a friend over or going out to visit someone. Margaret spent three quite happy years in that house in a way that could be considered mundane compared to all the years before. She continued to regularly attend the British Charitable Hospital, as well as to patients at the Anglican and London missions, and she maintained a small Chinese private practice. To augment her meagre budget she gave English lessons. She had to live economically, for, while she was in her sixties, retirement was not an option. Fortunately, Clifford's education and maintenance were no longer an issue as he had been taking care of himself since he was eighteen.

Her friends Olga Lee and Mrs. Thomas, from the British legation, visited every week. Margaret no longer sang with the Choral Society, so she used her available time to attend the Soroptimist club and meetings of the local chapter of the Eastern Star (the women's equivalent to Freemasonry), where she was eventually appointed Worthy Matron. Before retiring for the night, she might add a few stamps to her considerable Chinese collection, or play solitaire. If she felt fidgety, she plied her knitting needles or crochet hook; a number of her doilies are in use to this day. On Sundays she attended the Chinese service at the little church next door. During her last year in that house, Margaret took a small Sunday school class in her home.

♪※

THIS TEMPO OF LIFE CEASED on December 7, 1941. As a British subject, Margaret, now sixty-five, was considered by the Japanese to be an enemy alien.

On the morning of December 8, Margaret was listening to her radio at breakfast. The announcer agitatedly stated that people might have difficulty getting to their places of business because the streets of Shanghai were cordoned off. He had never expected to report such news, he added, and his voice broke. "I cannot go on," he said suddenly. "Goodbye."

Margaret rushed next door to tell her neighbour Miss Steven the news. Had there been a riot? Margaret returned home, and at ten o'clock she tuned in to London. At that hour, reception was often poor, but for once it was quite clear. The BBC announced the attack on Pearl Harbor. Simultaneously Hong Kong and Singapore were being attacked, and a naval battle was taking place in the Pacific. Margaret then learned that Japan had attacked the United States while negotiations were underway, and that Britain and America had declared war on Japan.

Again Margaret rushed to tell Miss Steven the news. She tried to telephone the British Charitable Hospital to say that she would not attend that morning, but the line was dead. So she put on her hat and coat to go and see Mrs. Thomas, who was scheduled to leave the country in two days' time. Just as Margaret was leaving, Bai arrived white-faced from the market and told her that the Japanese had taken over the Peking Union Medical College (PUMC). She told him the terrible news, then left. As she was walking past the Lockhart Hall, she saw some Japanese running to and fro, escorting a foreigner into the building, while the Chinese stood in groups, watching. Margaret asked to use the telephone at a grocer shop, and contacted the hospital to explain her absence, then called the Lindemans, leaving a message with their cook that she was coming to see them.

She carried on towards the Legation Quarter. Now and then she met a friend who warned her that she might not be able to reach the British embassy, but she continued on regardless. Japanese guards stood at intervals along Legation Street. A large notice posted on a wall announced that Japan was at war with England and America, and warned foreigners not to take any action against the Japanese. Otherwise, they could carry on their occupations as usual.

Margaret managed to get as far as the Wagon-Lits hotel, but there a Japanese officer stopped her. She told him she wanted to see her German friends, whom she thought she had just caught sight of in the distance walking back to their home in the Russian embassy. He told her to call to them, but they were too far away to hear, so she was instructed to turn back. Just then, Mrs. Lawless, wife of the British embassy constable (who was also chief of the Legation Quarter police), walked past escorted by three Japanese, who were taking her to her home in the customs compound. Her husband and other staff members of the British and American embassies (except the consul) had been taken to the US Marine Corps barracks, where they were detained for several weeks. "I'm under escort," she said to Margaret, who replied, "How grand."

Margaret returned home and had lunch, expecting to go as usual to the French school to give her English lesson, but a note arrived telling her not to—every place was under surveillance and the Legation Quarter streets were closed. She was just getting tea ready when four Japanese officers walked in, bowed, sat down and proceeded to interrogate her, starting with her name, age and place of work. One spoke English well and was quite polite. Why was she living in a mission house? He could not understand. She explained that she was the doctor to the mission, but not a mission member. All the furniture was her own, unlike Miss Steven next door who did belong to the mission, as did her furniture.

The Japanese soldiers walked through every room, placing paper seals on her telephone, radio and medicine cabinets. "Have patience for a few days," they told her, adding that she had better stay at home. She was refused permission to go next door, and a Chinese policeman was posted in the house to ensure that she did not leave and that no one came in. The policeman seemed more frightened than Margaret, who was, in effect, under house arrest. She would not have been surprised had she been carted off there and then to a concentration camp.

After the gendarmes left, Margaret relieved some of her tension by pounding on her piano and singing "Rule Britannia" and "God Save The King" at the top of her voice, hoping Miss Steven next door might hear.

The policeman was to have been relieved after a few hours. Although no relief came, a patrol called in to see whether he was on duty. Margaret wanted Bai to get something for him to eat, but the policeman declined. The following morning she gave the policeman some money, and he bought some food at the door which he cooked in her kitchen and so felt happier. He spent the second night again on the kitchen table, although Margaret was afraid of his being asphyxiated by fumes from the coal fire, which was banked down at night. As time passed and no one came to relieve him, he became more desperate. Eventually someone did arrive with some money for food, but by then he was too upset to eat.

The newspaper was delivered as usual, and though the Reuters telegrams had all been omitted, there was a full account of the Japanese attacks on Pearl Harbor, Manila and Hong Kong. Through a barred window in her bedroom, Margaret could see into Miss Steven's garden, and occasionally the two were able to speak through the bars. Both still expected to be carted off to some concentration camp, so Margaret spent the week in putting her things in order, packing her valuable ornaments, embroideries, and her best table and bed linens in a tin-lined box, which she hoped to entrust to the care of the Lindemans, who in this situation had diplomatic immunity. General Lindeman had originally come to China as artillery adviser to Chiang Kaishek's Nationalist army, and Margaret got to know Mrs. Lindeman through giving her conversation practice to improve her English. The general was strongly anti-Nazi and refused to return to Europe at the outbreak of war, so he remained in Peking. His political standing being fully established, the Russian compound in the Legation Quarter allowed him to rent a house and, he being a German national, Japan—as an Axis partner—could not touch him.

The Japanese barged into Margaret's house at any time. Sometimes they were friendly, and once a soldier asked her to play the piano. Margaret hated hearing them rattling her brass door-knocker, then *stomp-stomp-stomping* one after the other into her house and through her rooms, always asking the same question: "Whose is the furniture?"

One day two men arrived. The officer could speak very little English or Chinese, but his subordinate spoke Chinese. When Margaret rose to greet them, they ignored her and stood in front of the stove talking to each other. Thinking that they might be waiting for someone, Margaret sat down again and picked up her knitting. After a time the officer savagely motioned for her to stand up and stop knitting. In a menacing manner, he ordered her to stand in front of him. Margaret feared he was drunk. She had always been afraid of intoxicated people. Meanwhile, the policeman had come in and was standing in the doorway. It was hot by the stove and she began to unfasten her jacket, but the officer yelled at her, so she stopped. Afraid that he would order her to kneel down, she wondered what to do. Happily, there was a witness—the policeman at the door—and after a few more dreadful minutes, the two Japanese left. Margaret wept in relief. These two men were the only Japanese at the time who were not polite, and the policeman confirmed that the officer was indeed quite drunk.

One day Margaret's goddaughter Liu Meizhen arrived, and the policeman let Margaret come to the door to speak to her. She asked Margaret whether she needed money, but Margaret said that she had enough and told Meizhen that she was comforted by her concern. Another time a man, ostensibly from the Japanese Intelligence Service, visited Margaret in a commandeered car. He stayed for tea and assured Margaret that she had nothing to fear. Though he appeared to be appreciate her willingness to give him tea, she heard that he was later sent home by the authorities for looting and giving a false account of himself.

Margaret had no other visitors except the Lindemans, who forced their way in past the policeman. He followed after them, petrified with fear, begging Margaret to send them out. He was about to kowtow to her, so she asked them to go, taking the opportunity to give Frau Lindeman the Charter of the Eastern Star to take care of. They were most upset, and the general said he would go to the Japanese embassy to find out why Margaret was detained. That was Thursday.

♪✳

"WE'RE GOING FOR A WALK, Dr. Phillips." The Japanese soldier speaking these words had just come in with Miss Steven. It was about two o'clock on Sunday afternoon.

"What shall I take?" Margaret asked, thinking they were to be carted off.

"Nothing," said Miss Steven. "We're coming back."

Not that Margaret believed her. The three walked down the street to Lockhart Hall and went upstairs into a little room which was crowded with foreigners and Japanese. One after another they sat down to write out a statement that they would not sell or remove anything from their houses. Then they were taken home and told to return the next day at the same time, bringing a Chinese servant.

This time they went into a big room which gradually filled up with foreigners—all missionaries, apparently—who had been detained. Now they wrote down only their names and addresses, and had their finger-prints taken, as did their servants. Then a Japanese officer stood upon a table, with a foreigner on his right and a Chinese on the left, and gave a fiery oration—all Japanese speeches in those days were delivered in fierce and forcible tones—which was translated into Chinese and English by the interpreters on either side. By the time it was put into English, it was quite condensed: Japan had been forced into this war and meant no harm to the assembled company, who could now all return home and go freely about their occupations—provided they did not work against the Japanese.

So they were free! Margaret almost danced her way home with Miss Steven, and the two had a celebratory tea. Afterwards Margaret dressed to go out again, this time to rush off to see the Lindemans. She tried to get into the British embassy, but the sentry barked at her and sent her away, pointing meaningfully at the Japanese embassy across the way. At the Russian embassy, the Lindemans were overjoyed to see her and insisted she stay for supper. They told her that General Lindeman had first gone to the Japanese embassy, then to General Yasuji Okamura, head of the Japanese forces in North China, who sent word that he could not receive Herr General until Sunday. To his horror, as he waited to see the Japanese general, General Lindeman got mixed up with a group of German women who had been collecting parcels of comforts for the Japanese troops in recognition of Japan's entry into the war. A mass photograph was taken of the group, which stood close beside him. To his immense relief, he did not appear in the newspaper picture published the next day. When General Okamura heard that all the missionaries had been detained, he said that there had been a "mistake." (Margaret learned later that this was the standard Japanese excuse.) Only the heads of institutions were supposed to be "detained," and he was quite concerned about the "mistake." There was no doubt in Margaret's mind that it was owing to Herr General's intervention that they were released with an impressive alacrity.

"It was marvellous to be free," Margaret said. "In fact, it was almost worth being detained in order to realize the joy of freedom. I spent the whole of Tuesday rushing about to see my friends."

She went to the French school as usual, but never returned to the British Charitable Hospital, which had been closed down by Dr. Bai for lack of funds, although he had flour in hand and a good stock of drugs. He could have made it self-supporting had he wished, but he had recently opened his own hospital nearby, where he diverted the paying patients, while he lived rent-free in the hospital compound.

Margaret's telephone was never restored. Though the seal was removed, the line remained dead, and one day when Margaret was not home the instrument was taken away. A few days later a crew came to remove the wiring. As she would not open the door, they climbed over the roof. Margaret called to them, "Yes, that is the way for thieves to come in."

Several days later, she went to the Japanese embassy to register herself and her belongings: her furniture, camera, typewriter, piano, radio and so on. When she was reprimanded for coming so late, she answered, "How could I, when I was detained at home?" There was no reply. Apparently the embassy and the army were not on cordial terms.

Strangely, Margaret was able to keep her radio for more than a year, which was a great comfort, especially as she knew that others had their sets taken away. She could listen to London and San Francisco daily, and she particularly enjoyed the Sunday services. One afternoon, on her return home from the French school, she found a truck outside the door of the church next door. Two Japanese were loading a radio onto the vehicle, and they said that hers would be next. Following on her heels into the house, they somewhat apologetically demanded her set. As she had learned to do with the Japanese, Margaret played "simple" and asked why they would want to take an old long-wave set. Although disbelieving at first, they checked the radio, then left it. So Margaret possessed the only long-wave radio—which yielded Japanese newscasts as well as some music. She discovered that she could pick up a Russian radio station in Shanghai which told her a good deal.

♪❋

MARGARET WENT TO THE JAPANESE EMBASSY to apply for a pass to visit the British embassy, but this was refused. By mid-December she was tired of all this running around. She decided to stay home, unpack her suitcase and try to resume her normal routine as far as possible. How different Christmas was likely to be! But as it turned out, the main difference was the complete absence of mail—for many, the greatest hardship. A slight fall of snow made it feel seasonal, but friends entertained one another with a subdued spirit. Margaret attempted to listen to the king's speech, but signal interference allowed her to catch only the occasional word.

Finally, she was able to access the British legation, after Dr. Aspland applied for a pass for her to see Mrs. Aspland. On three further occasions she obtained a certificate as her medical adviser, enabling her to visit; the pass needed renewing every two weeks. Margaret felt that she could not draw the monthly allowance of relief money, for which she would have to sign a promise to repay. With so few paying patients, she had to live very frugally. She had her name added to a list of doctors who would charge a minimum rate for services rendered.

Meanwhile, a number of pupils applied to her for English lessons. Three were French, one from the barracks, and the Chargé d'Affaires and his wife from the embassy. They appeared to be quite pro-British, even after the collapse of the French army and surrender to the Nazi forces, which meant the withdrawal of the British troops at Dunkirk. However, when the Allies landed in North Africa, they decided to discontinue their lessons, declaring their sympathies with Vichy France. Margaret felt this was uncalled for, and she later heard that the French ambassador's wife agreed with her.

She also had several students from the Japanese embassy. After Pearl Harbor, once her freedom had been restored, Margaret asked them if it was appropriate for them to study under an Englishwoman. The reply was, "Why not? We are not fighting against you in our hearts." They seemed to admire England, and said Japan was similar. Margaret took this to mean geographically and constitutionally. Asked why they wanted to learn English, the students said that they must learn the language to be able to talk to the Russians. Margaret was surprised to discover that not one of her students had any education above high school. The Japanese had compulsory primary education but did not encourage higher education. Margaret's opinion was that the Chinese might wisely follow that example, as Chinese education was still sadly lacking. All things considered, she established a remarkable rapport with her pupils.

She was spared any further visits by the Japanese gendarmerie until March 30, 1942. That night, when she came home for supper, her faithful Bai said the "special police" had been to see her at seven o'clock, and would return at eight-thirty. Shortly before then, in marched two men without ceremony and sat themselves down. The spokesman said, in English, "Dr. Phillips, we want to know all your history since you came to China. Now begin." It was such a large order that she could only say "Oh" and wait for him to begin firing off questions: "When did you first come to China?" "Where…?" "When…?" and so on. Margaret answered question by question, but she did not volunteer any information.

The electricity had gone off, and they had only one candle to see by. The interrogator smelt strongly of wine, and he spoke rather indistinctly so Margaret was not always sure what he was asking. As the other man spoke no English, the interrogation was interpreted for him in Japanese, which he busily recorded in a tiny notebook. They presented no credentials and wore plainclothes, but she was interrupted when she tried to ask who they were and why they had come. They had come to ask the questions.

The main purpose seemed to be to ascertain her means of living, since she was not applying for the monthly relief. Margaret could not see the need for so much history, so what they did not ask she did not tell. Fortunately, they did not ask if she had worked anywhere except Peking, so that saved a lot of time. One by one they extracted the different sources of her income, adding them up till they amounted to about two hundred dollars per month—the amount foreigners were supposed to manage with, although it was a tight fit with the increases in prices. How had she managed on so little in such a large house? She replied that she had to be extremely frugal, and rarely rode in rickshaws. Finally, Margaret asked if they had any instructions for her. They replied "No" and explained that they were just going round to see how people were managing. If anyone could not cope, they would have to think of a plan. Margaret found it all very tiring. Towards the end they became a little jocular, then rushed away without further ado. The smell of wine was still strong in her room the next morning.

Early in April, Margaret went to the office of Dr. Hoeppli, the Swiss representative, to again register the reasons why she wished to stay in China:

Ethel Margaret Phillips, female, English, aged 66. I do not wish to evacuate Peking because:

1. I have lived here consecutively for 26 years and have nowhere to go if I leave here.
2. I have no foreign funds or deposits, and no means of living if I go away.
3. I possess only my furniture and the things in my house.
4. The Peking climate suits me very well, and I have had better health here than anywhere else.
5. My present means of support is by English teaching and a little medical practice.
6. I expect to be able to support myself in future as I am doing now. I have never had to apply for pupils. They have always applied to me.

ON APRIL 26, Bai's spoilt only daughter got married. Now aged twenty, she had refused two positions Margaret had found for her. She had also turned down every suggested offer of marriage because she would not marry a workman, or a carpenter, or a shoemaker, or a servant. Unattractive and uneducated, it was unlikely that Miss Bai would have married but for the war. A friend of the policeman who had been guarding the house for eight days was looking for a wife. After two interviews the daughter agreed, although many arguments and quarrels occurred before all the details were arranged to her satisfaction.

The bridegroom supplied her trousseau along with the wedding expenses, but the bride's parents had to entertain their own friends and relations at a restaurant, and pay for the carriages to take them to the bridegroom's house for the wedding ceremony. The wedding gown was hired. An old-style banquet for the groom's friends followed. Towards evening the bride and groom came to her parents' home (which, of course, was Margaret's house) to pay their respects. This usually took place on the third day, but as the two carriages were hired for the whole day it was decided to do it then, for the sake of economy. Several relations attended, and the cooking and feasting went on for two or three hours. The food for this feast had arrived in the morning as a present from the bridegroom's parents to the bride's parents.

In May, the English-speaking "plainclothes policeman" returned. The previous day Dr. Houghton, Mrs. Bowen, Dr. and Mrs. Snapper from the PUMC and Dr. Leighton Stuart of Yenching University had all been moved into Mr. Hemmings's house next door. This official was going round the adjoining houses to see who the new neighbours were.

ƒ✲

ON AUGUST 10, 1942, the members of the diplomatic corps representing the Allied nations were evacuated, after which there was unrestricted access to the British embassy compound, as the sentry had been removed.

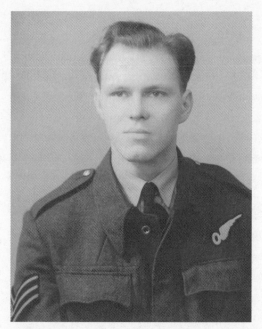

Clifford in his uniform as a sergeant in the Royal Air Force, 1942.

A large number of civilians were also evacuated, including four mission-aries: Mrs. Thomas, Miss Bowden-Smith, and Dr. and Mrs. Snapper.

Now Margaret fully recognized her precarious circumstances. Having established her independent status in Peking for the past twenty-odd years, she had deprived herself of the protection of any responsible institution. The Japanese situation had virtually eliminated her livelihood. As an enemy alien, she could scarcely be in a more tricky situation. She returned once more to Dr. Hoeppli to reiterate her wish to remain in China, which negated any chance of evacuation.

She had no way of contacting Clifford, nor did she wish to return to England any more than she had done during World War I. Clifford was now in the Royal Air Force, flying as a navigator on Coastal Command operations. His being a serviceman on active duty made it virtually impossible for Margaret to contact him via the International Red Cross. And although Clifford could send, through the Red Cross, an anodyne letter of thirty words to his mother once a year, there was no way of knowing whether it ever reached her. Security and censorship prevented Margaret from knowing, until after the war, about Clifford's forced landing in the North Sea on the first anniversary of Japan's attack on Pearl Harbor, spending nearly thirty-five hours afloat before rescue. And only afterwards did he learn what his mother underwent during the last thirty months of the war.

Inevitably what Margaret feared occurred: she received three days' notice of evacuation from Peking. Hastily she called on the Lindemans, who had kindly promised safekeeping for her few remaining valuables for as long as possible—Margaret's only recourse, otherwise she would have lost everything. General Lindeman called round in a car to collect the sizeable tin trunk containing her portable treasures. Mrs. Lindeman accompanied him to bid Margaret Godspeed and prayerful wishes for her safety. Not until after the Japanese surrender, nearly two and a half years later, were they to see each other again.

Somewhat terrified, Margaret prayed as she packed, relying on God to see her through, as He had always done. She was allowed no more than two pieces of luggage—the most she could carry. She wore her bulky warm coat, thankful it was cold. A crowded bus arrived early in the morning of March 29 to take her to the station. There was an emotional farewell with Bai and his wife. Margaret felt awful not being able to pension him off in some small way, as would be customary, but she consoled herself that he would most likely help himself to whatever he might get away with. Remarkably, at the station to see Margaret off were three of her Japanese students.

As the train departed, Margaret repeated to herself, "Goodbye, Peking; goodbye, Peking," thinking she might never return.

♪✳

THE NEXT DAY, entering the gate of the Weixian (Weihsien) internment compound, Margaret thought, "Goodbye freedom." Realistically, she expected to remain there for years, although she hoped for some form of repatriation. The Weixian internment camp in Shandong

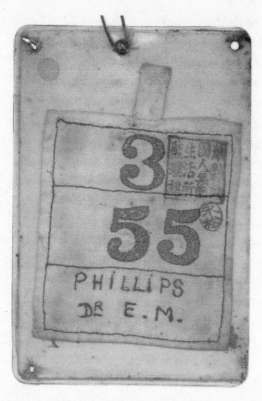

Dr. Margaret's war-time identification while she was interned in Weixian.

Province, otherwise referred to as a civil assembly centre, was rated the best of the civilian camps in China; compared with what was subsequently reported about similar camps in Shanghai and elsewhere, this may well have been true. It provided accommodation for eighteen hundred men, women and children collected from various cities in North China.

For two and a half years, the only people who saw the outside of the gate were the men who carried out the garbage boxes. In the early months this was done by Chinese coolies, who were only too willing to oblige in taking out letters or bringing in eggs. When the Japanese guards realized this, they made the male inmates do it instead. Nobody minded; in fact, there was a good deal of competition for the job in order to get to the right side of the gate once a day.

Despite Japanese efforts, a degree of "black marketing" flourished. One cold spring morning, Margaret sat on her dormitory steps, warming herself in the sunshine. This building, which she referred to as "Aroma Place," faced the cesspools. Suddenly a coolie sidled up and, slowly opening his hand, revealed a lovely brown egg. Margaret asked "How much?" and he replied "Sixty cents." Then she asked "How many?" And he said "Six." Of course she bargained a little, then they went behind the building. He put his hand inside his coat and produced one egg after another, and she bought the lot for the vast sum of $2.50. Having not seen an egg for several weeks, she felt the deal was well worth it.

The scavenger coolies came every day to clean out the cesspools, and the Chinese-style squat toilets which they had to make do with, as other provisions were inadequate. Under the Japanese public health system, the primitive sanitation remained until the inmates took charge of the situation. The lack of privacy was eventually alleviated by affixing doors to the cubicles. Margaret thought that the men and women who acted as sanitary cleaners deserved the highest praise, for they did a most revolting job with great efficiency. At first this job was voluntary, but later every woman under the age of fifty, unless medically exempt, took her turn for a week at a time. It was especially difficult in winter when the floors were covered in ice; buckets of hot water had to be fetched and poured down before any cleaning could be done. Fortunately, most of them only had to do it once, as the release of the internees came just as they were starting on the second time around.

Although the Japanese authorities were not too unfavourably disposed toward the internees, they strove to keep the upper hand by refusing concessions or luxuries. Even permission to buy medical supplies was granted grudgingly. Margaret considered that, in medical terms, the Japanese acted criminally since they had made no provision whatsoever. Before leaving for Weixian, the internees had been assured that there was a fine hospital there. Actually, it was no more than a shell, with no furniture and all the pipes and plumbing removed. The only medical equipment and drugs were what the various doctors had brought with them. Any patients who went to hospital had to bring their own beds and bedding, which was often unclean—at least by hospital standards. Gradually a few beds and other furniture were collected from here and there in the compound. Later medical supplies were obtained through the Swiss consul in Qingdao, who fortunately visited the camp frequently. Only the basement and ground floor of the building were allocated for hospital use. The second and third storeys were used as dormitories for the Catholic fathers. After they were evacuated, this accommodation was consigned to Yantai schoolchildren.

♪✻

THE CAMP QUICKLY BECAME a self-governing community. There was great keenness over nominations, and voting was by secret ballot. Management was under a committee of nine, each heading a different department: engineering, medical, religious, quarters, supplies, canteen, discipline, education and recreations. Japanese approval had to be obtained for every meeting of more than ten people, yet they seemed anxious to avoid any camp disturbances or mutiny. Weekly meeting with the Japanese commandant and staff enabled reports, requests and complaints to be made. The committee chairman, who was also the general affairs officer, could contact the commandant whenever necessary, as well as the Swiss consul, who supported the internees as best he could, from time to time generously providing funds for essential expenditures.

On the whole, Margaret thought the people in the camp—disparate groups from a wide range of communities—were well behaved, of good moral fibre and extremely resourceful. Most arrived in camp ill prepared and unequipped for the life that lay ahead. But ingenuity and cleverness always found some way of meeting the need. Empty tins were turned into mugs, cups and saucers, small flower baskets, stoves and chimney pipes. (Later, exhibitions were held to display their numerous inventions.) Margaret had a couple of valuable items made for her from two large soda cracker tins. One became her water pail, just the right size for her to carry her water; the other, a tiny portable stove on which many people in her dormitory cooked their breakfasts.

Every dormitory and row of little rooms had a warden whose duty it was to round up people for roll-call, and to ensure that camp rules were observed. "Lights out"—when they had any—was at ten o'clock, but most people were tired and went to bed early. Margaret was the warden of a dormitory of thirteen, and she was happy that they all got on well, with only one exception.

LIFE IS VERY INTERESTING

Life is very interesting, don't you find it so?
There are so many beauties of Nature,
So many wonders of the sky and marvels of the sea.
How strange are the multitudes of living creatures!
What makes them alive?
In animate we can know, but whence comes animation?
Life is so mysterious.

Most wonderful is man, but how puny, how weak;
So easily killed by accident, by war
Or the murderous hate of an enemy.
Man's power is not in his body, it is in his mind,
In his mind which lives in his animal brain.
How extraordinary is life!

Man can read the secrets of Nature, but not the secret of life
As yet.

(E. M. P.)

Generally, a great sense of humour abounded, although less so as one year passed into the next. By 1945, nerves wore thinner, as did the people themselves. Nonetheless, a strong feeling of service persisted, with people carrying out their camp jobs in good spirit. Here the Jesuit fathers set a wonderful example, actually seeming to enjoy themselves. Everyone was

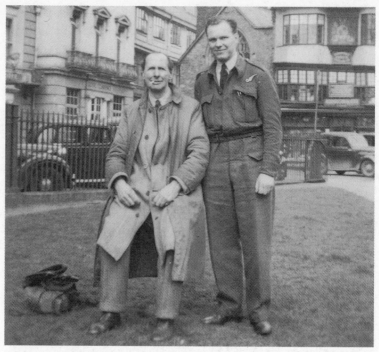

In 1943, on leave from R.A.F. Langham in Norfolk, Clifford joined his Uncle Bertie and his wife, Enid, in Exeter.

supposed to do a camp job, and as far as possible people could choose their jobs. Otherwise, a special worker allocated work suited to a person's capabilities. The jobs of stoking, cooking, pumping, shoveling coal, chopping wood and road sweeping fell to men, as did hauling and unloading supplies.

Typically, Margaret performed her full share of duties. For many months she counted heads as people passed into the dining hall for breakfast or lunch, a means of helping the servers to apportion the food and to prevent duplication or "visitors" from other kitchens. For seven months she was a sanitary policewoman, an easy job for weak people, she said. She supervised the showers for an hour every evening to ensure orderly behaviour and that no one stayed too long or used too much water. The best feature of camp life, showers were at first restricted to once or twice a week, but as things became better organized everybody could have a

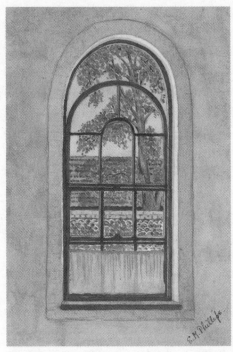

A watercolour of the view from Dr. Margaret's bedside at Weixian.

hot shower each day. Some found the absolute lack of privacy in the ablutions area difficult, but dormitory life soon accustomed people to that, and eventually the women took to it as naturally as Japanese women would.

As important as hygiene was the food supply, which Margaret considered to be not too bad, but failing in quantity rather than in quality. The Japanese provided only two meals a day, leaving the internees responsible for providing their own breakfast. The supply of bread was adequate and at first quite good, but gradually it became darker, turning sour and mouldy in the course of a day. As it was unrationed people became wasteful, often taking more than they needed, then throwing leftovers into the garbage boxes and even the toilets. The Japanese refused to supply any rice, millet or corn meal, but later issued small green beans or sorghum grain, which were hard to cook and rather indigestible. Milk, eggs and especially sugar were luxuries consigned to the hospital and small children.

The meat and vegetable ration enabled only small helpings, and much of the meat was unfit for consumption and had to be discarded. Men, women and children all received the same portions, with only men on heavy duties receiving an extra ration. Cooking facilities and methods were limited and stew was the usual result, although the cooks attempted to vary the meals as much as possible. Occasionally, sufficient joints were obtained and roasted in the bakery. The camp population ranged from eighteen hundred at first to about fourteen hundred later, after deaths or exchanges of prisoners.

Things improved during the last year in camp. The kitchens baked cakes for Sunday treats, and puddings of some kind were served twice a week. It was a great comfort to be able to buy honey and dates from the canteen, or peanut oil for frying black-market eggs. After a long wait, Red Cross parcels began to arrive as well as packages from friends, although many with some or all of the contents missing. Margaret lost one whole Christmas parcel, but the Japanese professed innocence, saying that there was no way of guarding against pilferage and perhaps the internees were guilty. Theft did occur occasionally, and the Japanese seemed quite shocked that foreigners would steal from one another, even if it was a case of survival. In these conditions Margaret learned was that no nation or race was morally superior and that theft was a prominent characteristic.

Anyone trying to evade work had to obtain a medical exemption, ousting the few attempted slackers. Even the many chronic invalids and elderly people preferred to do a job of some sort. Some needed looking after, and that task was also assigned. A camp job generally occupied two to three hours a day. Nearly everybody had to take care of their own daily living activities, such as housework and laundry, or fetching and carrying buckets of hot and cold water. To prevent waste, only half a bucket of hot water was provided at a time—hardly sufficient to wet a sheet and necessitating several journeys. A good portion of the day was spent in queues for one thing or another: meals, boiling water or tea, the canteen, entertainments, letters and parcels. The honour of the queue was well respected and strictly observed, though no rule was made. Most women had a "boyfriend" to do bits of carpentering or putting up stoves for them.

One shop repaired or patched shoes, and another mended men's shirts. Most mending was done by elderly women in their rooms, and Margaret was often requested to make or repair buttonholes. Mrs. Shoemaker advised on women's clothing, and she once helped Margaret to alter a coat. A missionary watchmaker made her watch run better than ever before. The tinsmith's shop repaired leaking buckets and kettles, charging only for materials used. No one received pay for a camp job, but the younger element earned pocket money by doing chores for the "wealthy"—laundry or making coal balls or chopping wood. For the first winter Margaret made all her own coal balls for use on the day when it was her turn to attend to the stove. However, the next winter the dormitory refused to let her do it.

People from Tianjin and Qingdao had been allowed to bring most of their books, so the camp enjoyed a good library of about six thousand volumes, which was so well patronized that four or five people were kept busy repairing book covers. Margaret acted as a librarian, working three hours one morning, then two hours the following afternoon. Although supposedly easy and suitable for the elderly, this job soon became quite strenuous as there were three subscribers to every two books, and they came streaming in every day or so to change them. Once most of the library staff were in hospital and Margaret had to recruit extra help.

Education buzzed. There was an American school from Peking providing a full curriculum for primary and secondary pupils, as well as an English grammar school from Tianjin, the China Inland Mission school from Yantai, and a kindergarten. Camp policy was "Young People First," and everything possible was done to prevent their time in camp from hindering their future prospects. There were Boy Scouts and Girl Guides, and evening clubs for the older teens. Adults could study English, French, German and Chinese, or attend art classes, music lessons, orchestral practices, a choral society or a dramatic society. Except in the coldest weather, Saturday nights featured some special entertainment—usually a play or a concert, which entailed endless preparation and brought people together in a common interest.

Church services of all kinds were held all day Sunday. The Protestant denominations united harmoniously in a Christian fellowship and planned their services to suit all, while still holding several forms of worship. Catholics were greatest in numbers, so they had first right to the assembly hall on Sundays.

Despite the best attempts, over this long period of confinement, the strain was tremendous. Health was inevitably impaired by the lack of nourishment, and people became woefully thin. Like many others, Margaret developed symptoms of beriberi, and her normally erect posture had become a sad stoop. Mr. Lawless, formerly a giant of a man, lost more than twenty kilograms (50 pounds) during internment. Many people of all ages died in Weixian, and the survivors worried how many more would meet that fate. Added to this was the misery of not knowing how the war was progressing. A bush telegraph was hard at work, but it brought little better than unconfirmed rumours.

All speculation came to an end when, on August 17, 1945, the first group of liberating American paratroops dropped from the sky. The entire camp streamed past the guards at the gates to welcome their liberators. At last World War II was over!

From her remote viewpoint, Margaret had speculated from time to time what had brought mankind to this desperate situation with all its ghastly ramifications. She could never bring herself to question why God permitted people to degenerate to these extremes, but she summarized her thoughts with the following words:

How frail and puny is Man, yet he rides the waves,
Dives down to the depths, and flies through the air.
Difficulties but stimulate, no obstacles deter;
He shuns not death.
Whence comes this power that nought can quell?
This force is God Himself, who lives and moves through all.

(E. M. P.)

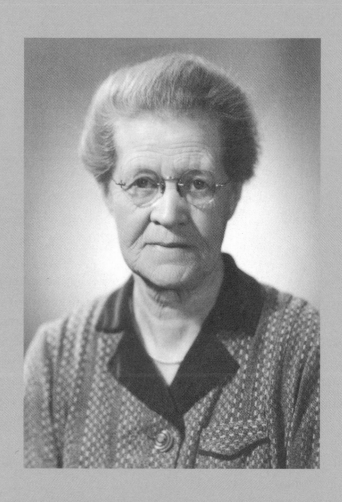

Aftermath

✿ AFTER THE WAR, the Chinese seat of government was re-established in Nanjing—a name signifying "Southern Capital." Hence the name Peking, the anglicized form of Beijing (signifying "Northern Capital"), was no longer appropriate, so the city was renamed Beiping, meaning "Northern Peace." The diplomatic services also set themselves up in the new capital, where they had been before war broke out. When the Japanese surrendered, Flight Lieutenant C. H. Phillips, Royal Air Force, was in Chongqing, the wartime capital of China, having just flown in from Calcutta. The Air Ministry had posted him to a Chinese air force staff college in Chengdu to utilize his Chinese qualifications, but due to the events, he was rerouted to Beiping.

By October, the British consul had allocated Margaret rooms in what was previously the students' accommodation in the British embassy compound. These were not salubrious but certainly a vast improvement on what she had endured hitherto, and she reveled in the privacy. On his arrival, Clifford headed straight to Margaret's accommodations, but, as luck would have it, she was not home. He sat, somewhat tensely, on a bench nearby, hoping she might return soon. When finally she came into sight,

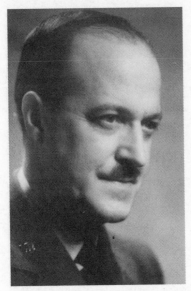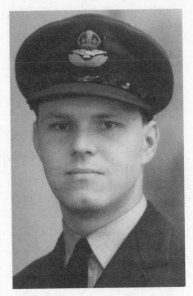

Left: In his first year at university, Clifford was told to report to Squadron Leader Hill, unaware that he had misheard, and that he was actually reporting to his godfather, Uncle Arthur, Squadron Leader A.J. Heal, R.A.F. V.R.
Right: Flt. Lieut. C.H. Phillips.

he could scarcely believe his eyes. It had been nine years since mother and son had been together. At first, he hardly recognized the elderly woman walking up the road, but she knew just who it was sitting there in an airforce blue uniform, and she was stretching out her arms to him before he got to his feet. Tears flowed, as they had done the last time the two were together, but this time, tears of joy.

Being together at last, safe and sound, caused strong emotions. Margaret was delighted that here was her son, all resplendent in his smart uniform. Clifford, on the other hand, was profoundly disturbed to see what the past three years had done to her. Holding her in his arms, he realized the effects of malnutrition at close hand. She had aged twice the number of years they had been apart. She had a sadness about her expression and a weary stoop to her shoulders, and she had obviously lost a lot of weight.

It took a while to feel completely at ease, and at first they spoke only in generalities. Initially Margaret was no more inclined to discuss her experiences in Weixian internment camp than Clifford was to discuss his wartime experiences. But within a few days they became relaxed and were talking nineteen to the dozen, frequently interrupting each other while trying to fill in the gaps of their long separation. Margaret was especially pleased when Clifford assured her that sending him to England was one of the best things she had done for him. He was married now, having met Enid Turner after volunteering for flying duties in the Royal Air Force.

When Margaret and Clifford were first reunited, his most delicate task was to persuade her to indulge herself at the best hairdressing salon. The ravages of camp life had taken its toll on all the women. Margaret, like many others, needed a luxury treatment to enhance her self-esteem. She accepted Clifford's advice and soon felt much better for it.

At first, nowhere in the embassy was particularly livable, if only because there was three years of dust to be cleared away. Four places in the compound had been made inhabitable, and a major cleanup operation lay ahead. Clifford, however, had comfortable accommodation at the Wagon-Lits hotel through his official capacity as an attaché. At the time he was the sole British officer in uniform in Beiping. As much as he wished otherwise, for now he could do little to give his mother better comfort. In any case, she was adamant about maintaining her privacy.

Air Ministry in London assigned Clifford the task of setting up a services' language school in the former British embassy compound. Several service officers would be joining him by year-end, and he was to prepare their accommodation. He and the consul responsible for the compound selected one of the largest buildings and began the cleansing process by sweeping large quantities of sawdust and damp old tea leaves over the floors to get rid of the dust, supplemented by buckets full of snow. To the consul's surprise this worked rather well, and it became the means for dealing with the remaining houses. Once he moved in, Margaret and Clifford were only about five minutes' walk apart.

Then came the demanding task of selecting staff. The domestic staff was easy, for when the word got around, Clifford virtually had the pick of the town. With Margaret's advice a suitable selection was made. Selecting the teaching staff called for more delicacy, but in due course three Chinese scholars were chosen and terms agreed. Margaret's resettlement took a little longer, for, apart from the barest essentials in her temporary accommodation, she had practically no possessions. Fortunately, her apartment was furnished. The Lindemans returned the trunk that they had so kindly looked after. Included in this was her old typewriter, which was to prove most valuable in the days ahead. There was no need for a servant, since Clifford made one of his available on an "as and when" basis.

Regrettably, because the outrageous wartime rate of inflation continued to depreciate accounts, Margaret's holdings with the Hong Kong and Shanghai Bank were practically worthless. Clifford was little able to supplement her financial needs, but he persuaded her to accept a relief allowance, which he promised to reimburse when the need arose.

In a surprisingly short time, life in Beiping was restored to its normal tempo. Previous treaty rights became anomalous and so were abrogated. To an extent the city was almost a garrison town. Now that China had been recognized as a wartime Ally, most Allied troops were gone, but numerous American troops remained to restore communications throughout North China. Between the army PX and the black market, little was lacking— for those who could afford it. Fortunately, Clifford and his colleagues regularly received bonded supplies from Hong Kong. Occasionally these came in useful for bartering purposes.

Clifford had a service vehicle at his disposal, making it easy to get around and to help Margaret locate and visit friends, many of whom had been in camp with her. People were eager to compare notes and see how others were settling. Some had known Clifford in his boyhood, and Margaret was proud to show him off. One day Clifford was surprised by a connection from the past. A middle-aged Chinese woman called at his hotel. Neither she or he knew each other, but she knew Margaret well, and that Margaret's son had recently returned to China.

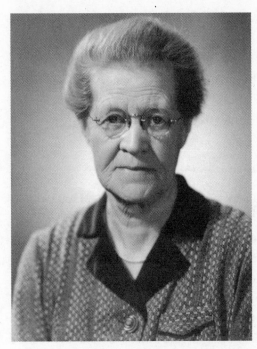

A care-worn Dr. Margaret Phillips after enduring the Weixian internment camp,
c. 1946.

She told Clifford that she was one of Margaret's former TB patients, and had had a lung removed. A second operation became necessary to remove a portion of the remaining lung, and the prognosis was far from promising. Then a faith healer visited the sanatorium. Drawn to this woman, she requested Margaret's permission to visit her regularly. Margaret, who fully supported faith healing, encouraged her to spend as much time with her as possible, saying "There is nothing more that I can do. She is in God's hands now." More than ten years later, this very patient was now calling on Clifford, slightly plump and rosy-cheeked, looking the picture of health. Wishing to show her gratitude but too humble to approach Margaret, she presented him with a gift: two pairs of hand-knitted, grey woollen socks.[1]

Another remarkable meeting had occurred before Clifford left England. During his briefing on duties in China, he was instructed to report to Squadron Leader Hill in Intelligence. At first he didn't recognize the man behind the desk, who was quite amused to announce that his name was not Hill but Heal—it was Clifford's godfather, Uncle Arthur. Neither of them had seen each other for ten years.

∫※

At the start of his tour of duty in Beiping, Clifford was required to update air force training material, and he began compiling a glossary of aeronautical terminology for the use of RAF personnel engaged in liaison or intelligence duties. Margaret assumed secretarial duties in typing approximately seven thousand general service and technical terms in English and Chinese romanization, about three times over. For this assistance, the air attaché authorized an honorarium, which pleased her no end, as did her involvement with Clifford's first publication. A Chinese tutor inserted all the Chinese characters by hand in the manuscript, as no Chinese typewriter was to be had.[2]

In the New Year, five service officers arrived in Beiping, with the promise that their families would follow. In March 1946, Clifford and Enid's first baby was born, and Margaret became a grandmother. In China, the paternal grandmother is called *Nai-nai* and the maternal grandmother, *Lao-lao*. Clifford decided to apply Chinese usage—a novel idea that was accepted all round, and to this day both Margaret and Enid's mother are remembered in this fashion. Six weeks later Clifford returned to London for a conference, and happily he was able to spend time with his wife and new daughter. Lesley's christening was arranged, and she was given the second name of Margaret after her *Nai-nai*. After his return to Beiping, Clifford waited impatiently, like the other husbands, for the grand reunion with his family.

For political and bureaucratic reasons, this did not happen for another year. Two married officers, unwilling to wait, resigned their commissions and returned to England. Clifford consoled himself with social activities. He was a member of the Peking Club, and for the midsummer celebration of the king's birthday, he brought Margaret to the club. Club rules did not permit women to enter the bar without a male escort, so Margaret was quite interested to look around while Clifford went in search of drinks. He returned with what he fancied might appeal to her: a nice long glass of iced orange juice. She took one hard look at it, then demanded to know what Clifford held in his other hand. Told it was a popular drink consisting of gin and vermouth, generally referred to as a "vergin," she immediately insisted on exchanging glasses, assuring him that, after two and a half years in camp, she was not about to accept anything so innocuous as orange juice, especially for toasting His Majesty.

Eventually the glad news came that the families were about to arrive, and in May 1947, the men waited at quayside in Hong Kong to welcome the troopship *Strathnaver,* with their loved ones onboard. After a couple of days in Hong Kong for shopping, an RAF York aircraft airlifted the families north, stopping in Nanjing to see the ambassador and the air attaché. Margaret was so happy to meet Enid and baby Lesley at long last. Lesley had just learned to walk, and it did not take long for Margaret to express her delight in the toddler's presence:

CONFIDENCE

She looked up to my face
with a smile like sunshine.
She slipped her hand in mine
so lovingly.
She knew no fear, for she had not met
unkindness yet.
My love went out to meet her trust
in sympathy.

(E. M. P.)

By now it was possible to provide families with individual accommodation. Fortunately, the second-floor apartment allotted to the Phillipses was more than large enough to house Margaret as well, as from then on she was a part of her larger family. As she regained her strength, her vitality improved very well for someone just turned seventy. During this period, she composed several poems on different topics. To Clifford she dedicated:

A MOTHER'S LOVE

Shall I tell you why I love you?
I love you because you've endured,
Because you're manly and true;
I love you because you're you.

Do you know why I love you, my son?
When you do right, when you get it wrong,
Whenever you smile, whenever you frown.
When you are angry (but not with me)
I love you, my son.

When you bring your troubles to me,
When you tell me your joys,
When you tell me your hopes
I love you, my son.

You are never angry with me,
You are always patient,
You take thought for me,
You are gentle to me.
I love you, my son.

(E. M. P.)

Now that the Phillipses were a whole family unit, it behove them to participate in the social round. Thanks to Margaret's help, Enid soon adjusted to the social whirl, and she began playing her part in returning hospitality. Unless she excused herself, Margaret was usually included in the parties—on one condition. After dinner she could stay as long as she liked, but when she wanted to retire she was expected to withdraw unobtrusively rather than to go round saying goodnight to everyone. Margaret considered it only courtesy to formally take her leave of the party, but the result was that others felt they too should retire—which tended to kill the evening stone-dead.

Margaret's portion of the apartment was self-contained off the landing, ensuring her desired privacy and enabling her to receive her friends independently. She had two pet cats. After taking time to recover from her long ordeal, she soon felt well enough to get back into the swim of things, although regrettably, she could not totally eradicate the signs of damage to her health. Her normally erect figure had given way to a slight stoop not solely due to her age.

She did not consider it worth trying to recover her medical practice, which had been completely ruined. Instead, she took on a new venture: a position with Radio Peking, delivering three weekly half-hour programs. Her listening public included many American troops and the officials and families from several international organizations, such as the United Nations Relief and Rehabilitation Administration (UNRRA) and the World Health Organization (WHO), which had based their headquarters in Beiping to assist the Chinese in restoring their country after the ravages of World War II. Margaret's on-air talks, covering various aspects of life in and around the city, earned her a large and appreciative audience. Her program lasted nearly a year, and the preparation alone kept her busy.

Although she no longer taught English, she parlayed her long experience into a 120-page paperback entitled *Useful English Conversation*, which contained twenty-four lessons, selected prose and some poetry. That winter, Enid was invited to teach English at the Railway College of Administration, and she ably put *Nai-nai's* work to good purpose.[3]

Margaret then decided that there was a likely market for an up-to-date guidebook on her hometown. A local publisher encouraged her to undertake the task. Clifford had already shown Enid some of the more obvious places, such as the Summer Palace and the Great Wall, but Margaret assured her that was not the half of it. She invited Enid to come along on her research trips, and both enjoyed these twice-weekly jaunts. Since her return from Weixian, Margaret constantly felt fatigued, yet after those outings, it was usually Enid who seemed more weary. Margaret sometimes described the high spots in other than standard prose:

THE ALTAR OF HEAVEN

This is no earthly place; this Altar to Heaven.
Appraise it not with worldly eyes for grandeur or size.
You who visit this Altar must see it with eyes of the spirit.
Majestic in simplicity and serenity it stands,
Fashioned by the humble hands of man.

Conceived in spirit at the inspiration of the Great Architect
To assist man's approach to the Supreme God of Perfection.
Here on this pure white marble, purified in body and soul
The Mediator pleads for clemency for his subject children.
Here in mystic communion Man draws nigh to his Maker.

(E. M. P.)

Due to post-war events, Margaret's guidebook was never published.

∫※

RUMOURS OF CIVIL WAR were rife, yet few foresaw the eventual outcome. Even fewer realized that this was, in effect, the result of what was known as the Xi'an Incident. Late in 1936, Generalissimo Chiang Kaishek was forced by the Warlords, led by Zhang Xueliang, to consent to collaborate with the Communists in fighting the Japanese. Nonetheless, Chiang Kaishek deliberately withheld the better half of the Nationalist army. They had been trained by General "Vinegar Joe" Stilwell of the US Army, who was only too eager to put his crack Chinese troops to the test. Due to internal politics, Chiang chose to rely on General Claire Chenault and his Flying Tigers (*Fei Hu*) to provide air cover in an attempt to establish air superiority over the Japanese. This suited the American strategists, at the same time allowing Chiang to harbour his ground forces until they could be used against the Communists when World War II was over. For at least three years, under the leadership of Mao Zedong, Communist forces had conducted a heroic war of resistance against the Japanese invasion without the promised help from the Nationalists.

Soon after the war Chiang Kaishek showed his hand and a civil war began, to establish ascendancy of rulership. Despite the intervention of US General George Marshall, and all the American military support, the Nationalist army was unable to resist the onslaught of the Communist Eighth Route Army, *Ba-Lu Jun*. The *Kuomintang* (Nationalist) government was corrupt in the extreme, and it had alienated such a large proportion of the population that the Communists had little trouble winning their support. By 1948, the Communists had routed the *Kuomintang* forces, and the Nationalists retreated to Taiwan.

Although the turmoil throughout China again seemed to have little impact on Beiping, it was time pull out. In late August, orders from the air attaché in Nanjing arrived to prepare to return to England. Clifford and Enid were anxious that Margaret should accompany them, and this time she agreed. At last she was reconciled to the fact that she would have to leave her home in China. Clifford negotiated with the embassy to grant her a free passage to England as a returning refugee, while the air attaché used his influence with air headquarters in Hong Kong to secure her a berth on the troopship that would take them to the United Kingdom. In the meantime, the language school was closed down and severance arrangements were made with the staff at the shortest possible notice. By September 3, an RAF York aircraft had arrived from Hong Kong, and all service personnel and their dependants flew out the following day.

While preparing to leave her beloved Peking, Margaret composed a final poem:

A SUMMER STORM

Darkness falls while yet it is day;
A covering of grey hides the blue sky;
There is an ominous calm.
Suddenly a wild wind comes raging by;
Any change is welcome from the sweltering heat.
Hark! The muttering of distant thunder.
Now a few raindrops patter down.
Some aircraft come flying low.
Soon the wind drops, the thunder is nearer;
The vivid lightning flashes are followed by loud rumbling.
We hear the soothing sound of falling rain
And feel a freshness in the air.
It will not last long; there is sunshine in the west.
We shall sleep well tonight.

(E. M. P.)

After forty-three years, Margaret left the country she considered home. Initially, both she and Clifford were somewhat depressed, for China was partly home to him too.[4] But spirits rose once all four Phillipses were onboard the troopship *Lancashire*, heading for England. After a brief stop in Aden, the journey continued via Naples and through the Strait of Gibraltar—significant landmarks to Margaret, who first saw these places when heading in the opposite direction into the unknown. So much had taken place in the intervening years, and she sadly realized that this return trip represented the end of the most meaningful part of her life. Regretfully, this was a compulsory move—not one she would have made voluntarily, had conditions been different. However, she thought, it was not just to please the family, for if this was God's will, so be it.

The homecoming ended in Liverpool, and Frank was there to meet Margaret and take her to his home in Birmingham. Clifford bid her farewell after what seemed three such short years. This time circumstances were much happier, for they were all together and within easy reach, only a phone call away. Clifford was posted to Kinloss in Scotland for a refresher course on flying duties, while Enid returned to London, where her mother received her and little Lesley with open arms.

♪﹡

BY THE FOLLOWING SUMMER, Margaret had left Birmingham to stay with Bertie; an unhappy rift had developed between her and Frank. During the late 1920s, when it appeared that the students' political agitation in Peking might get out of hand, the British consul had advised all British subjects to be prepared for evacuation at short notice. Bearing in mind what had happened during the Boxer Uprising, there was no way of knowing whether evacuation might be for a short or long period. Margaret had learned from earlier experiences how easily she could be parted from much of her worldly goods, so she packed a sizeable crate with her most valuable possessions and freighted it to Frank for safe-keeping.

Now it appeared that this crate no longer existed. Frank claimed he had been unable to accommodate it in the house so he had placed it in a garden shed, where it was subsequently destroyed by fire during an air raid. Margaret did not accept Frank's story, since no mention of this calamity had come up before, and, feeling badly let-down, she moved out. Clifford would have been unsurprised had Margaret gone to Bertie in the first place; the only contact he ever had with Uncle Frank was at their initial meeting in Liverpool. Margaret settled comfortably in Bridgwater with Bertie, who was only too happy to give her a home, as he had done some twelve years earlier for Clifford.

For the next while, Margaret was busy contacting old friends, occasionally accepting invitations to visit. She was finding it difficult to adjust to the English diet. Clifford winced at her remark that conditions in

England were not much better than in camp, although what she meant was that the rationing was poor compared to what had been available in Peking after the war. It was true that after the war, food rationing in Britain was even leaner than during the war years. A Labour MP, Aneurin Bevan, once proudly boasted something to the effect that: "Britain is an island consisting largely of coal and surrounded by fish. It would take an organizing genius to create a shortage in coal and fish at the same time." Yet before two years had elapsed, the Labour government had achieved precisely that.

Margaret was violently allergic to seafood of any sort. When fish was plentiful in England, most people welcomed the substitute for the meagre meat ration—mostly sausages—but she could not touch it. Becoming heartily tired of eating anything resembling a sausage, she, like many others, was heard to say, "Thank God for Spam."

Often Margaret had remarked that, if she were to have her time again, she would have concentrated on medicine of the mind. In 1950, she was delighted to receive a visit from her goddaughter, now Dr. Liu Meizhen, who she had last seen in Peking while under house arrest. After the war Meizhen moved to Taiwan, and now she had just arrived from Hong Kong to do postgraduate study in psychiatry at Birmingham, thus completing the circle arising from Margaret's care and direction.

Meanwhile, Clifford was called to the air ministry to receive new orders. Until then he had been serving as a volunteer reserve officer, as did all wartime aircrew. Now he was awarded a permanent commission, which meant that he could make the RAF his career. The immediate result was a three-year posting with his family to Melbourne as a liaison officer with the Royal Australian Air Force, leaving in September, with time only for a quick visit to Bridgwater to say goodbye to Margaret and Bertie. Enid was pregnant, and Deborah Jane was born in Melbourne on April 17, 1950.

Margaret was still suffering from the effects of the lean days in Weixian, and the ravages of past ill health were slowly pulling her down. By early 1950, she was noticeably weaker, fatigued and under constant medical care. She had developed severe oedema, which rather limited her mobility.

Bertie got word of a home organized by Rotary International, and he secured her accommodation at Badgworth Court in Axbridge, Somerset—not far from Bridgwater, and with a good interconnecting bus service, so he was able to visit often. Bertie was her only relative at her side; possibly shame kept Frank away.

True to character, Margaret soon settled into the new routine, and she became very friendly with the matron. By making herself useful she did not feel too restricted. But in early May, it was increasingly apparent that she had not a lot longer to live. Bertie was becoming more and more concerned that Clifford was unaware of this development. Margaret had flatly refused him permission to tell Clifford, saying that he had his duties to attend to and she did not wish him to be distracted. As letters were rarely exchanged more than once a month, it was not hard to leave the impression that everything was normal. When it became necessary for Margaret to take to her bed, Bertie ignored her wishes and via the air ministry sent word of her condition. Clifford was notified immediately and given top priority to fly home, but alas, events moved too quickly.

In mid-afternoon Margaret had difficulty breathing. Bertie sat beside her and held her in his arms so that she could speak quietly. She spoke randomly about her life and expressed no regrets—except that she would have liked more time to know Clifford as a man. Her conscience was clear since she had consistently obeyed what she believed to be God's will, and she assured her brother that God had plans for her. He had called her to do his work in China. He had restored her to her family and friends in England. Now Margaret felt that it was God's will that she return to Him. After a brief pause, she said, "Goodbye, Bertie," and with a sigh, she passed away. On the evening of Thursday, May 17, 1951, Ethel Margaret Phillips died of congestive heart failure.

The night before Clifford was to take off, a second signal arrived, expressing regret that his mother had just died. It was too late, although he had been given top priority to fly out. A week later the enormity of his loss struck home, and Clifford broke down. The three years spent together from 1945 to 1948 seemed such a short interlude in both their lives.

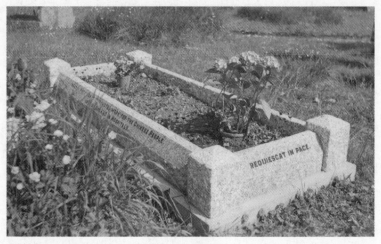

The last resting place of Dr. Ethel Margaret Phillips is in the churchyard of Axbridge, Somerset.

From what she wrote not long before her death, her family was convinced that Margaret died a happy woman:

Some people seem to think that happiness and pleasure are the same,
But this is not so.
Happiness comes from within, and pleasure is from without.
To live for pleasure gives little true satisfaction,
And often leads to discontent and moral deterioration.
Happiness is found in the love of what is right and beautiful.
I think that true happiness is only known by those who are in touch
    with God.

(E. M. P.)

Bertie was gratified at how many friends attended Margaret's funeral. He had supplied an obituary notice to two national daily newspapers, so Margaret's passing quickly became public knowledge. In due time he arranged for a headstone and curb to surround the grave. Engraved along the left-hand side is the message: "Well done, thou good and faithful servant."

♪✻

AFTER JUST OVER SEVENTY-FIVE YEARS, Ethel Margaret Phillips, a remarkable person, passed on peacefully from life in a world that had not always treated her very kindly. She bore no rancour, knowing full well that life for most people is seldom fair.

During Clifford's final visit with Margaret before leaving for Australia, mother and son had their last heart-to-heart talk. She congratulated him on his new career, and expressed disappointment over not having been totally successful in any of her many endeavours. While proud, Margaret was by no means vainglorious, so Clifford took this to mean that she felt she was never able to attain any particular pinnacle. The acclaim she had received for her achievement in Pingyin over St. Agatha's Hospital was heady stuff forty years earlier, but since then, in contrast, her efforts had not been well rewarded. Kaifeng was a phase she could well have done without, and she seldom referred to it. In Peking, her social service work and her efforts to combat tuberculosis were monumental, yet after the Japanese aggression, it all seemed to have been for nothing, and the paltry sum she eventually received as reparation was derisory. But she humbly accepted that this was God's will, and that her reward was to be in heaven.

Years later, Clifford discovered her poetry, expressing many of her views on life, including her feelings on her perceived lack of achievement:

FAILURE

I have come to the evening time
And now am content to rest.
I look back on my thwarted life
Without remorse or even regret.

I never achieved my ambitions,
I never reached my aims,
But I know it was better by far
That I tried to be—just myself.

(E. M. P.)

Apparently Margaret had not considered the widespread effect that she had wherever she went. After all, fifty years later, her memory lives on. Her influence may pass even further into the future—for, of all the seed she sowed, much undoubtedly fell on fertile ground. Good fruit may yet be recognized.

CYCLES

After day comes night and after night returns day.
After summer comes winter, then summer again.
After life comes death and after death new life,
For death releases the soul to join with other souls
In the great Soul of God.

(E. M. P.)

Chinese Pronunciation and Romanization

♪* THE WRITTEN CHINESE LANGUAGE uses charac-
ters, sometimes referred to as ideographs. These do not provide any
alphabet or guide to pronunciation. All characters have a sound and tone
value which varies in different regions of China, but the meaning remains
the same. While Chinese dialects vary, the one written form serves them
all. The national dialect of China is based on the sound values used in
its capital, Beijing. In English this is known as Mandarin, but in Chinese it
is called *putonghua*, meaning "common language."

To assist foreigners in learning the sounds and writing the characters,
various systems of romanization evolved. In the nineteenth century, the
Wade-Giles system, named for its originators, gained widespread usage
as a standardized spelling and was adopted by the post office for place-
names, giving rise to spellings like Hoang Ho and Yangtse Kiang, which
were commonly used in English. This also resulted in anglicized forms
such as Peking and Canton.

Fifty years ago, the Chinese People's Republic devised an official form
of romanization known as *pinyin*, which means "spelling sounds." This
style, now used universally, can cause some confusion: Hoang Ho is now

Huang He; Yangtse Kiang, Yangzi Jiang. Though the new convention may take some getting used to, it has the advantage of presenting the correct Chinese pronunciation, albeit without the tones. *Pinyin* is shown in italics throughout this book, except for place-names and names of persons, which are displayed in roman. To avoid confusion, place-names are accompanied by the alternate spelling in parentheses at first mention.

In pinyin, the sound of *q* is the same as *ch* in Wade-Giles (Qing, Ching); *x* the same as *hs* (Guangxu, Kuanghsu); and *z* as *ts* (Yangzi, Yangtse). These changes were made mainly to indicate the approximate formation of the lips caused by the different vowels succeeding the initial letter. The fact that Wade-Giles made use of the apostrophe for aspirated sounds was often ignored, and *pinyin* puts this error to rights. A rough indication of these features follows:

CONSONANT	EXAMPLE
c, as in *ma<u>ts</u>*	*cai* (wealth)
ch, as in *<u>ch</u>arge*	*chao* (damp)
h, as in *<u>h</u>ail*	*hao* (good)
and occasionally as in *<u>wh</u>en*	*hui* (assembly)
j, as in *<u>j</u>inx*	*jin* (strength)
p, as in *<u>p</u>utt*	*piao* (ticket)
q, as in *<u>ch</u>ew*	*qian* (money)
sh, as in *<u>sh</u>ow*	*shao* (burn)
x, as in *<u>sh</u>eep*	*xiang* (sound)
z, as in *ad<u>ds</u>*	*zai* (again)—cf. *c* above
zh, as in *<u>j</u>aw*	*zhong* (bell)

All other consonants may be pronounced according to usual English usage, and be readily understood. Vowels, on the other hand, require more explanation than this work justifies. Close attention to the way the Chinese speak should suffice.

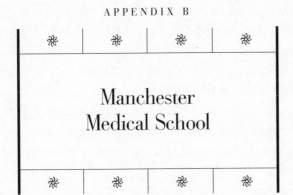

Manchester
Medical School

♫* IN 1905, Ethel Margaret Phillips became the third woman to receive a degree cum laude from the University of Manchester Medical School.

The history of the Manchester medical school goes back more than 150 years. A brochure entitled "Medicine at Manchester" states that "by the time the Owens College, the origin of the University, began life in 1851, there were two privately owned medical schools in the city." In 1874, Thomas Huxley opened the new medical school as part of Owens College. It now carries the name Stopford House. Items of Dr. E. M. Phillips's memorabilia, including her eight bronze medals (catalogued no. 1982.1), are on display in a showcase in the foyer, along with gold medals of exalted Manchester medics such as Sir Harry Platt (1921) and Dr. Eugenia Cooper (1923), to name but two.

Also on display is a large blue silk embroidery—an award Dr. Phillips received in 1915 from the Chinese provincial government (see note 1, Chapter 12)—donated by the author, together with his translation of the Chinese text.

APPENDIX C

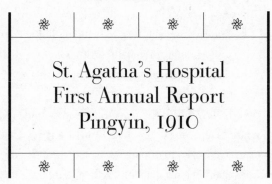

St. Agatha's Hospital
First Annual Report
Pingyin, 1910

♪✳ [IN] 1910 WE CELEBRATE the completion of the first year of regular hospital routine...

The situation too is not so central for dispensary work, and the numerous "medicine shops" within the city must save many would-be patients an uphill journey to St. Agatha's. Still there is a mental and physical gain in the purer, bracing air of the new locality, which is a very great aid to medical treatment of the inpatients, now the most important branch of our work.

...Outpatients are seen every day at noon, after listening to the preaching by the Chinese catechist. No charge is made for medicines, but each patient pays at the gate the sum of 40 cash (rather less than ½ d.) for the first admission and is given a numbered ticket on leaving. For subsequent attendances...he pays only half the original fee, but should he lose the ticket he comes as a new patient and must pay the full fee again...Besides name and number of the patient the tickets now bear on one side a text in Mandarin from the New Testament. After 12 o'clock the gate money is raised to 100 cash (about 1 penny). Any patient who seems a suitable case for admission is invited to stay for better treatment than can be carried in his or her own home. Only too often the patients most willing to stay are cases quite beyond our help…those who could most certainly be relieved, even if not always cured, will not consent to trust themselves to our care…[T]he real cause is…the prevailing ignorance and consequent suspicion of foreign ways and the fear of bringing ill luck upon themselves and their families, often perhaps the ridicule from their heathen neighbours, for everyone is deeply concerned in the affairs of everyone else, and secrecy is impossible.

We have two small wards in the dispensary compound, and with the help also of a large shed…for open-air treatment we are able to accommodate ten or even a dozen men patients who cannot be admitted into the Women's Hospital. The men patients each pay a fee of 500 cash (about 5 d.) on admission and are expected to subscribe towards the expenses of their compound when leaving. They provide and cook their own food and bring their own attendants. We do not profess to have a hospital for men, though we cannot refuse to help them…since there is no other foreign medical assistance . . .

The main hospital building, which is situated in the inner compound, is intended for women and children. Here we try to carry on as far as possible on foreign lines. Food and attendance for Chinese nurse probationers are provided free. Each patient pays an entrance fee of 1,000 cash (about 9–10 d.), quite a considerable sum for the Pingyin people to produce, and a subscription on leaving,…proportionate to the length of stay as well as the means and gratitude of the sufferer. There is no very great fear that patients will be attracted for the free food only, for conservation is strong here, and those who trust themselves to our care probably stand to lose prestige and fair name from their temporary association with the foreigners and Chinese Christians…Should they wish to leave before…their…treatment is completed they are required to pay the full cost of their board during the whole time of stay in hospital…This money has several times been paid without a murmur by the friends of patients when they wished to take them home.

[O]ur patients are usually in the chronic or convalescent stage… [y]et we are expected to perform the miraculous and complaints are many if recovery does not set in at once. Sometimes we are ourselves surprised at the speedy improvement in apparently hopeless cases as soon as they are placed under better conditions. We have some sort of a reputation for the treatment of abscesses; the native doctors here being evidently unsuccessful in this branch of their practice. Their universal method is the application of a black adhesive plaster, which is left *in situ* as long as the wearer pleases, and the discharge, unable to escape, spreads underneath and infects the surrounding areas. In the springtime we had an unusual number of abscesses of all kinds and suppurative joint infections. The joint cases are usually hopeless and amputations are never consented to, but chronic ulcers and other abscesses, cases of cellulitis, enlarged glands, etc., do very well, so we hope our reputation is growing by degrees and that confidence in other directions will follow in time.

Eye cases of course are many, but usually hopeless…they never possess the necessary patience for prolonged treatment. Two severe eye cases admitted both escaped the following day. A few cases of cancer remained for observation and relief, but were too far gone for hope of any but very temporary improvement. One young woman came in to try and break off the opium habit, but made her escape over the compound wall on the second day. She seemed so extremely docile…one never expected a small-footed Chinese woman to climb a wall with a drop of 16–17 feet on the outer side into the road.

Four cases of rheumatism have received very marked benefit. Of seven consumptive patients admitted for treatment two improved most wonderfully…Another one, greatly misled by the improvement in her health, left us, against our wishes, after a very short stay…she died a few months later. The others were at a hopelessly advanced stage…One in fact died in the hospital; her home being too far for her to return, but the others were taken home by their friends, who always prefer their sick people to die at home and not under some unlucky foreigner's roof. Two beggars found a last refuge with us and died here (of the results of years of starvation and exposure) because they had no friends to take them away. One was an excommunicated Christian, who turned to the church for help in his last days…Whether he was repentant we do not know, nor whether (for one cannot expect the beggars in China to be good!) he ever had a real chance of mending his ways. The other poor heathen man was buried by the magistrate, as we had no wish to get into trouble later should any friends ever turn up and accuse us of a hand in his death and burial.

Four…patients [needed]…needles removed from different parts of the body…they were difficult extractions. One was who was employing on himself the Chinese method of acupuncture for an indigestion pain when the needle (which was 1¾ inches long) slipped beyond his reach and entered the small intestine. Having prepared the way for a suppurative peritonitis by their own septic and unavailing measures…his friends brought him to us to remove the needle and undo the mischief they had already done…[A]lthough seriously ill for a time he eventually made a good recovery.

Another example of dangerous procrastination was a case of pyopneumothorax, a man who was stabbed in a quarrel by a friend at his wedding feast: the knife entering his chest just below the collar bone, and he did not come to see us until three (or more) weeks after the injury because he had to win his lawsuit first! We hesitated about admitting him, but he made a surprisingly good though not complete recovery. He stayed here for many months and has at last taken our advice and gone to Tsinanfu for better operative treatment than we can give our men patients.

One of our most gratifying cases was that of a man who suffered from attacks of obstinate and excruciating indigestion, and after several weeks' treatment obtained complete relief. The children have generally responded promptly to our measures…it gives us the greatest satisfaction to send them away fit and well after the emaciated condition in which they are brought to us. We should have this pleasure very much more often and save many more lives were it not for the ignorance of their elders. The parents usually profess the greatest willingness for the children to stay, but they must first gain the consent of the children themselves and then from the grandmothers and grandfathers, and sometimes even the great-grandparents also! Sometimes...after a few days' treatment the parents come and demand their children again. This is resisted as long as possible, but there are many times one must give way. In the case of one little patient with acute hip disease, whose parents demanded his withdrawal at the most serious stage of the disease shortly after the operation had been necessary, we held firm, knowing that to send him home would mean certain death. It was an anxious decision, for he might have died here and caused a good deal of trouble, but he is now walking about the hospital compound and only waiting to get a little fatter before being restored to his parents.

The mother professes gratitude now, and I hope she will remember to tell her neighbours her better opinions since she seems to have circulated those of the other kind freely.

One of the greatest difficulties...is the utter ignorance of foreign ways, medical or any other...We need to make the people...trust us more, and we can only hope to do this by keeping (as we try to do) the missionary aspect of our work always in full view. It was quite as much for the sake of the evangelistic work as for the medical that we built the hospital... [C]onventional courtesy requires their attention while they are actually receiving benefits from us, but it is most encouraging to find them willing to listen. So very few of our patients can read that we cannot give away much literature, but...[t]hey have almost all learnt the long easy prayer which we read every morning in chapel, and nearly everyone learns the hymn we sing. Both...are...expressed in the very easiest phrases of this most difficult language, and...we hope every patient will be a missionary to her own people...Several of the patients went on from the prayer to the catechism...singing it aloud until the hospital sounded like a school... All the Christians in the compound (servants and nurses) attend service at least once on Sunday, and sometimes the patients ask to go too...but the distance is a drawback to small-footed women...We...must have a Bible-woman to teach the women patients and help the nurse probationers to live up to a higher standard of duty. There are three nurse probationers in training...quick and helpful in many ways, but [they] dislike the drudgery of nursing, the daily cleaning and the actual tending of patients...However, for Pingyin, we are beginning the profession of nursing with very favourable material!

...Three or four villages are visited by one of us each month. The greatest number of patients seen in the villages in one day in 1910 was 174...[T]he real motive of itinerating is the missionary one, for medical relief cannot often be satisfactorily rendered at monthly intervals.

[T]he monthly At-Home for Chinese women...has been continued throughout the year...The Yamen ladies attended one of these At-Homes, and by special invitation we returned their call, when they entertained us with a luxurious repast and a wheezy gramophone by way of orchestra.

We conclude our report with grateful acknowledgment to all our kind friends and helpers and an earnest request for their continued help... alas! We...have exceeded our income this year, chiefly from a desire to make our work of the very best, and partly because we did not know how much money we could count upon. Our work, if it is to continue, MUST CONTINUE TO GROW, and for this we need additional support and not diminished expenditure.

E.M. PHILLIPS
St. Agatha's Day, February 5, 1911

Statistics for 1910

INPATIENTS		OPERATIONS	
Men	39	Major	25
Women	34	Minor	87
Children	27		
Total	100		

OUTPATIENT ATTENDANCES

Pingyin	3,877
Villages	1,038
Total	4,915

ATTACHMENT II

List of Inpatients

	No. of Cases
Abscesses, Ulcers, Cellulitis, Enlarged Glands, Sinuses, etc.	22
Joint Affections	10
Fractures	4
Hip Disease	1
Spinal Diseases	2
Amputation of Finger	1
Necrosis Superior Maxilla	2
Pulmonary Tuberculosis	7
Tubercular Peritonitis	1
Emphysema and Bronchitis	1
Pneumonia	1
Pyopneumothorax	1
Gastritis	1
Cirrhosis of the Liver	3

List of Inpatients

	No. of Cases
Anaemia and Marasmus	11
Ulceration Throat and Tongue	4
Salivary Fistula (same case admitted twice)	2
Cancrum Oris	1
Eye Diseases	4
Heart Disease	1
Postdipheritic Complications	1
Postscarlatinal Nephritis	1
Phosphaturia	1
Obstetrical	1
Removal of Needles	4
Removal of large Cyst, Upper Lip	1
Rodent Ulcer	1
Lipoma	1
Papilloma Foot	1
Multiple Epithelomia Face	1
Carcinoma Breast	1
Stricture of the Oesophagus	1
Melancholia	1
Attempted Suicide	1
Opium *Habitué*	1

Balance Sheet–1910

RECEIPTS		EXPENDITURES	
£20 Grant from N.C.M.S.*	$216.89	Debit Balance from 1909	$19.95
Bed Money, etc. per S.P.G.†	568.47	Chinese Staff wages	
Per S.P.G. Donations to		and Food	282.60
Building & Furnishing	677.52	Food for Patients	262.05
Inpatient Fees &		Fuel and Lighting	198.65
Subscription for Board	150.94	Itinerating	79.46
Dispensary Entrance Fees	64.50	Miscellaneous	71.06
Balance	92.05	Customs, Freight,	
		Transit Drugs from	
		England &	
		Supplementary	
		Drugs from Shanghai	125.19
		Medical Necessaries	
		(Soap, Milk,	
		& Dressings etc.)	48.32
		To Making Furniture	
		(part) for New	
		Hospital and Dispensary	357.56
		Building New Kitchen	
		& Bathroom	325.53
	$ 1,770.37‡		$1,770.37

N.B. *This refers to local expenditure only and does not include drugs (£42.11) bought in England.*

* NCMS = North China Mission Society

† SPG = Society for the Propagation of the Gospel

‡ In 1910, the pound sterling was the equivalent of about fifty pounds today, making the budget equal to approximately twenty thousand Canadian dollars at the time of reading.

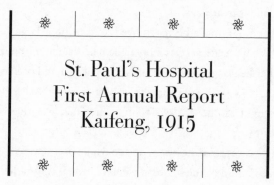

St. Paul's Hospital
First Annual Report
Kaifeng, 1915

♪* [W]E OPENED QUIETLY, without ceremony, during the cold and windy season of November 1914, [with no] rush of patients anxious to try something new, but...the months have marked stages of progress both in development and efficiency, and in the number of patients coming for treatment.

The first inpatient was an old woman of 72, her only son a cook in a military camp. She had broken her leg, and the hospital was to her a veritable haven of rest...The elderly in China are usually full of complaints and hard to please, but placid ease and contentment could be seen in every line of her face.

Another early patient was an old woman upon whom we operated for cataract—happily a very satisfactory case. Here the eyes are usually hopelessly spoiled with trachoma and all varieties of inflammation, and are unsuitable for treatment. It was good to hear the greeting she gave her son whom she had not seen for many months (if not years) when she left the Hospital, the proud possessor of a pair of foreign spectacles.

Abscesses...have been many and severe, but the worse they are and the larger, the more striking and gratifying the results. Carbuncles, dangerously large, have also been completely healed, and one of the most rapid and satisfactory cures was that of a woman with extensive and deep ulceration of the leg for years (to a degree almost incredible) which healed like magic under treatment.

Several tumours have been removed, one being a large post-rectal tumour which it was feared was inoperable. The state of the poor girl who could neither lie nor sit, and was a misery to herself and others, justified the attempt. Now she is a normal being and presumably her people are busily finding a mother-in-law for her, since that was their object in seeking treatment.

Operative cases have, however, on the whole been few as the women are too much afraid of the knife, so we have been trying rather to prove the efficacy of Western treatment in medical cases. At present they are apt to rely upon their Chinese charlatans, and it is only in a hospital run on Western lines that our methods can get a fair chance.

Three opium cases have been treated but…they nearly always revert to the habit as soon as anything occurs to vex them at home. As nearly all the women here, except the very poor, seem to have the habit it is a barrier to our getting many inpatients, for they are not willing to abstain while in hospital.

Many pthisical patients have been treated in the Tuberculosis Annex… the patients sleeping on the verandah in all weathers. Several cases of typhoid and also scarlet fever, of which there has been a severe epidemic in Kaifeng this year, have been admitted to the Isolation Hospital. One of our nurses contracted typhoid, but made a good recovery…Fortunately it did not get to the Girls' School, though we did have several of the school-girls for various other illnesses.

A poor slave girl who had swallowed corrosive poison some weeks before, came to us for a time, but as she was unable to swallow properly and would not be treated, we had to let her go. Another would-be suicide was a woman who had cut her throat in a neighbour's shop, with the desire to injure them, while absolutely reckless of the consequences to herself. We were called out to see her as her friends would not move her to the Hospital till the lawsuit was instituted. We found her lying on the mud floor in a pool of blood, with mud and rags stuffed into the hole in her neck. The shop was full of people, even though the windows were closely barricaded to keep away the crowd from the street outside. There by the light of a couple of candles (though it was broad daylight at the time) with wax dripping over our hands, we knelt on the floor and gave her chloroform. We stitched up her wound as well as possible by the light of the flickering candle which was held so close that we heard the crackling of singed hairs as we worked. A few days later she was brought into the Hospital and was making a good recovery when, her fright having passed over, her anger returned and she tore at the bandages and raved to go home. Such was the intensity of her rage, however, having secured her discharge she lost no time in making sure of her demise.

We had seven foreign inpatients during the year, and with them not only do we get appreciation but also the satisfaction of being allowed to do all we could for them. While we try to present the Gospel of Jesus Christ—the Gospel of Healing—attending first as our Lord did to bodily infirmities, we do not forget that He is the Great Physician of Souls. Every morning we read and talk of Him for a while, when all assemble for morning hymns and prayers. Every afternoon, for an hour, the nurses teach their respective patients to read the New Testament. Two of the Hospital women servants have asked to enter the Church to prepare for baptism, but without a Bible-woman or foreign Evangelist this work will be very slow since the nurses are not very willing evangelists. Few of the Chinese are, unless they make it their profession and livelihood.

[T]he Nurses' Training School is our chief work and…[s]ix nurses passed this examination, four of them doing extremely well (79% to 90%), and of the two who failed one came first of them all in practical work, but she could not write the papers. The examination consisted of written papers and practical, and viva voce tests in Physiology and Hygiene, Nursing and Dispensing. In practical nursing the nurses were examined in the making of beds, bathing and weighing patients, cleaning rooms, bandaging, and cutting out clothes, and in all subjects the year's marks were included in the final results.

Two new probationers have been admitted…We expect additions to this new class immediately, having had numerous applications. The second-year nurses are now studying Robb's *Nursing,* Halliburton's *Physiology* (all others being out of print), Midwifery (a simple and comprehensive survey of the normal and practical side of the subject, aided by some excellent models made by the Commercial Press), *Materia Medica* and English (this latter because we hope to have the patients' reports filled out in English).

…Night duty is taken in turn by the week, so too is the city Dispensary where a nurse accompanies the doctor every afternoon. The other work is taken for periods of four months at a time (e.g., Operating room, Consulting room, Dressing room, Dispensary, Public wards, Private wards, Tuberculosis Annex).

The nurses have two hours off duty every day…are allowed visitors on Saturday, and may go home for half a day (also a Saturday) once a month, and once a year they have a fortnight's holiday. They attend the city church by turns on Sundays. Every afternoon they teach the patients and ward women hymns and prayers, and they take turns to give the address at morning prayers. After the first three months' probation, they wear Hospital uniform (green in winter, white in summer) consisting of a Chinese coat piped with red, with a cross in red on the left shoulder. A skirt, apron and white sleeves, are all provided by the Hospital. They receive their food, but no salary is given until the first examination is passed. Then they receive $1.00 a month for the next year and $2.00 a month for the third and fourth years. They pay a guarantee fee of $10.00 on admission, to be refunded on graduation, or forfeited if the agreement is broken, in which case they must also pay for the cost of their food during the time of their stay in Hospital.

The nurses admitted so far have only received primary school education, though they prove themselves capable of learning anything and doing it well, but they are heedless and forgetful, and therefore not always reliable. Sometimes they are quarrelsome and their work suffers…but usually they enjoy it wholeheartedly. All but one are Christians and though faults are glaring, their intentions and efforts are clearly for the good.

At the beginning of June we opened a Dispensary in the city as a feeder for our inpatient work and because there is no other Medical Mission work there. As funds were short, we could not make it free and so have been trying an experiment of a small charge every time for medicines and dressings. We can only open for a few hours every afternoon on account of the work here. The results have been very satisfactory, both in the number of attendances and the appreciation by the patients of the convenience of a Dispensary in the city, and also in the fact that it brought several inpatients to the hospital. We have also started a Mothers' Union there and hold meetings once a month to discuss and teach the care of babies, and hygiene at home.

Looking back upon the year's work, we feel exceedingly encouraged both as to the actual results and statistics of the medical work...because the standard of work was attained so quickly, as well as the number and progress of the nurses in training. We have reason to believe that the training being given is equal to any in China (if not at home also, such being our aim), but of course we are handicapped by the shortage of our staff, which we meet by undertaking double work.

At the time of writing the future is uncertain, but we have tried to do faithfully the task which was committed to us.

E. Margaret Phillips
December 1915

Abscesses, sinuses, ulcers, etc.	12
Adhesions, elbow	1
Anaemia	5
Cut throat	1
Dysentery	3
Eyes, various	10
Fractures	2
Haemorrhoids	1
Heart disease	1
Hepatitis	1
Hysteric spasm	1
Joints (tubercular)	4
Malaise	1
Malaria	1
Mastitis	2
Nasal catarrh & eczema (child)	1
Neurasthenia	1
Neuritis	1
Obstetrical	2
Opium	3
Phthisis	16
Pneumonia	1
Post scarlatinal nephritis	2
Puerpiral fever	1
Rheumatic fever	1
Scarlet fever	5
Stricture of oesophagus	1
Tonsilitis (acute)	2
Tumours	9
Typhoid fever	4
Various	10
Total	107

GENERAL STATISTICS

INPATIENTS

Foreign (One Japanese)	7
Chinese	100
Total	107

OUTPATIENT ATTENDANCES

New	1,586
Return	3,469
City Dispensary	
(June to November)	864
Total	5,919

OUTCALLS

Numerous (record not correctly kept)

November 1915

Medical Superintendent	Miss E. Margaret Phillips, M.Sc., M.B., Ch.b. China 1905, Henan 1913
Assistant Director	Miss Agnes Tso (Diploma, Hackett Medical College, Canton)
Nurse-probationers	Miss Sia Ku Yu (2nd Year)
	Miss Wang Su Ch'in
	Miss Wang Hua Mei
	Miss Wang Hsiu Ch'ing
	Miss P'an Feng Kwei
	Miss Lo Ching
	Miss Wang Su Mei (1st Year)
	Miss Chang Ju Chin
	Mrs. Sun Kuei Chen
	Miss Chang Mei Chie
Visiting Clergyman	Rev. A. J. Williams, B.D.
English Master	Rev. N. L. Ward, M.A.
Writing Master	Mr. Tsung

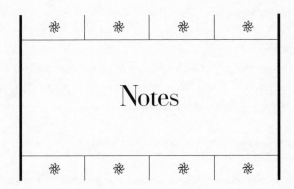

Notes

CHAPTER 4

1. The Middle Kingdom was the term used before China became a republic, being the direct translation of the Chinese name for China, Zhong Guo. Now that China is a republic (the Chinese People's Republic or CPR), the term *Zhong Guo* can be translated as "Central Nation," while still retaining the meaning of the Chinese characters.

CHAPTER 9

1. Labour costs were estimated at one hundred pounds sterling, which in those days worked out to at about a penny per foot, or barely one hundred "cash" (a round Chinese coin of infinitesimal value with a square hole in its centre). Today, this would amount to fifty pence or approximately one Canadian dollar per square foot (about nine cents per square metre).

2. It appears that the speaker, Rev. Mawson, representing the Society for Promoting Christian Knowledge (SPCK) from England, had overlooked the fact that Margaret's many accomplishments included a sound working knowledge of the Chinese language—both spoken and written—acquired over the preceding few years. Nonetheless, for the times, almost a century ago, this was a glowing tribute for a thirty-three-year-old woman.

3. See *China Medical Journal,* November 1909.

CHAPTER 10

1. James Burke, *My Father in China* (London: M. Joseph, 1945).

CHAPTER 12

1. Some seventy years later, this item was entrusted in perpetuity by the author to the University of Manchester with the rest of her memorabilia. With it is his translation of the presentation text:

LOVING KINDNESS SHIELDED THE STRICKEN

This inscription serves as an appreciation in praise of the English Lady Physician [Dr. Ethel Margaret Phillips], who treated all the victims who survived the disaster in the summer of 1913.

A special award from Henan, presented by Minister of State, Tian Wenlie.

June, 1915.

CHAPTER 13

1. Excerpt from a short article Margaret once wrote, entitled "My Peking Home," submitted for publication under the pen-name of Philippa King.

CHAPTER 14

1. Jean Escarra, *China Then and Now* (Peking: Henri Vetch, 1940).

CHAPTER 15

1. The traditional willow pattern, devised in England in 1780, depicts a Chinese legend in blue on a white background. The design portrays a river scene with willow trees, a zigzag bridge and a pagoda. Overhead two magpies fly towards each other, representing two legendary lovers who traditionally met once a year on the seventh day of the seventh month.

2. A free English rendition is "thunder [over] fertile fields." Thus, good came out of a sorry situation. The author could not apologize for his childish ignorance, but to this day he bears with pride the name Lei Houtian.

CHAPTER 18

1. The author wore these socks *inter alia* for more than ten years. During that time, his wife darned them again and again until they could be worn no longer. Enid and Clifford were extremely touched by this token of love, for undoubtedly this was what the woman felt for Margaret. The socks remained as a memento until several years after Margaret's death.

2. This eventually took the form of a book entitled *English-Chinese Handbook of Royal Air Force Terminology*, published in 1947 by Air Ministry under Crown copyright. It was used as a training manual for more than twenty years. The original manuscript took over a year to produce, the task enabling the author to travel extensively in North China.

3. E. Margaret Phillips, *Useful English Conversation* (Peking: Guili, 1948). The publication date is listed in the book as the "thirty-seventh year of the Chinese Republic."

4. Had Margaret been alive many years later, she would have been so proud to know that a Chinese professor at Yenching University had hailed Clifford as "*Jingzi hui xiang*," meaning "A son of the Capital returned home." This happened in 1996, ten years after the author retired from teaching Chinese at the University of Alberta, when he was conducting a tour of China with a group of senior Minerva sightseers from Grant MacEwan College in Edmonton, Alberta.

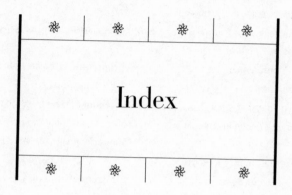

Index